The Art and Science of Thread Lifting Based on Pinch Anatomy and Moving Plane

Seung Min Oh • Giwoong Hong
Wu-Chul Song

The Art and Science of Thread Lifting Based on Pinch Anatomy and Moving Plane

Second Edition

Springer

Seung Min Oh
O.N Clinic Dermatology and Plastic Surgery
Seoul, Korea (Republic of)

Wu-Chul Song
Department of Anatomy, College of Medicine
Catholic University of Korea
Seoul, Korea (Republic of)

Giwoong Hong
SAMSKIN Plastic Surgery
Seoul, Korea (Republic of)

ISBN 978-981-97-5518-9 ISBN 978-981-97-5516-5 (eBook)
https://doi.org/10.1007/978-981-97-5516-5

This Springer imprint is published by the registered company Springer Nature Singapore Pte Ltd.
The registered company address is: 152 Beach Road, #21-01/04 Gateway East, Singapore 189721, Singapore

Preface

The first edition of *The Art and Science of Thread Lifting: Based on PINCH Anatomy* received widespread acclaim from numerous medical professionals. Translated into six languages—Korean, Chinese, English, Portuguese, Spanish, and Japanese—this book has been embraced by practitioners around the world. This acceptance has led to multiple presentations at international academic conferences and facilitated scholarly exchanges with esteemed colleagues. The publication of this book has significantly transformed my professional life, which was previously focused solely on clinical practice.

One particularly memorable experience occurred during a Q&A session at an international conference. An overseas physician, who introduced himself as a reader of my book, expressed a deep desire to meet me and ask specific questions. This encounter was profoundly moving and reinforced my sense of responsibility toward the content I create.

Since writing the book, I have felt an increased obligation to provide higher-level evidence beyond mere expert opinion. My goal has been to elevate the standard of evidence to support the practices discussed in my work.

The first edition enabled me to engage in knowledge exchange with many distinguished professionals. It also inspired new experimental results and research, leading to demands for an updated version of the book. As I continued to explore the discourse on thread lifting, I collaborated with Dr. Gi-Woong Hong and Professor Wu-Chul Song to prepare the second edition of *The Art and Science of Thread Lifting*.

Considerable time and effort were invested in this new edition, which incorporates fresh research findings. The core concept of the first edition, the PINCH concept, received positive feedback from many clinicians for its practical utility. In the second edition, we introduce a new core concept called the "moving plane" and detail its clinical application. We have integrated anatomical insights, clinical experiences, and various experimental results to elucidate this concept and its implementation for effective and safe thread lifting procedures.

Additionally, this edition explores the history of thread lifting, analyzes the types of threads, and discusses their respective advantages and disadvantages. We have examined newly developed threads and reflected on various experiments regarding their principles and application methods.

After years of dedicated effort, the authors are pleased to present the culmination of their work. We hope that this second edition will contribute to safer and more effective thread lifting practices for medical professionals worldwide. We also look forward to engaging in spirited discussions with global colleagues based on the new content presented.

With hope for the future,

Seoul, Korea (Republic of) Seung Min Oh
Seoul, Korea (Republic of) Giwoong Hong
Seoul, Korea (Republic of) Wu-Chul Song

June 6, 2024, Early Morning

Note of Appreciation

I would like to express my sincere gratitude to Dr. Bong Cheol Kim, who collaborated with me on the first edition of *The Art and Science of Thread Lifting*. Although he could not co-author this edition, his valuable participation in discussions and insightful feedback were greatly appreciated.

I also extend my heartfelt thanks to Mr. Doyeon Kim, CEO of Healux, for his invaluable support and collaboration on various thread lifting research projects. Without his dedication to research, this book would not have been possible.

To my parents and family, I owe immense gratitude and apologies. Despite my numerous commitments, you have always understood and encouraged me. Your unwavering support has been my strength.

I am deeply thankful to the professors, seniors, and juniors who have guided me and contributed to who I am today.

Lastly, I want to extend my sincere appreciation to the board members of the Korean Association for Laser, Dermatology and Trichology (KALDAT). Your encouragement and support have propelled me from the confines of clinical practice into the realms of academic research and scholarship. I am grateful to share this moment with all of you.

With heartfelt thanks,

June 6, 2024, Early Morning

Seung Min Oh
Giwoong Hong
Wu-Chul Song

Contents

Author's Profile

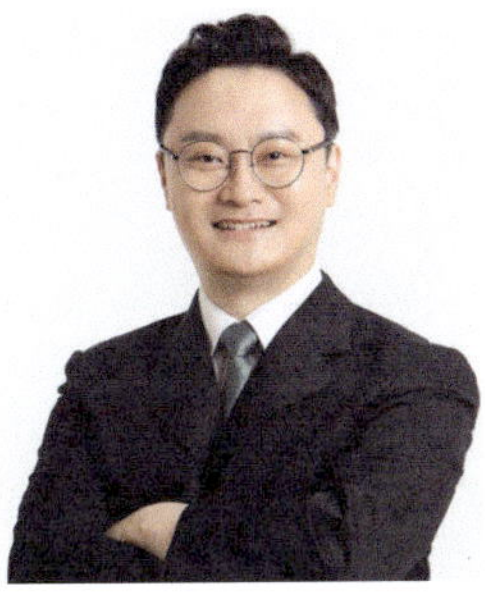

Seung Min Oh Aesthetic physician

Director of O.N Clinic Dermatology and Plastic Surgery
Graduated from Seoul National University College of Medicine
Trained at Seoul National University Hospital
Clinical Lecturer at Seoul National University Hospital
Senior Academic Director, Korean Association for Laser, Dermatology and Trichology
CEO of OK Medi Co. Ltd.
Advisory Board Member of HEALUX
Advisory Board Member of Medytox
Advisory Board Member of S.THEPHARM
Advisory Board Member of Galderma Korea

Awards

Best experimental paper award 2021, Plastic and Reconstructive Surgery

Books

The Art and Science of Thread Lifting. Springer Nature
The Art and Science of Filler Injection. Springer Nature

Articles

1. Changes in the neck tissue layers during pinch manipulation: implications for lipolytic deoxycholate injections for double chin. https://doi.org/10.1111/jocd.14696.
2. Tissue changes over time after polydioxanone thread insertion: an animal study with pigs. Journal of Cosmetic Dermatology 2018:1–7.
3. Changes in the layers of the temple during pinch manipulation: implications for thread lifting. Dermatologic Surgery 2019;00:1–6.

4. Development and usability of a virtual reality-based filler injection training system. Aesthetic Plastic Surgery. 2020. https://doi.org/10.1007/s00266-020-01872-2.
5. Comparative effectiveness of different interventions of perivascular hyaluronidase. Plastic and Reconstructive Surgery. 2020;145:957.
6. Comparison of hyaluronic acid filler ejection pressure with injection force for safe filler injection. Journal of Cosmetic Dermatology 2021;00:1–6.
7. Current practices and perceived effectiveness of polynucleotides for treatment of facial erythema by cosmetic physicians. Skin Research and Technology. 2023:29;e13,466.
8. Lateral facial thread lifting procedure with temporal anchoring in deep temporal fascia: Anatomical perspectives of superficial temporal artery. Skin research and technology 2024:30;e13,587.
9. Aesthetic doctors' perception and attitudes toward tolerance in botulinum toxin. Skin research and technology 2024:30e;e13,691.
10. Investigating the mechanisms of intradermal injection for easier "skin booster" treatment: a fluid mechanics approach to determine optimal delivery method. Plas reconstr surg glob open 2024;12:e5723; https://doi.org/10.1097/GOX.0000000000005723.

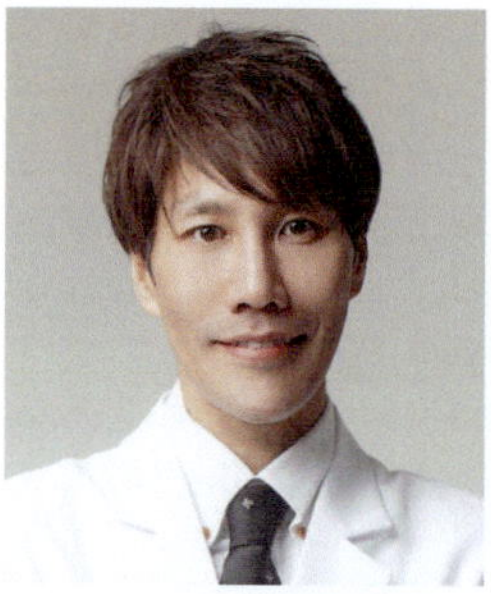

Giwoong Hong

- Board-certified Plastic Surgeon
- President of SAMSKIN Plastic Surgery Clinic
- Clinical Professor, Department of Plastic Surgery, Chung-Ang University Medical Center
- Member of The Korean Society of Plastic and Reconstructive Surgery
- Member of The Korean Society of Aesthetic Plastic Surgery
- Member of Korean Cleft Palate-Craniofacial Association
- Member of Korean Society for Microsurgery
- Member of Korean Association of Stem Cell Therapy
- Scientific Committee of Korean Association of Minimally Invasive Plastic Surgery

- President of ICALA (International Clinical Aesthetic Leaders Academy)
- Dissertation judge of Archives of Plastic Surgery
- Editor-in-Chair of Atlas Aesthetics (AA) Journal
- Advisory Board Member of Galderma Korea
- Advisory Board Member of HEALUX
- Advisory Board Member of Medytox
- Advisory Board Member of Hugel
- Advisory Board Member of S.THEPHARM
- Advisory Board Member of N-FINDERS
- Restylane Filler Global Key Doctor

Published Books

- ***Arteries and Veins of the Face* (2024), MDWORLD Medical Publishing Co.**
- ***The Art and Science of Thread Lifting* (Korean Version) (2024), KOONJA Publishing Inc.**
- ***All About Fillers* (2023), MDWORLD Medical Publishing Co.**
- ***HA Filler Guide Book for Restylane* (2023), MDWORLD Medical Publishing Co.**
- ***Minimally Invasive Aesthetic Surgery Techniques* (2022), Springer Nature Singapore Pte Ltd.**
- ***Nerves of the Face* (2021), MDWORLD Medical Publishing Co.**
- ***The Art and Science of Filler Injection* (2021), Springer Nature Singapore Pte Ltd.**
- ***Botulinum Toxin Clinical Usage* (2020), MDWORLD Medical Publishing Co.**
- ***Thread Lifting Clinical Usage* (2020), MDWORLD Medical Publishing Co.**
- ***Practical Guidelines for Effective and Safe Filler Procedures* (2019), KOONJA Publishing Inc.**
- ***Clinical Application of Thread Lifting* (2019), MDWORLD Medical Publishing Co.**
- ***Clinical Application of Botulinum Toxin* (2019), MDWORLD Medical Publishing Co.**
- ***Clinical Anatomy for Filler and Toxin* (2018), MEDICAL Observer**
- ***Practical Guideline for Effective and Safe Filler Procedure* (2018), KOONJA Publishing Inc.**
- **Filler.Toxin Practical Knowhow (2017), MDWORLD Medical Publishing Co.**

– ***Practical Knowhow of Minimally Invasive Aesthetic Surgery* (2016), Most M.D&PS Publishing Inc.**
– ***Minimally Invasive Plastic Surgery* (MIPS) Hand Book (2015), Medimembers.**

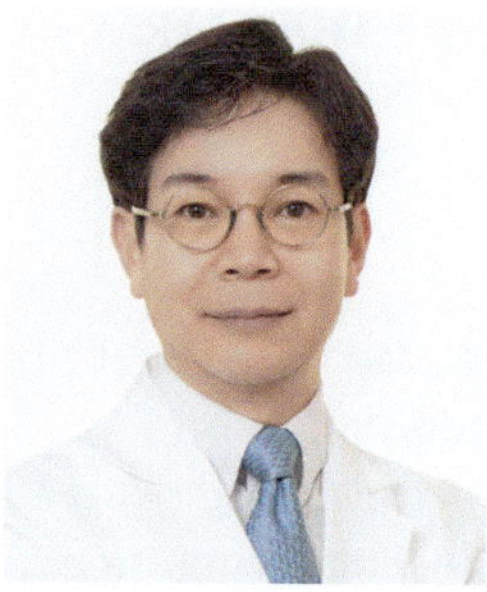

Wu-Chul Song
Department of Anatomy, College of Medicine, Catholic University of Korea
Prev) Full Professor in Department of Anatomy
Professor, School of Medicine, Konkuk University
Professor, College of Dentistry, Kyung Hee University
Advisory Board Member, Medytox
Advisory Board Member, Hugel
Advisor, Aesthetic Surgery and Laser Society

Awards

Best Paper Award 2020, Cosmetic, Plastic and Reconstructive Surgery

Paper

[PRS cover article] Park JA, Koh KS, Song WC. Are there other muscle fibers on the orbicularis oris muscle in the upper lip? Plast Reconstr Surg. 150(6):1314e–1321e, 2022

[PRS cover article] Lee SH, Ha TJ, Lee JS, Koh KS, Song WC. Topography of the central retinal artery relevant to retrobulbar reperfusion in filler complications. Plast Reconstr Surg. 144(6):1295–1300, 2019

[PRS cover article] Lee SH, Ha TJ, Koh KS, Song WC. External and internal diameters of the facial artery relevant to intravascular filler injections. Plast Reconstr Surg. 143(4):1031–1037, 2019

Park JA, Yeo IS, Lee HI, Shin HJ, Koh KS, Song WC. Lateral branches of the facial artery and its clinical implications. Clin Anat. 2022 Nov;35(8):1142–1146

Shin HJ, You JW, Koh KS, Song WC. Topography of the orbital part of the lacrimal gland for treating epiphora using botulinum toxin injection. Clin Anat. 35(7):861–866. 2022

Lee HI, Park JA, Yeo IS, Koh KS, Song WC. Topographic anatomy of the zygomatico-orbital artery. J Craniofac Surg. 33(4):1241–1244, 2022

Yeo IS, Park JA, Lee HI, Koh KS, Song WC. Anthropometric analysis of the growth proportions of the head and face in Koreans. J Craniofac Surg. 33(1):333–336, 2022

Park JA, Lee SH, Hwang SJ, Koh KS, Song WC. Anatomic, histologic, and ultrasound analyses of the dorsum of hand for volumetric rejuvenation. J Plast Reconstr Aesthet Surg. 74(7):1615–1620. 2021

Shin HJ, Lee SH, Ha TJ, Park JA, Koh KS, Song WC. Investigation of the orbital arterial distribution using image superimposition to determine safe zones for retrobulbar injection and to prevent filler complications. Plast Reconstr Surg. 147(6):1321–1328. 2021

Park JA, Lee SH, Ha TJ, Lee JS, Lee HI, Kim SH, Koh KS, Song WC. Location of the split line of the deep temporal fascia when reducing a zygomatic arch fracture. J Plast Reconstr Aesthet Surg. 73(6):1130–1134, 2020

Shin HJ, Song WC, Lee SH, Ha HJ, Koh KS. Consistency of the lateral canthus as an anatomic landmark and its clinical implications. Clin Anat. 32(5):630–634, 2019

History of Thread Lifting

1

Contents

1.1 Beginning and Backgrounds of Thread Lifting

The minimally invasive procedures in the field of cosmetic medicine, called petit esthetic surgery, have begun to gain popularity in the 2000s, and for successful procedural outcomes, esthetic, physiological, psychological, and anatomical approaches are required. Especially with regard to anatomy, the necessity of clinical anatomy for minimally invasive procedures arose, other than anatomy for purely academic purposes or surgery that have been conventionally taught in medical schools. So, we, the authors have discussed the anatomical considerations for minimally invasive procedures over the past several years, which are considered to be necessary for the clinicians with the cooperation of many other clinicians using the cadaver study. Based on these studies, the author first tried to sort out the clinical procedures for fillers and botulinum toxin procedures, which are considered to be the safest and most effective methods with consideration of the anatomical characteristics of Asians and Caucasians, rather than just surgical techniques. Then, the author would like to summarize a minimally invasive procedure using thread lifting, to correct the area where improvement only with fillers or toxins is limited. Various methods used for clinical minimally invasive procedures in Asia are briefly summarized as follows (Table 1.1).

Table 1.1 Various minimally invasive procedures for the esthetic field

1. Use of many kinds of filler and Botulinum toxin for face and body
2. Use of many kinds of thread for face and body
3. Various skin, hair, and body care products and devices
4. Subcutaneous and intravenous injection of various cocktail solutions for face and body
5. Use of different kinds of laser (CO_2, dye, multiwavelength, interstitial, picosecond, etc.), ultrasound, HIFU, and radio frequency devices for face and body
6. Other devices using flash lamp, air-jet, fluid-jet, dermojet, CO2 gas, plasma, etc.
7. Use of fat-derived PRP, adipocyte-derived stem cell, and many cell and tissue-stimulating factors

S. M. Oh et al., *The Art and Science of Thread Lifting Based on Pinch Anatomy and Moving Plane*,
https://doi.org/10.1007/978-981-97-5516-5_1

As one ages, various signs of aging appear complexly throughout the face, but there are specific symptoms that are commonly observed depending on each anatomical structure of the face with certain usage and features. Fillers, botulinum toxins, and thread lifting, the most commonly performed procedures among the various minimally invasive procedures shown in Table 1.1, can be simply applied to the face according to the most common symptoms of each facial structure. Firstly, with division of the face into three parts, from trichion to glabella, glabella to subnasale, subnasale to gnathion, toxins are mainly used for upper third of the face, which have main problems of wrinkles on glabella, bridge of nose and crow's feet, while fillers for middle third of the face, with main problems of tear troughs, midcheek groove (Indian bands), sunken cheek, and nasolabial folds. Since drooped facial tissues are concentrated to the lower part, enlarging the face squarely as one ages, thread lifting is most commonly used for the lower third of the face as a method of lifting the lower facial tissues to meet the needs of contouring the face to the shape that are found when we pull up the side tissues of our face artificially (Table 1.2).

However, even though there is a certain major minimally invasive procedure that is frequently used for each facial part, procedures are commonly performed together regardless of certain sites, and so is the thread lifting procedure, being used for the entire facial parts. Even though some minimally invasive procedures to lift drooped facial tissues are already available, including various devices such as laser, high-frequency wave, ultrasound, or air pressure, thread lifting would be the most effective and easiest method for lifting the sagging tissues, even when compared to fillers and toxins.

Table 1.2 General concept of facial rejuvenation

1. Main complaint of upper face—wrinkle and crease of forehead, periorbital area, glabellar, and nasal root area
2. Main complaint of midface—volume restoration of periorbital groove and hollow, flat malar area, midcheek groove and hollow, buccal and lateral cheek hollow, nasolabial fold
3. Main complaint of lower face—perioral static and dynamic line, marionette line, jowl and prejowl sulcus with irregular jawline, drooping of redundant tissue

Many clinicians of plastic surgery have studied on how to lift drooped tissues easily using threads and there are several studies done on the efficacy of lifting procedures on crow's feet, malar fat pads, nasolabial folds, or even jowl lines using suture threads after making a small incision inside the hairline of the temporal region. The basic principles of thread lifting procedures using a small incision, which is still used by some clinicians, are usually based on the surgical methods of lifting the drooped facial tissues with minimal incisions on temporal regions using conventional suture threads.

It was early 2000s when the thread lifting procedure, which has currently growing demands, became popular. Advanced from conventional procedures of simply threading the tissues and lifting them with preexisting suture threads, some clinicians have personally attempted to lift the tissues more effectively by using cogged threads, finally releasing the cogged threads as a product in many countries around the same time. However, the cogged threads were initially used for the main purpose of pulling the tissues by suturing the tissues, rather than simply inserting them and lifting the tissues. Therefore, the threads were used to facilitate suturing the open incision site by pulling the resected tissues together. Some clinicians have come to use the cogged threads for purposes other than this, to pull and sew up the facial tissues around the eyes, cheeks, jawline, tissues of the neck, and body tissues on the breast and buttock on an incision site from the surgery. However, as many clinicians have got to use the threads, various methods using these threads simpler than suturing were suggested and that was how the thread lifting procedures began to be performed.

Many clinicians, including Sasaki, Cohen, Keller, Buncke, Alcamo, Sulamanidze, Isse, Ruff, and Wu, have devised and developed various types of threads and methods of usage over the decades, many of which have actually become commercialized. It was not until the first import of bidirectional cogged threads, developed by Dr.

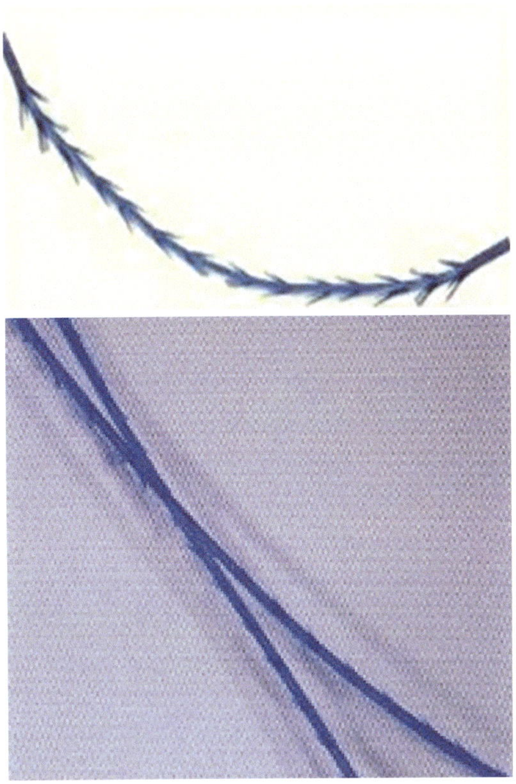

Fig. 1.1 Image and physical photos of the early models of the APTOS thread

Sulamanidze from Georgia and named APTOS in the 1990s that the methods of thread lifting began to attract attention in Korea. APTOS, the name of which is derived from antiptosis, was the first cogged thread developed for tissue lifting procedures performed only with the insertion of cogged threads, not including even a single incision (Fig. 1.1).

When the cogged threads were first introduced in Korea as a method of lifting the skin with the cogs on the threads after its insertion, the fact that the skin could be lifted even without a small incision interested many plastic surgeons, including the author, myself, attending a demonstration of thread lifting procedures using APTOS for the first time at a seminar of a hospital in Seoul.

However, as I remember, when the APTOS thread was first imported and made public, many of the clinicians in Korea, just as when Botox was first introduced, were dubious about the efficacy of the procedures, by which facial tissues are lifted with threads without even a single skin incision. Also, since the import price of the threads was expensive, some clinicians questioned whether there are any differences between using the thick nylon suture threads on which the cutting thorns were personally made and using the commercially released products. Some of them have used the conventional suture threads with personally made cogs by densely cutting the surface of nylon thread partially. As the APTOS threads became increasingly known to people, some vendors even sold tools to make cogs on the threads, insisting that general nylon threads can also be used for lifting by making regularly positioned cogs on the thread by hand. From the present point of view, which emphasized various variables for lifting, such as number, shape, lifting angles, tensile strength, and force of cogs of the threads, that could be considered as a time of lack of knowledge on thread lifting procedures. It is astonishing how much things have changed these days, in that various types of lifting threads are imported from all over the world and even produced by many domestic companies. Cogs of initial lifting threads, whether the threads were absorbable or nonabsorbable, were manually produced by a human hand at that time and therefore, the lifting force of some threads got lost too soon or the tip of the thread often got protruded once the thread breaks, due to irregular angles and strengths of the cogs.

The lifting threads released later were produced by a fully automatic automatized process to make the angles, strengths of cogs, and tension of threads constant, but the quality of the threads was still inconsistent due to the nature of the microfabrication process requiring precision. To compensate these technical defects, some Korean products are manufactured partially by hand to retain the sharpness and invariable depth of cogs, which had been impaired by the fully automatized process, while maintaining the constant spacing and depths with ancillary instruments. With products properly selected among various products available, it is possible to expect a certain degree of lifting effects.

A method of inserting the threads into the skins of the hairline or anterior part of ears, pulling the inserted threads out at the site of nasolabial

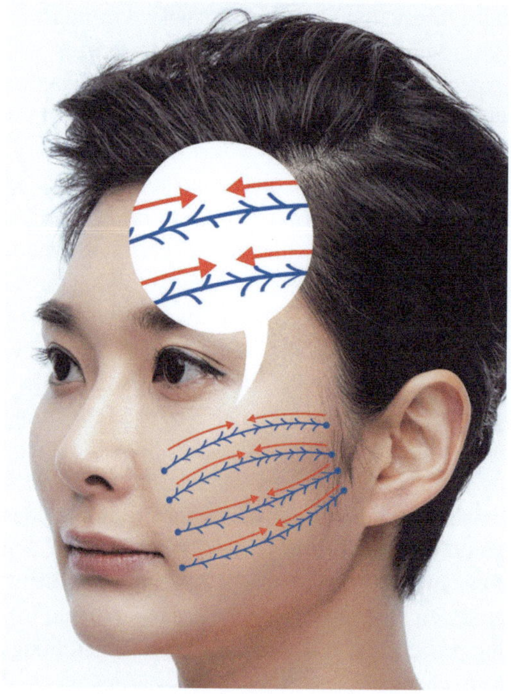

Fig. 1.2 Gathering of subcutaneous tissue toward the center of the thread

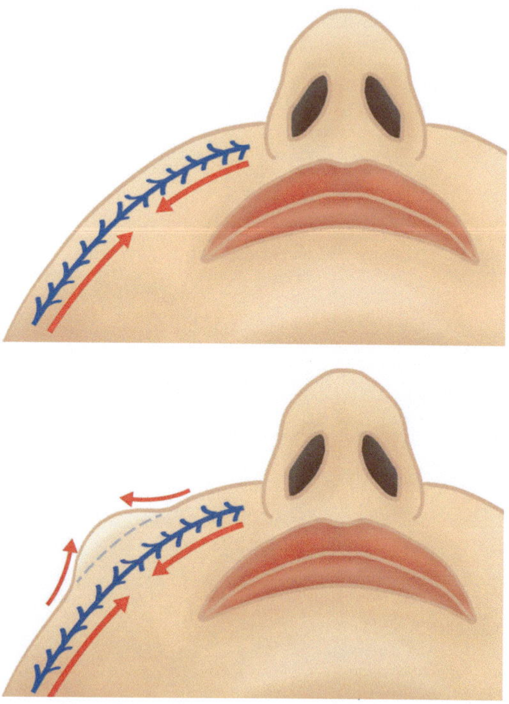

Fig. 1.3 Augmentation of malar and cheek area toward the center of the thread

folds or around the mouth and resultantly, gathering the skin and subcutaneous tissues at both ends of the threads toward the central part of the inserted threads is generally used for APTOS, which was a typical method used for bidirectional cogged threads (Fig. 1.2).

The APTOS threads considered its action mechanism, by which the tissues are held by the cogs on lateral sides of the thread that are positioned to be in opposite directions to each other and gathered toward the central noncogged part of the threads, advantageous, resultantly forming the apple cheek which is more preferred by Caucasians. However, for the Asians, many of whom have their malar eminence protruded, many had complaints of more prominent cheeks after the procedure (Fig. 1.3).

Despite its initial sensational popularity, APTOS threads had some limitations of insignificant efficacy and short duration of retention, compared to the high cost of the product. Also, the APTOS threads gradually lost their popularity due to many postprocedural insatisfaction caused by discordant postprocedural expectations between the Asians and Caucasians and frequent exposure to the threads.

Several years later, new products that complemented these defects were released. As Quill lift thread was first imported to Korea, the U- or V-shaped long bidirectional cogged thread, which has no cogs on the central part, was first introduced. Since then, with the introduction of the EZ lift, the initial domestic model of U- or V-shaped long bidirectional cogged thread, there have been a lot of discussions about the cogged thread lifting method suitable for anatomical features of Koreans that lifts the lower facial tissues upward and the author also have regained interests in thread lifting procedures.

However, since most of the lifting threads that are initially manufactured in Korea were mainly made of nylon, which is nonabsorbable, there always were problems in removing threads due to various accompanied complications including inflammation or sense of foreign bodies with the increasing number of procedures performed.

After overcoming the technical difficulties, absorbable thread lifting became widely known in Korea as cogged PDO threads, like Quill lift thread, also became available in Korea. In addition, as absorbable monofilament thread lifting, which has no cogs and can easily be accessed by less experienced clinicians due to its manageability, has become more popular among clinicians, as well as the cogged threads, the publicity of thread lifting has also naturally increased. Even though the monofilament thread itself may have less lifting effects on the facial tissues when compared to the cogged threads, the collagen produced at the periphery of the inserted monofilament thread may induce skin tightening effects. The popularization of monofilament threads has paved the way for the vitalization of the thread lifting market. Also, surgical methods with threads have made remarkable progress, with the improvements of type, shape, and quality of the cogged threads, being applied to various indications beyond simply lifting the drooped tissues of the cheek. Recently, the procedure with the lifting threads has rapidly increased, as it is used in combination with other minimally invasive procedures including filler, botulinum toxin, procedures with energy-based devices such as laser, high-frequency wave, and ultrasound, liposuction, and fat transplantation.

1.2 Nonabsorbable and Absorbable Threads

Among the various minimally invasive lifting methods that are usually performed without a large incision of skin as opposed to the conventional surgical approach commonly referred to as face lifting surgery, there used to be no active use of threads in petit esthetic surgeries at the beginning. But nowadays, noninvasive thread lifting is the most popular minimally invasive lifting procedure. Even though it is difficult to list all kinds of lifting threads with the more than several hundred types of threads all over the world, all threads can be roughly categorized as absorbable and nonabsorbable.

Table 1.3 Nonabsorbable lifting threads

1. Sasaki—2002 Used Gore-Tex, Vicryl, polypropylene
2. Keller—2002 Used modified Sasaki method using 4-0 polypropylene
3. Sulamanidze—2002, presenting magic lifting Used aptos threads, the first cogged polypropylene
4. Contour thread lift—2005, USA
5. EZ lift—the first Korean U-shaped bidirectional cogged lifting thread
6. Silhouette lift—2007 Lifted the soft tissue with cone and fixed at a temporal area with mesh
7. Tess and ribbon lift, raise me up—used both cylindrical mesh and cog thread
8. Misko, Misju lift—the first Korean I-shaped cogged lifting thread

There are various types of absorbable threads, but all can be summarized as follows in the aspect of the components of the threads: Silk, Nylon (aka Ethilon), Polybutester (aka Novafil), Polypropylene (aka Prolene), Polyester (aka Dacron, Ethibond). Among them, the first introduced lifting procedure with nonabsorbable threads is "magic lifting" using APTOS thread, the cogged polypropylene thread first introduced in 2002. After the contour thread lifting was introduced in the USA, EZ lift, Silhouette lift, Tulip lift, Quick lift, Feather lift, Miracle Frame thread lift, TESS lift, Ribbon lift, Misko and Misju lift, Raise me up have been developed and used (Table 1.3).

Surgical gut, Polyglactin 910 (aka Vicry), Poliglecaprone 25 (aka Monocryl), Polydioxanone (aka PDS II), Polytrimethylene carbonate (aka Maxon), and Glycomer 631 (aka Biosyn) are currently used absorbable threads classified by the materials. Due to the limitations in the duration of retention which is less than that of the nonabsorbable threads, the monofilament threads that have no cogs and mainly used to improve the quality of skin rather than the actual lifting were more frequently used in Korea at first. Lifting procedures using monofilament thread lifting that has no cogs were first derived from thread embedding therapy used in oriental medicine. In oriental medicine, a chromic catgut, which is used to suture the subcutaneous tissues during surgery, was inserted into the skin layer using a needle to stimulate the acupuncture points and induce a meridian effect, promoting or changing certain body energy thereby, inducing the natural improvement and correction of the body and face. The main purpose of using embedding therapy in oriental medicine was to control chronic pain, but it became known that the inserted absorbable thread may stimulate the fibroblasts of the skin inducing the production of collagen and elastin to improve the wrinkles and tighten skins and also stimulate the subcutaneous fat to produce the effect of lipolysis. Doctors who still use monofilament thread insist that the effect of embedding therapy is the main role of the monofilament thread lifting procedure.

For absorbable lifting materials, PDO (polydioxanone) threads are the most widely used and domestically produced PDO threads including Ultra V lifting, Omega lifting, and twister lifting. The early polydioxanone threads were not very popular because the actual lifting effect was insignificant due to the absence of cogs and only limited effects of improving and firming skins could be expected. However, over time, as, with the absorption of threads, its efficacy of tissue tightening effect, reducing the fat tissues and synthesizing collagen, which may clarify and firm the skin, got accepted, the procedure has become popular with people who want to improve their facial shape and skin.

After that, domestic manufacturers started to produce lifting threads that could be used for actual lifting by making cogs on the thick absorbable threads, modeling after the Quill lift, which were commonly used to suture skin and tissues in other countries. Since then, various types of PDO threads from various manufacturers with improved functions of cogs and threads such as N-Fix, N-Cog, Phoenix, Super cobra V lift, Blue Rose, Diamond, Mint, Miracu, C-cogs, M-cog, VOV line, Puff-V lift, and QT-lift have been developed and used. Also, products made of different materials from the conventional PDO threads became available, such as V-loc thread, which is made of polytrimethylene carbonate and has cogs.

Table 1.4 Absorbable lifting threads

1. Monofilament-type polydioxanone (PDO) threads N-scaffold, ultra V lift, omega lift, tornado lift, phoenix, super cobra V lift
2. U-shaped cogged polydioxanone threads Quill lift, blue rose, diamond, mint, C-cogs line lift, i-THREAD
3. I-shaped cogged polydioxanone threads N-fix, N-cog, M-cog lift, C-cogs line, ultra V lift, omega lift, VOV line Super cobra V lift, phoenix thread, miracu thread, cobra V lift, puff-V lift QT-lift, anchor thread, ultrafill thread, i-THREAD
4. Trimethylene carbonate barbed thread V-loc
5. PCL (polycaprolactone), PLLA lifting threads Silhouette soft, marionette lift

In addition, advanced from the conventional Silhouette lift, which consists of absorbable cones and nonabsorbable thread, Silhouette soft doesn't require fixation of threads on the temporal region that consists of threads made of PLA (Poly-lactic acid), the main component of Sculptra, and cones made of PLGA, a mixture of poly-lactic acid and glycolic polymer, is introduced and now being used in Korea. By inserting the threads using the needles integrated to both ends of the thread, the threads were used as a cell stimulator accompanying various tissue regenerating effects that are induced in the process of threads being slowly absorbed as well as repositioning effects induced by the lifting of cones, rather than actual lifting effects. Also, domestic manufacturers are currently producing products made of PCL (polycaprolactone) and PLLA (poly-L-lactic acid) materials instead of PDO (Table 1.4).

1.3 Development History of Lifting Threads

It can be assumed that various types of lifting threads have been imported or produced in Korea, in that the trend of lifting threads in Korea naturally reflects the history of the type of threads used worldwide.

After the Botox and Restylane HA (hyaluronic acid) fillers were first introduced in the late 1990s, the thread lifting procedures were introduced a little later than botulinum toxins and fillers, gaining the public interest in the early 2000s. Especially, in 2002, APTOS thread, developed by Dr. Sulamanidze from Georgia, was first imported to Korea, attracting the interests of many clinicians and the procedures became more generalized.

The very first version of APTOS thread was a nonabsorbable 2-0 polypropylene thread with cogs on each side positioned to be in opposite directions to each other. It was a typical initial model of bidirectional cogged threads, which are inserted into the subcutaneous fat layer and gather the drooped skin and tissue toward the central part of the thread. Polypropylene, which is used as a material of the initial thread, was promoted for its little foreign body reaction and tissue-firming effects induced by the formation of fibrous tissue around the cogs of the threads. But nowadays, it is astonishing that various absorbable threads that induce the actual tissue reaction are generalized. At that time, there were several adverse effects of APTOS thread that the author experienced: asymmetry, pain, edema, and hematoma. Also, since it was an early model of lifting threads, the threads were found to be often protruding into the oral cavity or from skins. It is assumed that, even allowing for the unestablished procedural methods or techniques, the initial product was not as effective as current products in holding or fixing the tissues due to the shape, number, and position of the cogs.

In addition, there were always concerns about continuous pain due to inserted threads, displacement of the threads caused by the gradual loosening of the cogs, inflammation due to foreign body reaction, and formation of granuloma. Also, some clinicians were reluctant to perform the procedure since, when a patient wants to remove the threads for any reason, it is inevitable to make an incision to remove the threads, unless the outline of the thread is visible or can be touched from the outside.

APTOS thread had succeeded in gaining popularity when initially introduced to Korea, by virtue of some clinicians who were involved in the process of importing and distributing the product actively promoting the APTOS thread through live seminars and other activities. However, due to many problems mentioned above and the basic designs of the bidirectional cogged threads which gather the tissues toward the center and resultantly, protrude the tissue of central part, complaints were raised since the procedure made the malar cheek stand out. Since Koreans have malar eminence that are already naturally protruded unlike that of Caucasians, who are generally satisfied with the outcomes of the procedure, the apple cheek, the procedure was considered to be inappropriate for Asians.

In addition to these problems, the effect of the procedure was relatively insignificant, despite the high cost. As a result, the popularity of the APTOS threads gradually decreased and even the newly introduced other lifting methods had failed to gain popularity. After that, the methods of lifting the lower facial tissues and fixing them to the upper part of the face, maximizing the lifting effects by making a small incision on the temporal region, exposing the deep temporal fascia. Then the nonabsorbable threads that are holding the lower facial tissues are tied together and fixed on the hard fascia using an anchoring device such as a cone or mesh. Although the lifting effect of the procedure and the retention period was satisfying, the disadvantage of making an incision was a cause of concern about the surgical scar and hair loss.

Currently, the APTOS thread is not available in Korea but it is used in more than 50 countries including China. Also, the threads mainly composed of polycaprolactone (PCL) and polylactic acid (PLA) are produced in addition to the polypropylene (Fig. 1.4).

Various designs of products integrated with cogs, springs, and wires are now available, so that a clinician may select a proper product for various purpose of the procedure depending on the target site including breast, abdomen, arm, thigh, and knee as well as face (Fig. 1.5). Thus, it seems that this cogged thread could have gained more popularity if the products were introduced a little later.

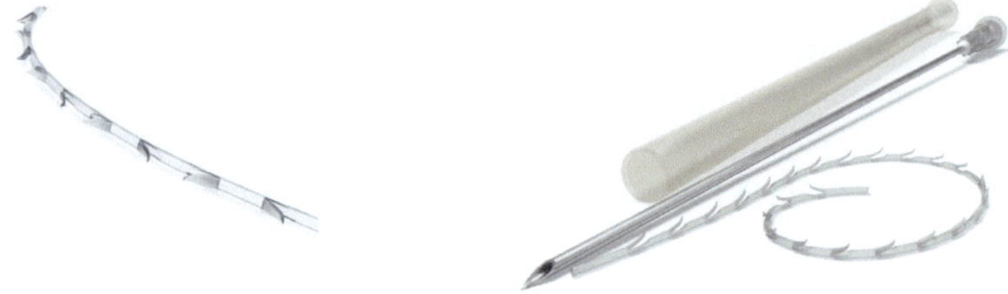

Fig. 1.4 Absorbable and nonabsorbable APTOS threads for the face

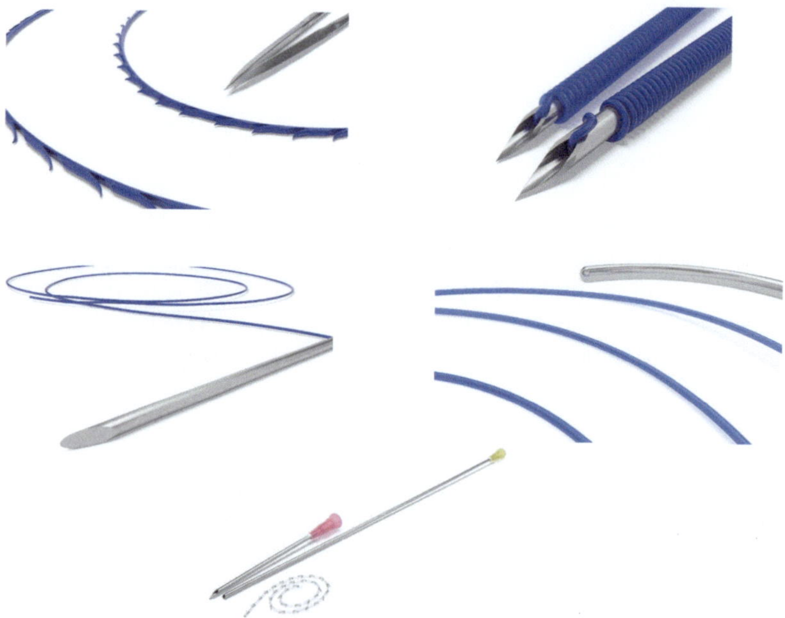

Fig. 1.5 Absorbable and nonabsorbable APTOS threads for the body

The author has come to lose interest in the thread lifting procedures since the effect was not as much as we first expected, and, as explained above, several problems were found, using the APTOS thread.

Afterward, the U-shaped Quill lift with cogs made of absorbable PDO (polydioxanone), which was developed for suturing purposes in other countries, became available and it was the first absorbable cogged threads with actual lifting effects that the author got to use (Fig. 1.6).

The Quill lift thread was originally produced not for the lifting procedure, but rather for suturing purposes, which consisted of the central part without cogs and both sides that are made of cogs with opposite directions thereby strongly pulling and gathering the tissues to the central part. It was the first thread model produced with the principle of U- or V-shaped lifting threads, which are widely used types of lifting threads these days. However, when compared to the current models, the initial model was considerably thicker and rougher, causing many discomforts in patients, such as irritation or stabbing pain when the threads are broken.

Since an absorbable thread with cogs that can make a significant lifting effect was not yet released, Quill lift was used despite the many problems it caused. Then, the EZ lift, a U- or V-shaped cogged thread developed with principles of Quill lift, but purely for lifting purposes, was released for the first time in Korea. Although there was an inconvenience caused by the unabsorbable nature of polypropylene, it was more effective in lifting than existing products, gaining much attention from the clinicians and mainly being used for the procedures.

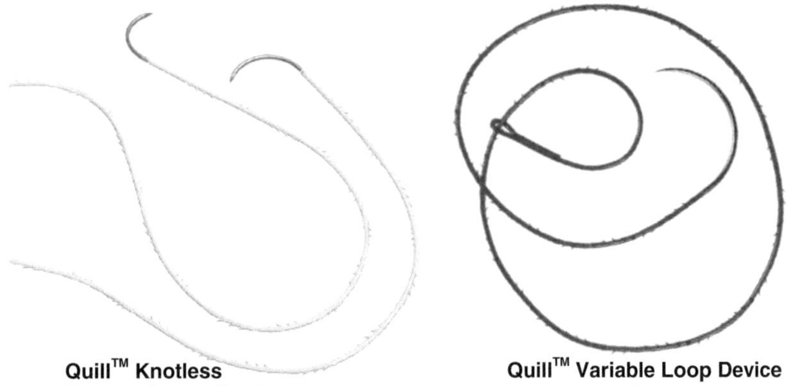

Fig. 1.6 Quill lifting threads

Unlike the initial APTOS thread lifting, this lifting method using U- or V-shaped cogged threads was not only effective in lifting the drooped tissues of the cheek and mouth but also in making slimmer facial shapes. With lifting procedures, it was possible to improve the squared facial shape with decreased skin elasticity with age and to intensely lift the drooped skin and tissues on cheeks and chins even in young patients, making the face smaller and slimmer.

However, while the procedure had the excellent effect of lifting the tissues of the lower facial part and the neck, patients got to feel severe headaches, when the thread was fixed too deep, instead of precisely on the deep temporal fascia. On the contrary, when fixed to a superficial layer, the cogs of both sides of threads lose their balance, since the noncogged central part may not play its role as a buffer zone by firm embedding and finally, the threads often get pulled out toward the side where the force was concentrated.

In addition, when using certain products for the first time, the main concern was the efficacy of the procedures. While the product had a strong lifting effect, when the procedure was mistakenly performed or the barbs held the targeted skin too superficially, adverse effects such as skin dimpling or unevenness were found, which lasted more than one or two months and were not relieved by massage. In the aspect of materials of threads, since the nylon threads were not absorbable, when moving the face or making facial expressions after the procedure, the threads displacement or irritating sense were increasingly reported as the procedures were more generally performed. Also, as with the case of the APTOS thread, even when a patient wants to remove the threads for any reason, there is a real problem that there is no easy way to remove them.

For this reason, since the late 2000s, the lifting method using the absorbable PDO thread, similar to the Quill lift, has been developed and used in Korea. Among the various types of absorbable suture threads used in various surgical operations including plastic surgery, PDO has been widely used as a material for absorbable lifting threads because it has a relatively long half-life and less tissue reaction than Catgut or Dexon.

These absorbable PDO threads were used based on the findings suggesting that a short monofilament thread without cogs may improve skin tone and elasticity when inserted under the skin. With the first introduction of short PDO threads with fine cogs, the technique of contouring the thread shape also developed. Various designs were developed, including a straight type, mainly used initially and gradually converted to the bundling of two lines; a twin type; a twist type, which is made by twisted monofilament threads; a coil type, coiling the monofilament threads on the needle; and water drop type that is embossed like water droplets (Fig. 1.7). Recently, a product that is made by braided multiple strands of monofilaments has been developed and can be used as a scaffold for the skin and tissues.

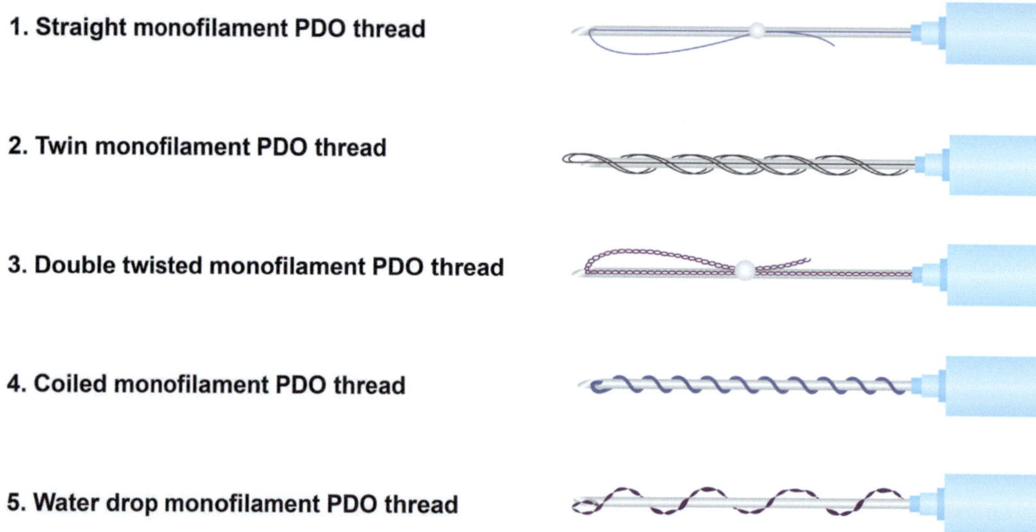

Fig. 1.7 Various types of monofilament PDO threads (i-THREAD, HEALUX)

In addition, as the technique of making cogs on the absorbable thread has also been developed, diversifying the number and shape of the cogs and the thickness of the threads, products with strong tensile force cogs are now available and thus, the actual lifting effect of the absorbable thread that naturally pulls the tissue also improved.

It still seems that monofilament thread lifting, for which several PDO threads without cogs integrating the needle are inserted to improve skin tone and resilience, is commonly performed among the various lifting methods and it is assumed to be due to its simple procedural process, manageability, and decreased risks of post-procedural complications or swelling. In addition, considering the materials of the thread, there is an immediate wound-healing process in the tissue in terms of the physiological effect on the skin when using the absorbable threads. As a result, new connective tissues are increased and new capillary blood vessels are formed. Since the retention period of the thread is more than 6 months, it is gradually absorbed, continuously stimulating collagen production and activating skin regeneration. As a result, the skin gets to look younger. For the physical effects, the absorbable thread helps skin tightening, firming, and shaping, which makes the skin healthier and more elastic. It naturally smoothens the lines of the cheek and jaw, which helps reduce wrinkles and make elastic and narrow facial features. Concomitantly, the thread serves as a scaffold in the skin, which enhances the effect and duration of the accompanying procedures such as filler and toxin injection, fat transplantation, laser therapy, and so on. Nowadays, these types of monofilament threads have become very diverse, and many methods of treatment have been developed, monofilament thread lifting procedures have established a solid foothold in the esthetic markets.

In the mid-2000s, gold threads, which were popular in Japan at the time, were introduced to Korea and also became prevalent, with some domestic companies starting to manufacture gold threads themselves and some groups of clinicians studying the effects of gold thread lifting. The authors used to perform gold thread lifting frequently, based on the findings on gold thread lifting that shows improvements in skin tone by stimulating collagen proliferation, which were even better outcomes than that of simple PDO threads, and its prevalent usages in Europe. Because the inserted gold threads of the initial model tend to be pulled out easily, due to the stiff nature of the material, the pure gold, the product that was designed to insert the PDO threads and

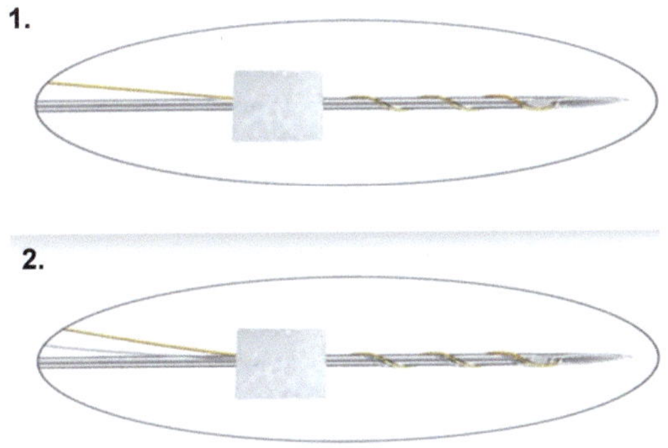

Fig. 1.8 (1) Gold thread, (2) gold and PDO combination thread

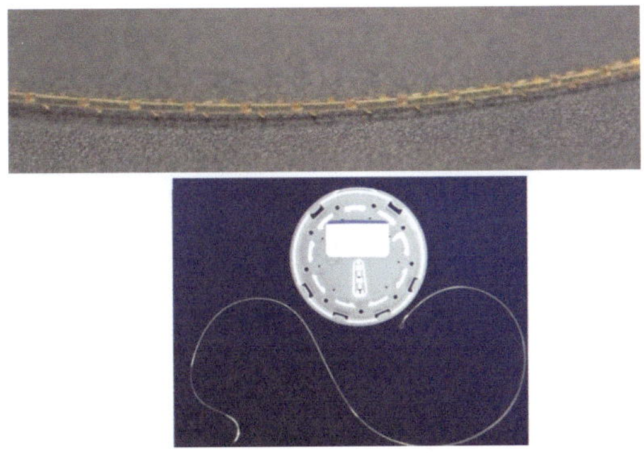

Fig. 1.9 V-loc lifting threads

the gold threads at the same time was developed. The PDO threads inserted with gold threads helped the settling of gold threads to the skin without being pulled out easily, facilitating the insertion of gold threads. It compensated for the disadvantage of the gold threads of the delayed effects when compared to the PDO threads, playing an auxiliary role in stimulating skin tissue (Fig. 1.8).

Nowadays, the product has been changed for easy usage, coating the PDO thread with gold on the outside to achieve the effects of the PDO thread and the pure gold thread simultaneously. Although any form of a product containing gold may have a lasting effect, the metal that remains in the body may disturb the results of many medical radiologic evaluations. Also, in patients with a lot of laser procedures, the gold threads inserted superficially on the surface of the skin may cause pigmentation, so the author does not perform the procedure, but some clinicians still prefer gold thread lifting.

Even though absorbable monofilament threads without cogs are frequently used for the natural outcomes, due to Koreans' thicker and firmer skin properties and heavier weight of the tissue per unit of lifting area, compared to that of Caucasian people, it is necessary to use absorbable lifting threads with more strength to pull the tissue. Since the author initially focused on lifting the tissues visibly using lifting cogged threads rather than monofilament threads, looking for the threads with definite lifting effects, we have come to have interests in other imported thread products after experiencing the EZ lift.

After experiencing various imported products, the author has come to use V-Loc, which is an I-shaped suturing thread with multiple cogs (Fig. 1.9).

V-Loc thread lifting is a lifting method using polytrimethylene carbonate (Maxon) material rather than PDO, the most commonly used material of absorbable threads, with the advantages of being not slippery like PDO, but softer and more resilient due to its material properties, facilitating the process of tying. It is also manageable and a clinician can feel more comfortable with pulling the threads. The number of cogs per unit length is larger than other existing threads, and the shape of the cog is not as sharp as the tip of the initial cogged threads, but rather made in the shape of the cogged threads of the press type nowadays. As it is known that the dual-angle cogs allow the area of contact with the tissue to be widened and the threads to be more effectively fixed, it is suggested that there is no necessity to fix the thread on the side of the temporal head but rather fixing on the front of the hairline. The author has come to choose the method due to the advantages of no need for fixing the threads on the temporal region like U- or V-shaped long cogged threads (Fig. 1.10).

However, since there is a hook on one side and a needle on the other side due to its usage for suturing, when not using the hook part, there was an inconvenience of removing the hook part and then bundling the threads together to pull the tissue and fix it. Using a method of inserting a thread into the skin and soft tissues in a V-shape,

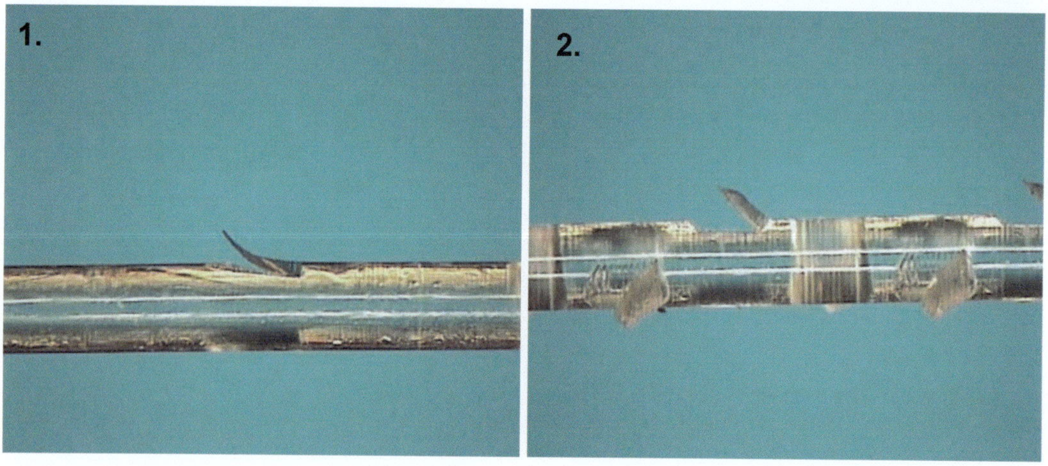

Fig. 1.10 (1) Single-angle cogs, (2) dual-angle cogs

pulling them together, and then tying them together, was used to lift tissue around the cheek and mouth, to improve the jowl of the mouth, and sharpen the jawline. Not only in elderly patients but also those who have relatively thin skin and want slimmer and taut faces, it was better to use the front of the hairline to pull the tissues rather than fixing threads in the temporal region which can cause headaches in patients.

In addition, due to the properties of the thread materials, the threads under the skin were not expected to only play the role of skin lifting but also to play the same role as reinforcing steel into the cement as if constructing the building. In addition, the procedure also has shown some effects of stimulating the skin and dermis broadly to promote the collagen production of the dermis, resulting in improved skin tone and elasticity after the thread lifting procedure, making the face more lifted and resilient. However, as the quality of the cogged threads that are integrated into the cannula produced in Korea has been improved, the demand for the thread lifting method of bundling the threads has gradually decreased.

There were some attempts of lifting tissues with other methods other than simple cogs. To make the fixation firmer and to extend the maintenance period, various products of nonabsorbable threads such as Tess, Ribbon, or Raise me up, which were fixed with a mesh in addition to cogs on the deep temporal fascia were developed (Fig. 1.11).

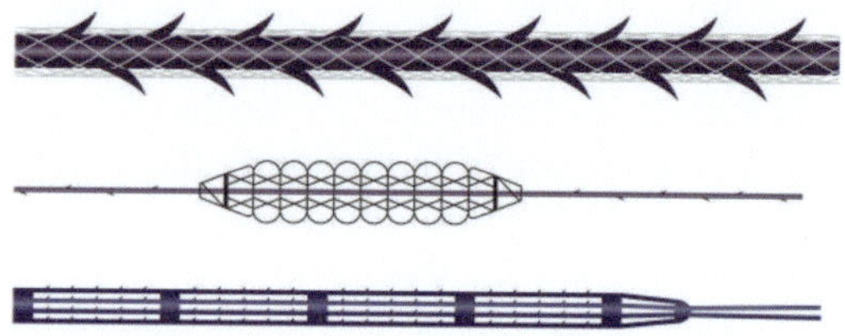

Fig. 1.11 Various types of lifting threads that combine cog and mesh

An elongated cylinder-shaped mesh surrounding the thread is known to be able to maintain the lifting effect by strong adhesion created through the mesh even after the tensile strength of the cogs is eliminated. However, these products were not widely used despite their efficacy, because of the burden of incision in the temporal region.

Also, another method of threading, bundling, and fixing the tissues with a silicone band, which was made as a rubber band rather than the general thread that easily breaks and once, the band gets loosened, the inserted area is incised and cut and lifting the drooped part again is possible. The lifting using a silicone band called M-sling has been developed by a domestic clinician and is still being used by some clinicians. It has been widely used as a material for vaginal molding and tightening in obstetrics and gynecology especially because of its elasticity. In recent years, Elastic

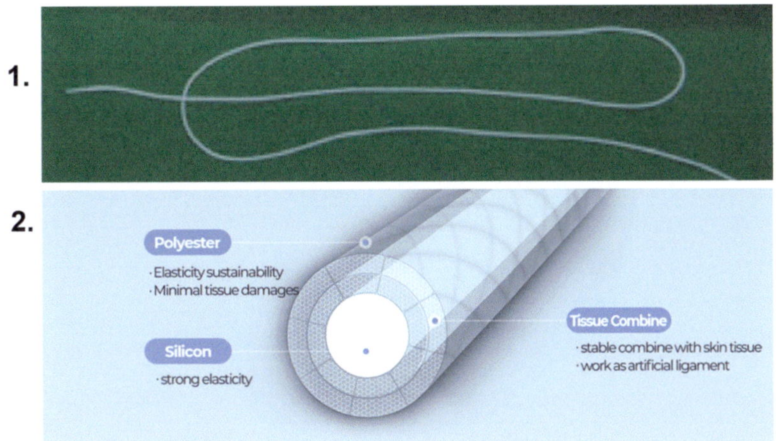

Fig. 1.12 (1) M-sling silicone band, (2) elasticum band

thread lifting using Elasticum, a nonabsorbable suture thread that is wrapped in a form of sheath by polyester weaving in the middle of a silicone monofilament, called Elasticum lifting, has been introduced and used in some clinics. It can be said that it is a lifting method using an elastic band with elasticity like M-sling (Fig. 1.12).

These methods commonly require a small incision to insert the materials due to difficulties in implanting with completely no incision, which is different from the basic method that we commonly use with nonincisional thread lifting. Of course, in thread lifting, a stab incision can be used to tie the thread to be fixed, but basically it is distinguished from normal nonincision thread lifting in that it requires a certain size of incision to manipulate the material. In addition, at first, the elasticity of the silicone band is good, so the pulling effect is strong, but since it is made of nonabsorbable material, some people may feel uncomfortable. In addition, if the elastic band fixing the tissue is tied too tightly, the tissue can be torn due to pulling force, and the possibility of inflammation or foreign body reaction over time is also higher than when using the suture-type cogged thread.

The histories of trends in lifting threads in Korea since its first introduction have been discussed above. Nowadays, since various kinds of lifting threads are manufactured and imported, instead of a certain type of thread being recommended suitable for lifting, it is preferable to select threads that meet the purpose of the procedure according to the overall condition of the patient, the operation site, and status of patient's skin and tissues.

2 Basic Considerations for Thread Lifting

Contents

2.1 Definition of Terms

For effective and systematic learning of thread lifting procedures, it is important to start by clearly defining the terms used to describe the procedure. There are three basic terms in thread lifting: the first is the Fixing Point, the second is the Hanging Point, and the third is Directionality.

2.1.1 Fixing Point

The fixing point refers to the location on the face that receives the pulling force when a thread is used to lift a specific area. It does not mean that the thread is physically anchored at that specific point; rather, it represents the area that receives force in the direction of the thread lift's orientation. To understand this concept, consider bungee

S. M. Oh et al., *The Art and Science of Thread Lifting Based on Pinch Anatomy and Moving Plane*,
https://doi.org/10.1007/978-981-97-5516-5_2

jumping. When jumping, the body is connected to the jump platform with a cord. The jump platform, where the cord is attached, can be thought of as the fixing point.

2.1.2 Hanging Point

The hanging point refers to the location on the face toward which the thread is pulled, based on the fixing point. When assuming that a barbed thread is inserted toward the area of the face that needs lifting, the hanging point is where the end of the thread reaches. The hanging point may or may not coincide with the area the practitioner intends to lift. For example, when lifting sagging cheeks, the hanging point could be anywhere between the fixing point and the sagging cheek flesh. The procedure can still be effective even if the hanging point does not exactly match the intended lifting area because the tissues below the end of the thread can still be lifted. This is possible because the facial soft tissues are interconnected by subcutaneous connective tissue and various ligamentous structures. In certain areas of the face, like below the zygomatic arch or at the border of the anterior part of the masseter muscle, the subcutaneous fibrous tissue is dense and firm. When the thread is anchored in these areas with dense fibrous tissue and pulled, it can lift tissues even at a distance from the point of anchorage. For instance, lifting the marionette lines toward the head does not necessarily require the thread's end to reach the marionette lines. In some patients, inserting and pulling the thread near the dense fibrous tissue beneath the lateral cheekbone can achieve significant lifting effects (Fig. 2.1).

2.1.3 Directionality

In thread lifting procedures, directionality refers to the direction of the pulling force generated from the hanging point toward the fixing point. True lifting, in its real sense, requires clear directionality to achieve the desired effect. For example, in the early days of thread lifting, procedures involving the insertion of smooth, absorbable threads could create weak fixing points and achieve some degree of skin tightening but could not establish a clear directionality between the fixing and hanging points, thus failing to produce sufficient lifting effects. In such cases, the effects of thread lifting were attributed merely to the chemical reactions occurring when the absorbable threads interacted with the body's tissues.

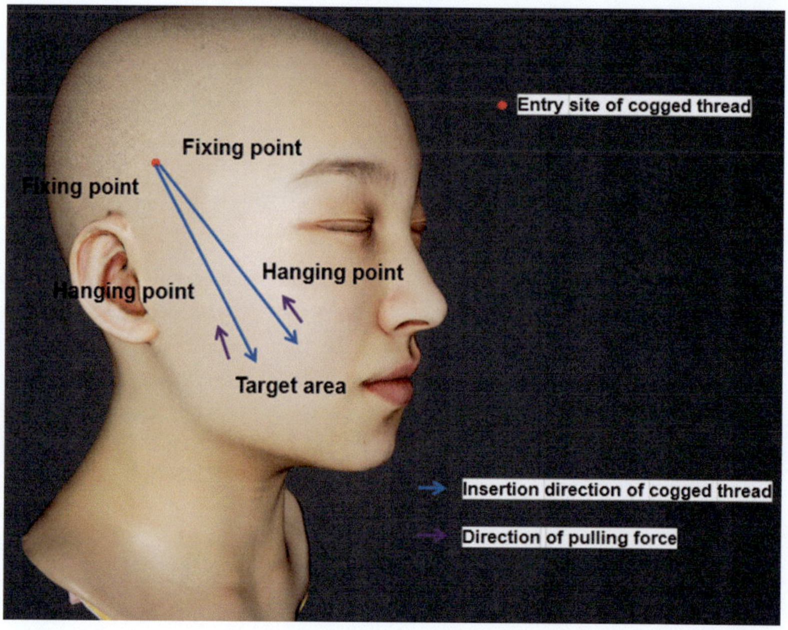

Fig. 2.1 When the target area to be pulled and hanging point are different

Therefore, to be considered a meaningful thread lifting procedure, it must clearly demonstrate the directionality of thread lifting, enabling visible lifting effects.

2.2 Importance of Fixing Points

The difference between thread lifting procedures that create a fixing point and various other treatments that do not (such as thread lifts without a fixing point, and treatments using ultrasound or radiofrequency devices) lies in the presence or absence of clear directionality in the results. Generally, treatments lacking directionality can still achieve a degree of lifting effect by contracting the skin or atrophying the fat layer, making the face appear tighter.

This is related to the changes in the face due to aging, as every component of the face undergoes changes over time. The combination of skin laxity, fat reduction or sagging, and the stretching of fibrous tissues surrounding the fat contributes to the appearance of an aged face. By contracting the skin or the subcutaneous fibrous connective tissues, or by atrophying the subcutaneous fat layer, these treatments can tighten loose skin and facial tissues, thereby producing an effect similar to lifting.

However, these methods fall short of the actual lifting effect achieved by barbed thread lifting procedures that strongly form a fixing point. The concept of the fixing point is not new. Sulamanidze et al. have discussed the existence of both floating and fixed types of threads in thread lifting. Mendelson et al. have divided the face into two major areas: the mobile inner part and the static, fixed outer part, suggesting that the outer part of the face, which is firm and less mobile, can be utilized as a fixing point in lifting procedures and surgeries.

Hyen Ho Han et al. have reported good results by using fixed-type thread lifting in the outer parts of the face and floating-type thread lifting in the more mobile anterior parts of the face. The fixed-type thread lifting mentioned here, which involves forming a strong fixing point in the SMAS (superficial musculoaponeurotic system) area, underscores the importance of the fixing point (Fig. 2.2).

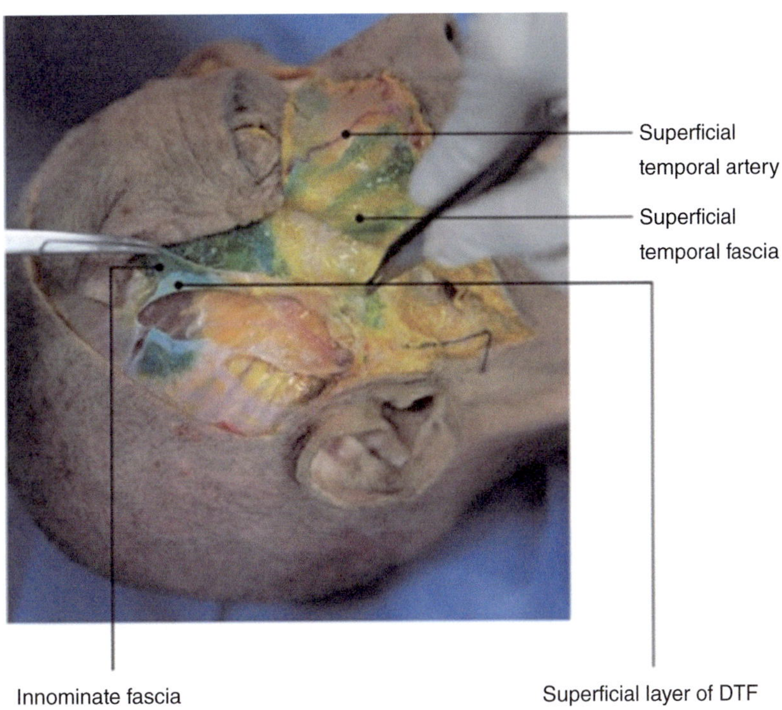

Fig. 2.2 Superficial and deep temporal fascia of the temple region

Therefore, to maximize the lifting effect, there must be a solid fixing point in the direction the tissue is being pulled. This is because a force that pulls in the opposite direction of the sagging caused by aging and gravity must be created and sustained.

While there is a relative difference in strength, all thread lifting techniques implicitly involve the principle of a fixing point or something that serves a similar function. Some have evidence from animal or clinical studies, while others lack substantial evidence. A solid fixing point can be created by passing the thread through or over the firm fascial areas of facial tissues. However, anchoring the thread in the fascial areas is not technically easy, and bleeding can prolong the procedure. Improper handling of bleeding can lead to complications such as hematoma.

Therefore, if anatomical knowledge that minimizes the possibility of side effects like bleeding while securely creating a fixing point is established, along with standard procedural methods based on this knowledge, safe and effective thread lifting can be expected. This is also why the discussion of fixing points is often the starting point for considerations in thread lifting procedures. In the book, the authors plan to present various studies conducted to understand the mechanism of thread lifting, which will greatly assist readers in fundamentally understanding thread lifting.

2.3 Basic Method of Forming Fixing Points

The principle of the first generation absorbable monofilament noncogged PDO thread lifting, which was used in the past, is illustrated in Fig. 2.3. During the era when mono-thread lifting was popular, techniques that involved inserting a greater number of threads on the side where lifting was desired were utilized, taking into account the direction in which lifting was hoped to occur. Initially, it was difficult to provide evidence-based answers to why this was done, but subsequent studies on absorbable monofilament thread lifting have been conducted, allowing for a scientific explanation of the reasons. Among

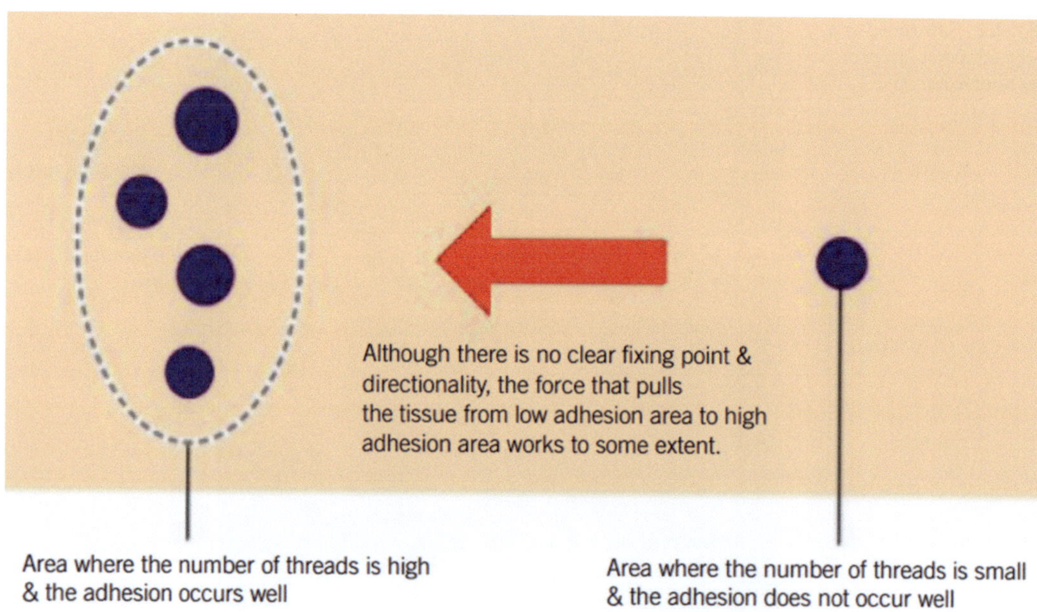

Fig. 2.3 Principle of pulling force and directionality in monofilament non-cogged thread lifting

these, the histological changes such as tissue contraction and fibrous tissue proliferation that occur when the PDO component of the threads enters human tissue provide theoretical support for the use of monofilament threads in thread lifting. However, as previously mentioned, monofilament thread lifts without barbs cannot create distinct fixing and hanging points. This results in weaker tissue traction compared to barbed thread lifts, leading to a lack of clear directional effect, which is a significant drawback.

With the advent of absorbable barbed threads, the methods and principles of creating fixing points in barbed thread lifting procedures have become well-known. The most commonly used thread lifting technique today involves short, straight, bidirectional cogged threads. This method pulls and gathers tissue from both directions toward the middle section of the thread, which lacks barbs. Therefore, this technique is more aptly described as soft tissue repositioning rather than lifting using fixing and hanging points. However, by tying the ends of the threads at the same entry point after inserting short, straight, bidirectional cogged threads, a weak fixing point can be created, allowing the tissue at the opposite end of the thread to be pulled.

However, when using medium-length I-type cogged threads for thread lifting, it is advisable to anchor one end of the thread in the firm and fixed tissues on the outer side of the face, such as the head or ear area, or in the tough fibrous ligamentous tissues, thereby serving as a fixing point. The opposite end of the thread should be anchored in the tissue of the area to be lifted, creating a clear directionality toward the firm tissue and pulling the tissue in that direction. The ability to form a solid fixing point by catching one end of the straight barbed thread in the SMAS layer, where there are firm ligaments or fascia, has been proven through anatomical studies. If the practitioner understands the principles of fixing and hanging points and has sufficient anatomical knowledge of the face, they can achieve good lifting effects.

2.4 Basic Classification According to the Purpose of Lifting Threads

In the past, the usage of threads to lift drooped facial skin and tissues were mainly for the subsidiary role of surgery or suturing, lifting, and fixing tissues to firmer tissues with minimal incision. As cogged threads made by cutting out the threads, maximizing the tissue-holding effects of threads became available, it was feasible to lift the tissues using threads with small cogs even without a single minimal incision, but until then, the products introduced in Korea were made of unabsorbable materials. Other than some foreign products, the initial absorbable thread models from domestic manufacturers were mainly used to enhance skin tone and elasticity by collagen generation induced by tissue reaction in the absorbing process of threads rather than actual lifting effects.

Therefore, even until the mid-2000s, when selecting the threads for facial lifting, unabsorbable threads were mainly used for lifting drooped tissues of the lower third of the face to maintain the effects over time, while absorbable threads were used on a limited basis for purposes of retaining elasticity of skins or contouring jawlines.

However, with the development of thread and cogs production techniques, many manufacturers have come to produce various types of absorbable threads with actual lifting effects and advanced shaped cogs, facilitating convenient application of the product, especially with significant improvement in qualities of product from domestic manufacturers.

With these improvements in the quality of the product, lifting effects of PDO-cogged threads also have improved with prolonged periods of maintenance, resultantly gradually increasing the demand for absorbable lifting threads. One of the important changes due to these tendencies was overall changes in perceptions toward the efficacy of unabsorbable threads and absorbable threads.

In the author's personal view, with an increase in patients undergoing thread lifting procedures, it seems that there are no significant differences shown in clinical maintenance duration between absorbable and unabsorbable threads. In addition, in many cases that undergo facelift surgery and have a history of thread lifting procedures in the past, it is shown that fibrosis induced by collagenesis is more likely to be found in patients with procedures using absorbable threads when compared to those with unabsorbable threads, which may result in prevention of skin drooping and improvements in quality of the skin.

Nowadays, since procedures to lift the drooped skin and tissues are popularized, it has become the main concern whether to use absorbable threads which are processed to be manipulated with cogs, cones, or meshes or absorbable monofilaments without any processing. However, in order to accord with the original purpose of "lifting" the targeted tissues or skins, the authors suggest that the lifting threads which are processed to be manipulated with some tools to hold and lift the skins or soft tissues directly be selected.

Focusing on the differences in morphological characteristics of the cogged threads for lifting, there are two types of threads that are most commonly used: 30–40 cm long-length U- or V-shaped cogged threads, a long thread bent to act as two strands of threads, and short- or medium-length I-shaped cogged threads, a shorter thread that is inserted as one strand.

Long-length U- or V-shaped cogged threads are manufactured in a bent form, which are divided bidirectionally by relatively long central parts that have no cogs, forming a single bidirectional type of cog whose strands are facing each other (Fig. 2.4).

Unlike the long-length U- or V-shaped cogged threads that are folded to be used as two strands, short- or medium-length I-shaped cogged threads are products that are shorter in length to be inserted in a straight line without folding. I-shaped cogged threads are usually equipped in the cannula for convenience. The single bidirectional type of I-shaped cogged threads basically has the same position and direction of cogs and mechanisms as U- or V-shaped cogged threads, but U- or V-shaped cogged threads just have a longer length and manufactured in bent form (Fig. 2.5).

Unlike the long-length U- or V-shaped cogged threads on which only single bidirectional type of cogs that concentrate the strength to the central part can be equipped, various types of cogs with different positions and shapes such as single or double bidirectional type, multiple bidirectional type, and twin or spiral bidirectional type can be used for short- or medium-length I-shaped cogged threads. As mentioned above, the shape of the initial cogs for lifting thread was also simply sharp, but as the technique of cogs production developed, curved cogs with the shape of the cobra's head, rose thorns, or triangular shape of arrowheads became available and recently, even cogs with the shape of reversed trapezoids by inner punching, which may enable clinicians to use the cogs freely regardless of the direction also became available.

It is also possible to use the long-length U- or V-shaped cogged threads in various forms such as L-shaped, V-shaped, and I-shaped threads cen-

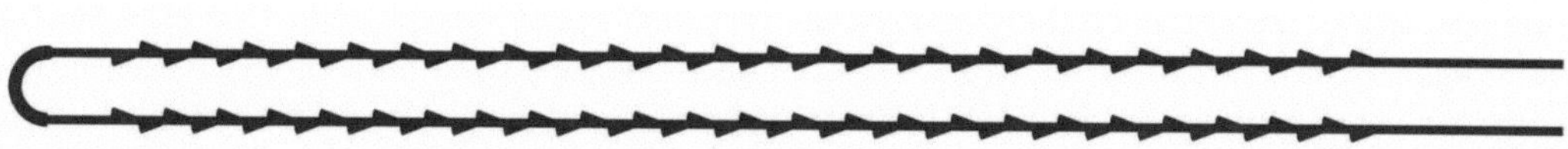

Fig. 2.4 Long-length cannula-guided U-type cogged thread

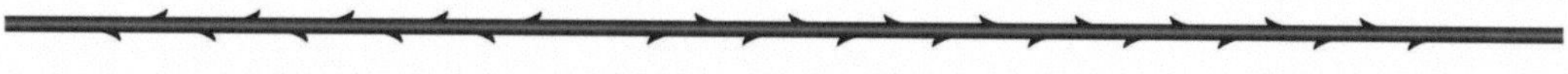

Fig. 2.5 Short- or medium-length I-type bidirectional cogged thread

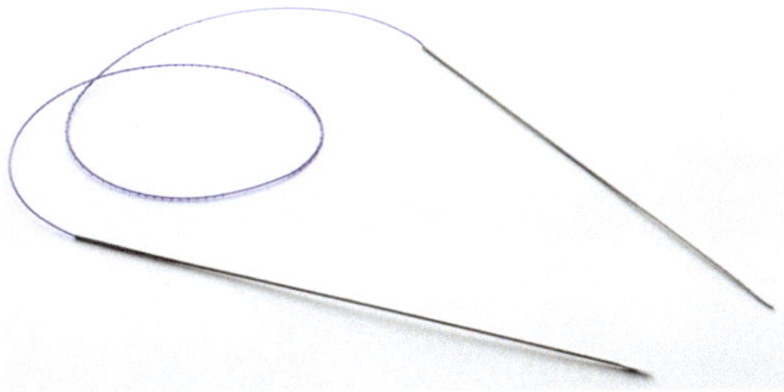

Fig. 2.6 Long-length double needle V-type cogged thread (i-THREAD Magic Plus, HEALUX)

tering in the parts of threads with no cogs according to the goal and site of the procedures. Also, some products of thin cogged threads with integrated needles that can be used without the help of a cannula are being manufactured (Fig. 2.6).

In the case of thicker cogged threads, a cannula should be used to facilitate the movement of the threads without stimulating the tissues through which the threads protrude. However, since it is impossible to equip the long-length U- or V-shaped cogged threads with a cannula due to its procedural principles, products only packed with threads are manufactured and a cannula guide should be used in practice. These lifting threads longer in length are bent and manufactured in U- or V-shape to have lifting effects of two strands for one of the main goals to lift drooped facial tissues including the jawline. Each strand that is bent and facing each other is basically designed to gather the tissues of both lateral sides of the threads into the central part of the threads that have no cogs. Even though many procedural designs are possible to use with these long cogged threads, these threads have been named U-shaped cogged threads symbolically after the form of the most commonly used procedural design.

On the other hand, the short- or medium-length I-shaped cogged thread lifting, which is performed without changing the design of threads according to the purpose and site of the procedures, is a simpler method to lift the skin and tissues by inserting the I-shaped cogged threads into any sites near the hairline, around ears and mouth, rather than inserting into the temporal regions. I-shaped cogged threads that are relatively shorter than the U- or V-shaped cogged threads were initially considered to have much less lifting effects than the long-length cogged threads and thereby, mostly used to lift the tissues lightly, including the nasolabial folds, melolabial folds, crow's feet, and infraorbital wrinkles, which require natural lifting rather than lifting the lower facial tissues upward. However, with recent improvements in the production process of the cogged threads and the shapes and positions of cogs, the lifting effects of the I-shaped cogged threads have noticeably improved and resultantly, the procedures using this type of cogged threads have become more popular.

The initial I-shaped cogged threads for lifting the lower facial tissues, which have the same numbers of cogs in both the upper and lower sides of the thread, had the disadvantage of making the cheek more bulging in patients with large cheekbone by concentrating the strength to the center of the thread and gathering the tissue.

Afterward, the number of the upper cogs that are placed on the temporal region were reduced since its main role was to hold relatively tight upper facial tissues above the cheek to prevent threads from slipping rather than gathering the tissues. On the contrary, the number of the lower cogs that are placed under the cheek increased since it had to lift the loose lower facial tissues upwards including the drooped cheek tissues. In this way, it became possible to prevent the cheeks from standing out in patients with prominent zygomatic bone and lateral cheek hollow after the procedure by keeping the firm tissues of the upper facial part including the zygomatic arch evenly threaded and gathering the loose tissues beneath the zygomatic arch.

In recent years, the purpose of thread lifting has changed and the key to the procedure is to retain the lifted tissues in place rather than forcibly lift the tissues. As mentioned above, multiple or spiral directional cogged threads that are optimized to naturally reposition the drooped tissues that had moved to the site of firmer tissues in lying down with chin-up position and effectively

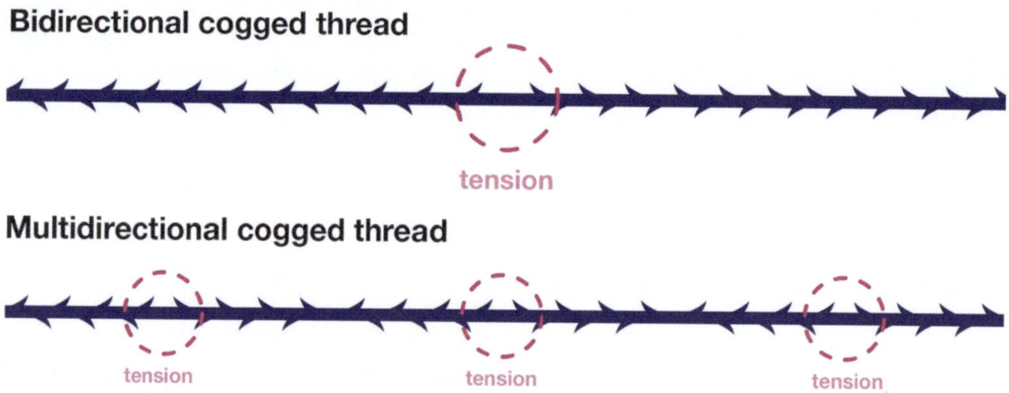

Fig. 2.7 Dispersion of tension in multidirectional cogged thread

stabilize them became available, which, unlike single bidirectional cogs, may distribute the tension rather than concentrating the tension to the center. These cogged threads, which are called zig-zag type cogged threads due to their shape, are manufactured to maximize the holding strength that the threads hold and fix the tissues on the spot rather than maximizing the anchoring strength, as described above (Fig. 2.7).

For these I-shaped cogged thread lifting, some clinicians have used a method of tying the threads of the upper entry point rather than cutting them, thus preventing the sagging over time as much as possible to lift the tissues more firmly and extend the duration of retention. However, with recent improvements in the shapes and types of cogs on the I-shaped cogged threads, products with improved anchoring strength for the immediate effect of lifting the tissues upwards and maximized holding strength that is considered to be important for the extension of the retention duration became available, the additional measures for fixing have become increasingly obsolete.

Particularly, the recently developed products have greatly improved fixing effects on the firm tissues of the upper facial part without making the entry point within the hairlines where hair exists. And they can be used with a method of embedding the thread in the tissue without making an exit point through which the tip of the thread penetrates the skin like a long-length U- or V-shaped cogged thread due to its procedural mechanisms, reducing the risks of bleeding in lower facial part caused by vascular damage or damages to the other structures such as nerves due to penetration of the skin.

Also, since I-shaped cogged threads are equipped with the cannula, it became easy to use the products with no need of using a cannula guide. In addition, the shape of the integrated cannula of the product is also designed to be much easier to use than that of the initial products, with products recently being manufactured with cannula whose shape of tips are designed for little damage to the structures and enabling pass smoothly through the tough ligamentous tissues firmly fixed to surrounding tissues. The various types of tips of needle and cannula products on the esthetic market so far are summarized as follows (Fig. 2.8).

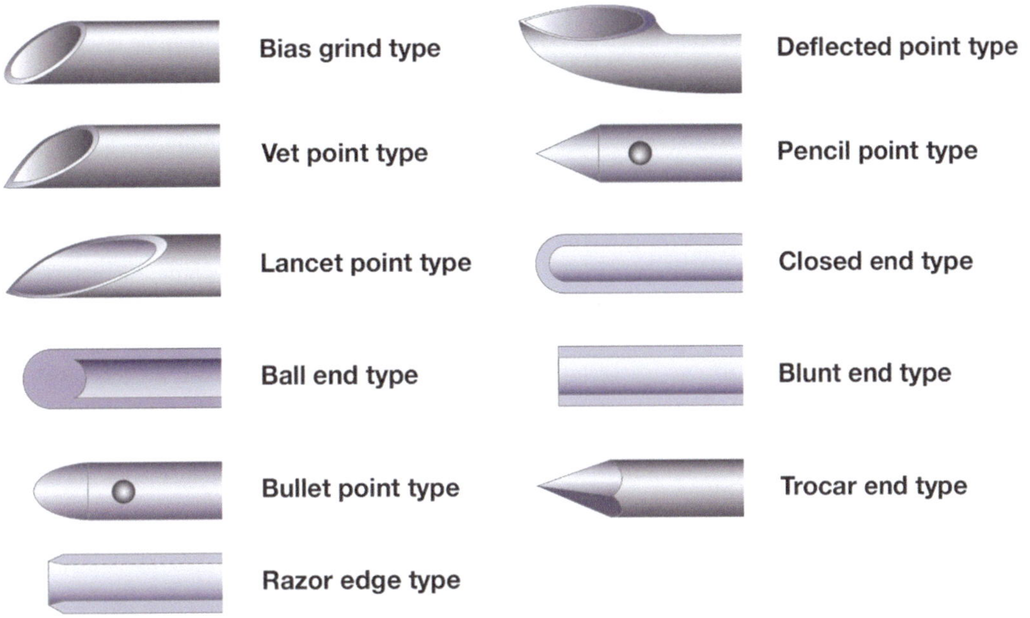

Fig. 2.8 Various types of needle and cannula tips

2.5 Influencing Factors on Outcomes of Procedure

Until recently, the main purpose of thread lifting was to improve the sagging of skin and soft tissue that appeared with the progress of aging. Therefore, anatomically, we studied why and how this sagging of skin and soft tissue occurs as aging occurs, and what structural changes in the face are particularly involved in this change, we are interested in making the face look younger by inserting the thread into a plane to improve the sagging of the skin and soft tissue.

But these days, Thread lifting is used to improve jowls around the mouth corner and sharpen the jawlines not only in patients with old age but also in those who want to have narrow and distinct facial features even without drooped skins. In addition, as threads that are effective in contouring the narrower face as well as in lifting drooped skins on the cheek or around the mouth are currently developed, demands for the procedure have increased, including patients in their 20s or 30s who want to make a slimmer face as well as patients with relatively old age who have widely changed face with inelastic skin. By intensively lifting drooped tissues around cheeks and jawlines, which are not sufficiently solved by botulinum toxin, the effects of sharpening jawlines can be found in patients of young age without too square and large jaw bone.

The author also currently uses cocktail contouring injections (named oval face injection) which may lessen soft tissues to make a slimmer face and lift drooped tissues, reducing the lateral volumes of the face as much as possible and then, additionally perform lifting procedures with cogged threads to lift drooped skin of cheeks, maximizing the slimming effect of the face by tightening the skin around jawline while reducing the bulges of the lateral part of the face.

Therefore, these days, doctors who perform thread lifting procedures should have their own procedural methods and concepts depending on the purpose of the procedures. You should be fully familiar with the techniques used basically for general thread lifting, the types and characteristics of threads from various brands made by various companies, and how to use them suitable for each thread.

When choosing a thread based on the degree of sagging of the skin and tissue, it is difficult to clearly determine which thread is appropriate for a certain degree of sagging. The reason for this is that when performing thread lifting, the selection can be different according to the doctor's pursuit of a degree of lifting or uniqueness of each patient. The pre- and postprocedural pictures of cases provided by the thread manufacturer, often are pictures of patients with ideal conditions. To give more credibility to the procedure to the patient, it is more advisable to provide information on indications of each product, properly explaining precise indications and limitations of procedures.

If some degree of personalized indication is established, cogged threads, which may cause less sense of irritation, can be used for slight tissue sagging that requires light lifting, but when stronger tensile and anchoring strength and stress are required, products that are specifically appropriate for the case should be selected. When not using a fixed type procedure that ties up from the top or fixes to the mesh, a long-length U-shaped cogged thread or short- or medium-length I-shaped cogged thread with good pulling force (considering the thickness of the thread, anchoring, and holding strength) can be used. However, it can't be said that a certain product is absolutely superior to the others, since, for example, when a long-length U- or V-shaped cogged thread is used in the temporal region, the lifting effects can be significant, but the degree of inconvenience due to the patient's unique feature or many complications caused by end of the thread penetrating through the skin should be considered.

The best option is a product that may minimize the inconvenience and side effects of the patient, but with significant effects. In order to achieve this goal, it is possible to use products in combination.

In case the lifting was performed forcibly, the adaptation period may last more than 1–2 months in severe cases, and the ruggedness of the skin can last longer than that. To solve these adverse events, some doctors lift the tissues upwards as much as possible and release them through massage, adjusting the pulling force, in this case, the excess massage after the procedure will loosen the lifted sites and the effect can be gone. On the other hand, in some cases, even with an intense massage, the sites don't get loosen, and the patient might strongly complain.

Therefore, it is necessary to establish the characteristics and the quality of each thread according to the type, so as to select the most appropriate type of thread for the condition of the patient and the concept pursued by the clinician. For that reason, the author will look at various factors that affect the results of thread lifting that we basically need to know in order to produce good results regardless of the actual product type of each company when choosing threads for thread lifting procedures.

2.5.1 The Materials of Threads

The material of thread used for thread lifting has a significant influence on the lifting effect and the duration of retention. In the past, polypropylene (Prolene™) nonabsorbable thread was widely used, but recently, polydioxanone (PDO) thread is the most widely used. Also, polylactic acid (PLLA) and polycaprolactone (PCL) threads are currently being used. Some absorbable threads are made of a single component, while others may be made of multiple components in combination with PGA (polyglycolic acid). Quill lift, for example, is made of a mixture of 75% PGA and 25% PCL, while V-loc is made of 60% PGA, 26% (polytrimethylene carbonate, Maxon™), and 14% PDO.

Unlike nonabsorbable threads such as single-component polypropylene, the mixture of multiple materials is used when manufacturing absorbable threads, because each material has a different tissue reaction, tensile strength, and absorption period. For example, threads such as chromic catgut can induce better tissue reactions, but have weaker tensile strength and shorter absorption period, while PDO thread may have the strongest tensile strength among the absorbable threads and it takes longer than six months for PDO threads to be absorbed, making the threads be widely used.

The components of the thread also affect the elasticity of the thread.

Elasticity refers to elastic force, which should not be viewed simply as a property of an elastic and flexible object, but elastic force refers to the force by which an elastic object returns to its original state.

Elastic force is calculated by Hooke's law, which is usually expressed by the formula $F = k\triangle X$. Here, F means Elastic force, K means Elastic modulus, which quantifies the hardness of each object, and X means the degree of deformation (elastic limit).

To explain the equation, Elastic modulus k and Elastic limit X are constants determined by the material and shape of the object. Therefore, when an object has a similar Elastic force (F), a material with a larger Elastic modulus and a smaller Elastic limit feels like a solid, and a material with a larger Elastic limit feels like a more viscoelastic object that has a more flexible and soft elastic property than a firm elastic material (Fig. 2.9).

For example, Silhouette soft, which is made of poly-L-lactic acid (PLLA), has a larger Elastic limit than other threads, so it can be better adapted to the contraction and relaxation of the skin and tissue caused by facial movements after the procedure. However, in any case, this soft elastic thread is not always good. In the case of threads with good firm elasticity due to their high Elastic modulus, such as PDO threads, this firmness can rather support tissues well at the beginning of the procedure and keep the lifted skin and tissues in place without movement. Therefore, if you understand the difference between the firm and soft elasticity of each material, you can choose the most suitable thread depending on the patient's facial condition and the purpose of the procedure, and furthermore, mix the threads well to produce the most harmonious result.

2.5.2 Thickness of Thread: Tensile Strength

Tensile strength of the thread can be determined by measuring how long the thread holds without breaking when applied with tension force, a force that holds and pulls the ends of the thread on either side of the thread, and the thickness of the thread is the most important factor determining the tensile strength of each thread (Fig. 2.10).

The thread used for thread lifting is usually made in a circular shape, and when comparing the size of a long object in this circular shape, there is a method of comparing the diameter of the circle formed by the object and the cross-sectional area of the circle. First, after measuring the diameter of the thread, the cross-sectional area of the thread can be obtained using the math-

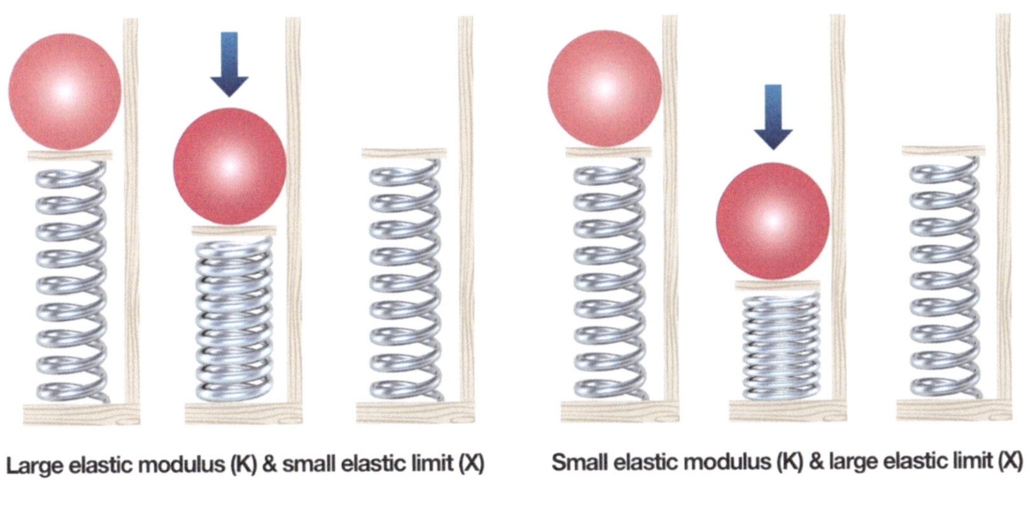

Fig. 2.9 Comparison of two springs with similar elastic force (F), but different elastic modulus (K) and elastic limit (X)

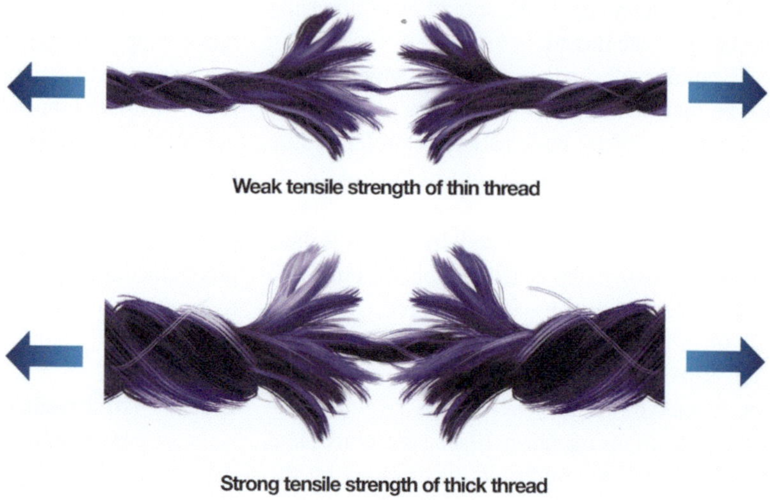

Fig. 2.10 Relationship between thickness and tensile strength of the threads

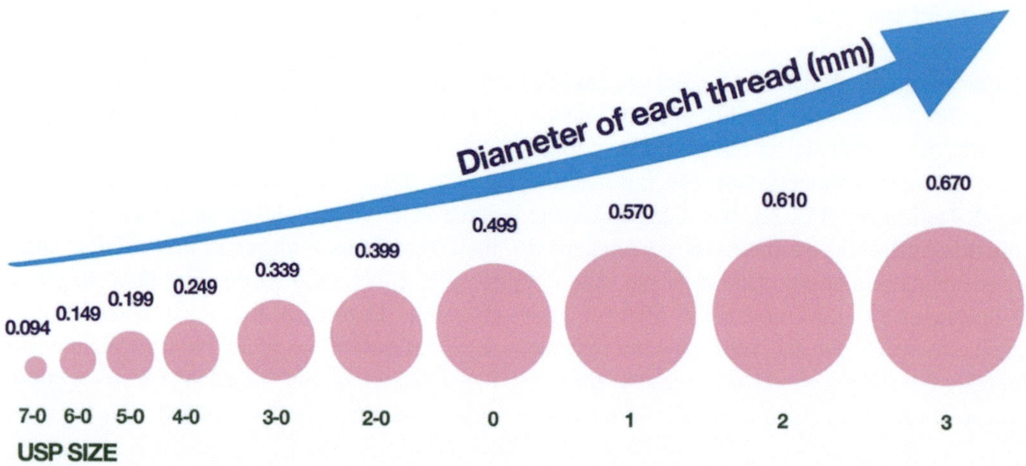

Fig. 2.11 Comparison of thread thickness based on diameter

ematical formula, which is calculated as the cross-sectional area of the circle = 3.14 × the radius of the circle^2. After measuring the diameter of the threads, calculating the cross-sectional area of each thread using this formula, and comparing the difference between the diameter and cross-sectional area, it can be seen that the cross-sectional area of each thread differs by the square of the diameter difference. For example, if the difference in diameter size of two threads is twice, the cross-sectional area of two threads is four times the square of two, and if the difference in diameter is four times, the cross-sectional area is 16 times the square of four.

Comparing the difference between the diameter of a thread and the cross-sectional area depending on the thickness of each thread after measuring the tensile strength of threads with the same material and shape, it could be seen that the difference in the cross-sectional area, not the diameter of the thread. If you look at the classification according to the thickness of the threads we usually use, you can see that the USP size based on the diameter of the threads is numbered as follows (Fig. 2.11).

According to this classification standard, if the difference in diameter between two threads is twice that of the same material and shape, the dif-

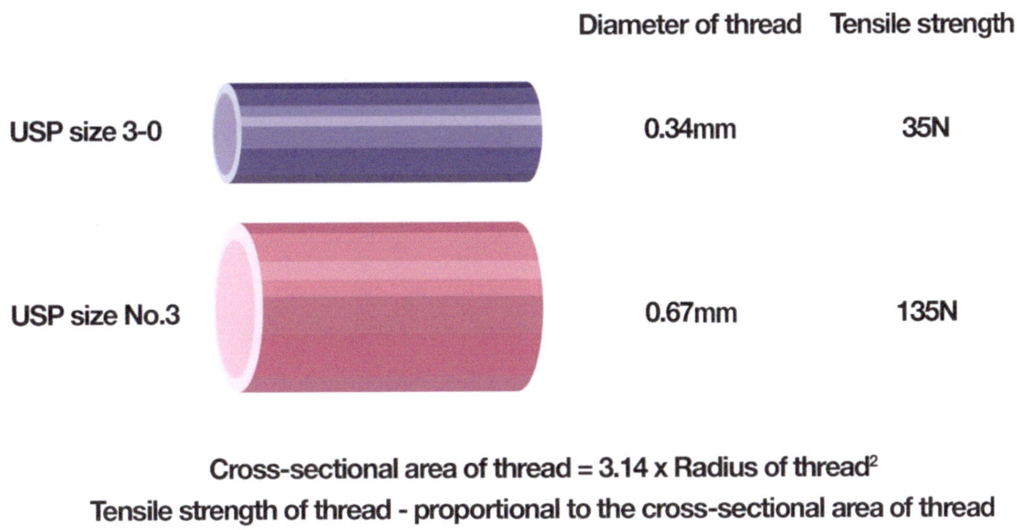

Fig. 2.12 Differences in tensile strength according to differences in diameters of threads

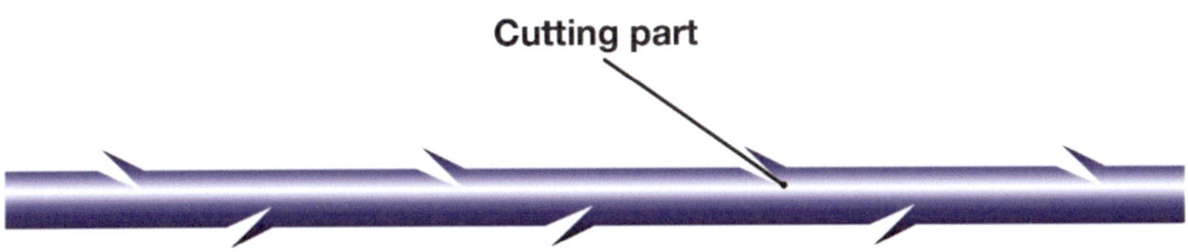

Fig. 2.13 Cutting-type cogged thread

ference in tensile strength between the two threads is proportional to the cross-sectional area, so it should be considered that the difference in diameter is four times. For example, comparing the tensile strength of USP size 3-0 thread of 0.34 mm diameter and USP size No. 3 thread of 0.67 mm diameter, the tensile strength of 3-0 thread is about 35 N and No. 3 thread is about 135 N, which is about four times the difference in diameter in tensile strength (Fig. 2.12).

What we need to think about here is that the actual tensile strength of the cogged threads for lifting is not the thickness of the original thread, but the thinnest part after the cogs are made in the thread. Another important consideration is how much heat treatment was applied to the thread to shape various thread products, including the cogged threads. In order to form a specific shape of the thread products, heat treatment is required, and at this time, heat given to the thread changes the basic properties of the thread and acts as a factor to reduce tensile strength. In addition, heat may be inevitably generated in the process of mechanically manipulating the thread to form a cog or a specific shape without intentionally applying heat, which may affect the physical properties of the material of the thread.

When comparing several clinically used cogged threads, cutting-type cogged threads that cut the thread with a machine blade first make a thorn-shaped cog by making a scratch on the thread, so the parts with the cog on top become thinner, reducing tensile strength compared to the thread as a whole (Fig. 2.13).

These days, molding-type cogged threads are increasing to maintain the thickness of the thread as much as possible, and these molding-type cogged threads do not have only advantages.

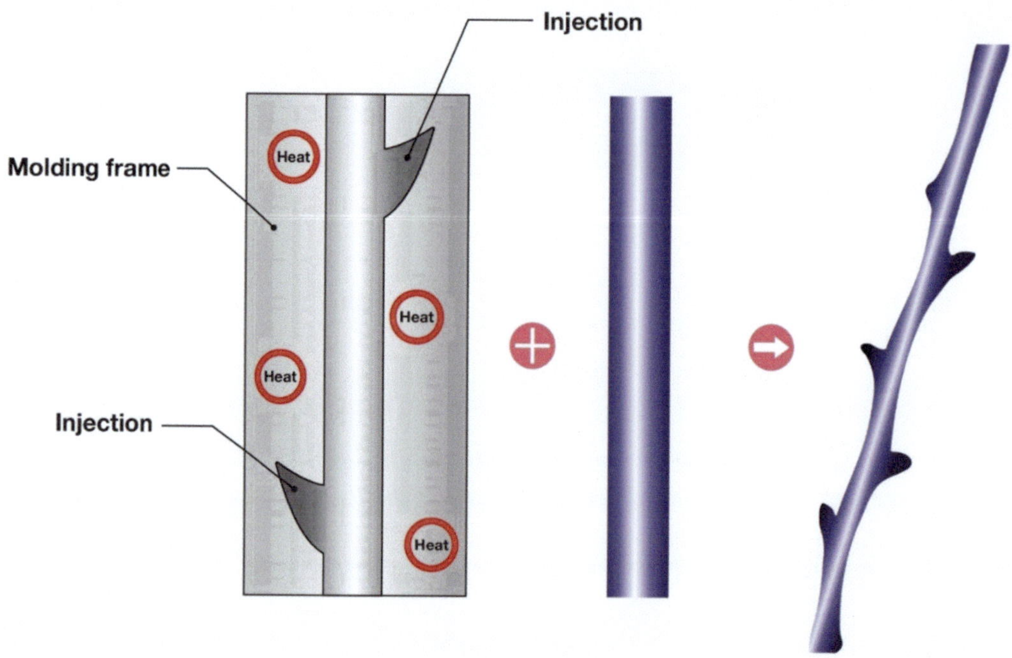

Fig. 2.14 Manufacturing process of injection molding-type cogged thread

Usually, these kinds of cogged threads are produced in two ways.

First, the thread is placed in a molding frame with a thread shape, heat is applied, and the cogs are attached to the injection molding system, and due to the heat applied during the manufacturing process, the shape may be slightly distorted (Fig. 2.14).

Another method is to cut unnecessary parts by pressing a thread thicker than the marked size of the thread with the press molding system with a sculpt cutter, and to print only the shape of the thread from the thick thread (Fig. 2.15).

Due to the nature of the manufacturing process of attaching the cogs when the thickness of the thread is the same as the cutting-type cogged thread, the cogged part may have a stronger tensile strength than the cutting-type cogged threads, but products heat-treated during the manufacturing process may have a weaker tensile strength.

These days, many so-called heatless molding cogged thread products are seen that press sculpt molding is performed without a heat treatment process to prevent the tensile strength of thread from decreasing due to heat treatment as much as possible. Of course, each company may differ according to the press molding method, but the author believes that heat is inevitably generated to some extent while carving the shape of the cogged thread using a machine. Therefore, it can be said that products that minimize the heat inevitably generated during the manufacturing process are good products.

Another clinical consideration when using a molding-type cogged thread rather than a cutting-type cogged thread is the size of the cannula required to insert the thread and the degree of discomfort during the procedure. If the thread parts without cogs are similar in size, it can be seen that the cutting-type cogs occur upward and the outer part of the cogs is slightly larger than the product size, but the difference is not as large as the molding-type cogs. In the injection molding-type cogged thread, as mentioned above, since a cog is added to the outer surface of the thread, it can be seen that the part with the cogs becomes considerably larger than the size of the product. Sculpt molding-type cogged thread cuts unnecessary parts of the original thread which is much

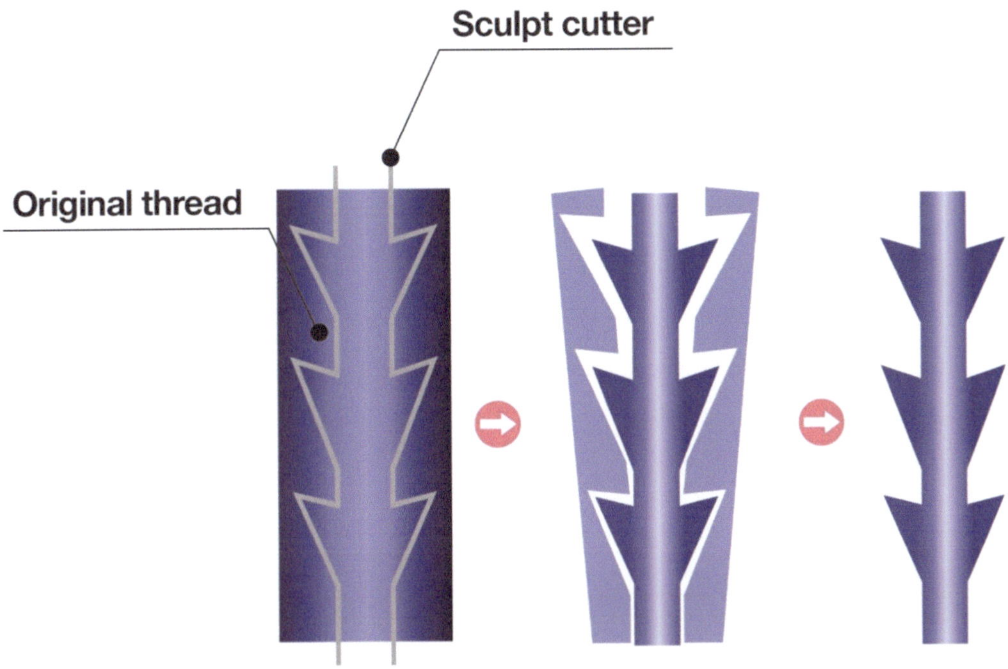

Fig. 2.15 Manufacturing process of sculpt molding-type cogged thread (i-THREAD Sculpt, HEALUX)

thicker than the size of the product and leaves only the shape of the cogged thread. Therefore, it can be seen that the thread part without the cogs becomes as thin as the size of the product, but the thread part with the cogs is as thick as the original thread.

Therefore, when performing procedures using a cannula, the thickness of the cannula required is larger than that of cutting-type cogged threads, which increases the discomfort not only for the operator but also for the patients undergoing the procedure. In addition, patients may complain of foreign material or discomfort when moving their faces because the thickness of the entire thread is thicker than the product size after the procedure, so the size of the thread should be determined in consideration of this.

So far, the author also has chosen the product based on the common sense we know, rather than directly measuring the tensile strength of each of the cogged thread. After simply checking the product size of the cogged threads and asking how it was made, I thought that for the same size, the cutting type would have the weakest tensile strength, the injection molding type would be better, and the sculpt molding type would be the best. However, even if the molding-type cogged threads feel thick, the tensile strength of injection molding-type cogged thread products, which have been heat-treated a lot in the manufacturing process, was actually measured compared to cutting-type cogged threads of similar product size, and it was confirmed that the tensile strength was weak.

The tensile strength was compared with products of similar size marked by the company, which are the cutting-type cogged thread and the sculpt molding-type cogged thread that does not generate maximum heat. Contrary to expectations, it was found that the average tensile strength of the two cogged thread types was similar. The product size of the sculpt molding-type cogged thread is not based on the thickness of the cogged part, but on the part where there are no cogs after press molding the cogs, so the size of the original thread before molding the cogs should be considered to be much larger (Fig. 2.16).

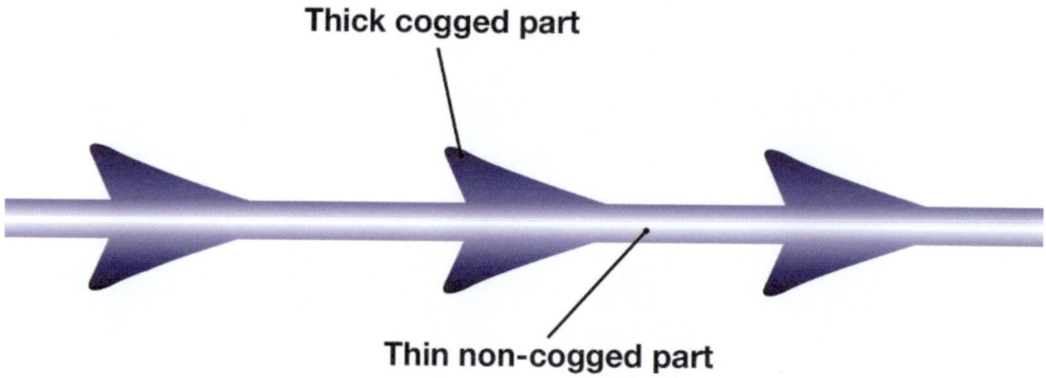

Fig. 2.16 Sculpt molding-type cogged thread

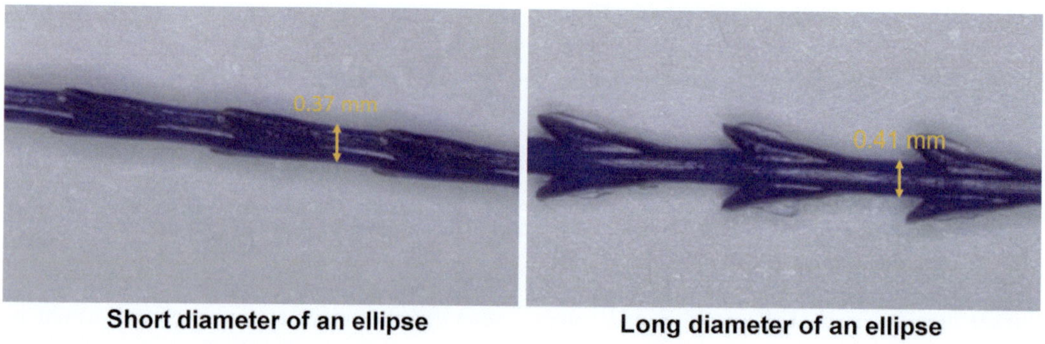

Fig. 2.17 Diameter of noncogged part of sculpt molding-type cogged threads

The cutting-type cogged threads are formed by cutting a thread having a thickness corresponding to a product size to form a cog, such that a part below the actual cog becomes thinner than a product size, and thus, the tensile strength would be affected. Therefore, when comparing threads of two types of similar product size, the tensile strength of molding-type cogged thread was expected to be much greater than that of the cutting type because the molding-type cogs were added to the part without cogs about the product size, but it was not. Accordingly, the author could assume that the heat generated in the process of press molding the cogs from the thick original thread using the sculpt cutter had this effect.

To confirm this hypothesis, the author asked a company that manufactures cogged threads to make two types of cogged threads, sculpt molding and cutting type, based on general manufacturing methods, and then measured the tensile strength of the two products to produce an average value. For objective evaluation, it is important to make the thinnest part of the thread that determines the tensile strength similar, and first, the USP size No. 2 original thread with a thickness of about 0.6 mm was used to make a sculpt molding-type and a cutting-type cogged thread product. In the sculpt molding method, the size and shape of the cogs were designed so that the diameter of the thinnest part of the thread without the cogs and the thinnest part of the remaining thread after raising the cogs in the cutting method was about USP size 2-0.

The cogged thread produced by the sculpt molding method was found to be slightly oval, not round, as the thread was pressed while pressing the cogs. When measuring the diameter of the ellipse, the short axis was 0.37 mm and the long axis was 0.41 mm (Fig. 2.17).

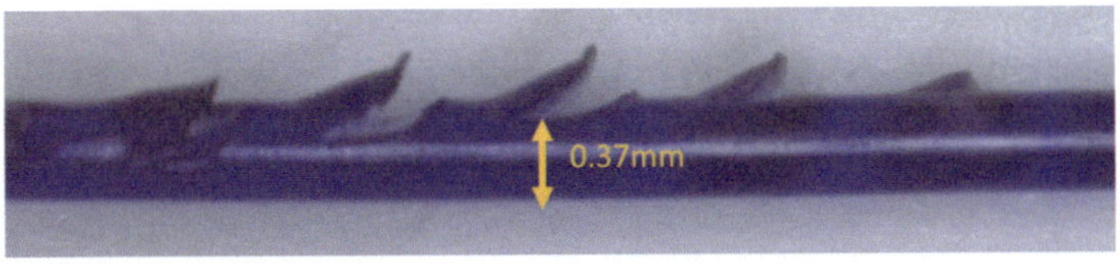

Thickness of the remaining part after making the cogs : 0.37 mm

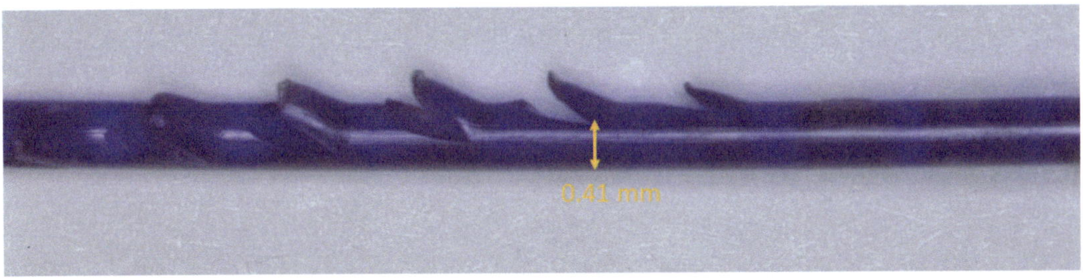

Thicknesses of the remaining part after making the cogs : 0.41 mm

Fig. 2.18 Cutting-type cogged threads of two thicknesses of the remaining part after making the cogs

In the cutting-type cogged thread, almost no heat was generated during the manufacturing process, so there was no pressing of the remaining part after the cogs were made. In order to make the same conditions as the sculpt molding-type cogged thread, two types of cutting-type cogged threads with diameters of thinnest parts of 0.37 mm and 0.41 mm were made to measure each tensile strength, as shown in the sculpt molding method (Fig. 2.18).

First, the tensile load of the sculpt molding-type cogged thread consisting of an oval with a diameter of 0.37 mm for a short axis and 0.41 mm for a long axis, which is a noncogged part, was measured (Fig. 2.19).

Next, after cutting the cogs in the cutting-type cogged thread, two types of cutting-type cogged threads were made so that the diameters of the thinnest part of the remaining thread were 0.37 mm and 0.41 mm, respectively, and the tensile load was measured (Fig. 2.20).

As a result of measuring the tensile load at the time when the thread was cut, it was found that the thread was cut at an average tensile load of about 53.72 N in the sculpt molding-type cogged thread. In the case of the cutting-type cogged

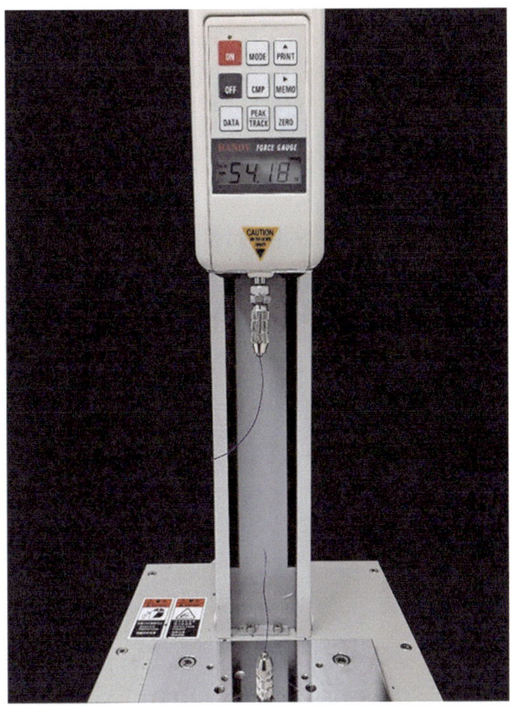

Diameter of non-cogged part of sculpt molding type cogged threads : Average 0.39 mm

Fig. 2.19 Measurement of tensile loads at the break of the sculpt molding-type cogged threads

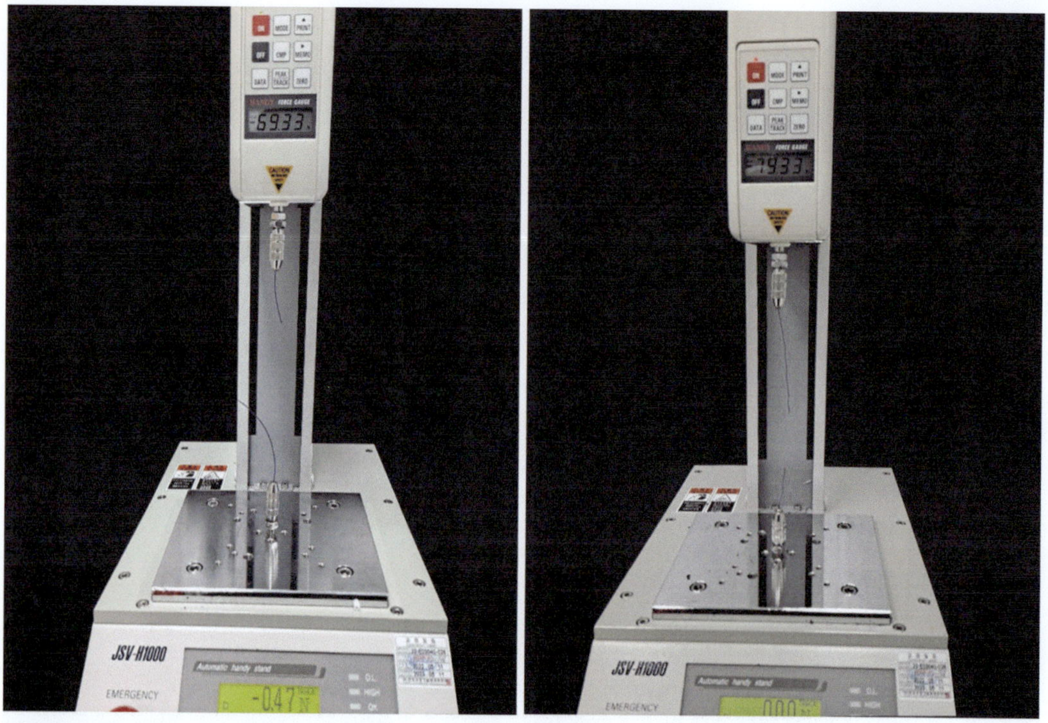

Thickness of the remaining part after making the cogs : 0.37 mm

Thickness of the remaining part after making the cogs : 0.41 mm

Fig. 2.20 Measurement of tensile loads at the break of the cutting-type cogged threads

Table 2.1 Results of tensile strength measurement for cutting-type cogged threads and sculpt molding-type cogged threads of the same size

Classification	Cutting-type cogged threads		Sculpt molding-type cogged threads	
	Thickness of the remaining part after making the cogs		Short diameter	Long diameter
Diameter (mm)	0.37	0.41	0.37	0.41
			Average 0.39	
Tensile loads (N)	69.33	70.47	51.06	
	71.68	71.06	56.51	
	72.38	78.22	54.18	
	70.76	79.33	53.12	
Average	71.03	74.77	53.72	

thread, the average tensile load of the cogged thread with a diameter of 0.37 mm was 71.03 N, and the average tensile load of the cogged thread with a diameter of 0.41 mm was 74.77 N, and the average value of the two threads was calculated as 72.9 N (Table 2.1).

In view of the above results, when cogs are made using the same original threads and the same thinnest parts of the threads are made, the tensile load of the sculpt molding-type cogged thread is 53.72 N and the tensile load of the cutting-type cogged thread is 72.9 N, showing that the cutting type is 35.3% greater than the sculpt molding-type cogged thread.

The results of the experiment showed that the cutting-type cogged thread had better tensile strength than we thought when comparing tensile strength after manufacturing the two types of cogged threads to have similar sizes. Perhaps, when the thread is pressed during the manufacturing process, the heat inevitably generated in the process of pressing the thread with a sculpt cutter changes the physical properties of the thread, weakening the tensile strength.

However, I said earlier that I compared the tensile strength of the two types of threads of similar sizes on the market and found similar figures. It seems that the reason for this is that the sculpt molding-type cogged thread is made of the original thread thicker than the product size, and the cogged part of cutting-type cogged thread is made thinner than the product size after raising the cogs using the original thread of the product size.

Many doctors have a negative image of the cutting-type cogged threads because the previous cutting-type cogged threads were so poorly manufactured that they break easily and have weak anchoring and holding strength of the cogs. However, through the results of this experiment, if the cutting-type cogged thread is manufactured properly, the tensile strength can be maintained better than the press molding-type cogged thread that generates heat during the manufacturing process.

Most recently, it has been said that it is possible to use ultrasonic waves to sculpt the cogged thread, and it can be seen that these threads do not generate heat until the final stage of manufacture, even though they are pressed, and we expect more and more of these kinds of products in the future.

Lastly, especially when doing the cogged thread lifting using the absorbable cogged threads, threads with a certain thickness and good tensile strength should be used because these threads are more likely to take longer to be absorbed. The absorbable threads enter the human body and undergo various tissue reactions during the retention period to regenerate collagen and connective tissue, because if the threads get absorbed before enough of this reaction, the effect of thread lifting disappears too quickly. Therefore, when choosing absorbable cogged threads, it is important to choose a cogged thread that may proceed slowly so that the degradation process may occur slowly and, as a result, remain in the human body for as long as possible.

2.5.3 Shape, Location, and Number of Cogs: Anchoring and Holding Strength

The tensile strength of the cogged thread is a value that shows how well the thread holds when pulled from both sides under the same conditions, regardless of how well the cogs of the thread are hung on the tissue or how hard the tissue is.

However, the anchoring and holding strength of the cogged threads are the forces that occur when the cogs of the thread are actually caught in the tissue, so it can be said that it appears only in the cogged threads. Anchoring strength literally refers to the force in which the cog of thread is easily caught in the tissue and plays a role in pulling and collecting the tissue, just as the cog of thread catches the tissue and anchors in place. Holding strength is a value that indicates how well these forces can be maintained without being released once the cogs are caught in the tissue and the force to pull and gather the tissue is exerted.

Even if a thick thread with good tensile strength but without cogs is put in the tissue, the tissue is not caught, so anchoring does not occur, and thus holding, which means the force to hold after the cog is caught in the tissue, does not occur.

Some people may think of anchoring and holding strength as the same force, or simply express holding strength without dividing the two, but the author personally thinks that dividing the two forces is more clinically useful when choosing a cogged thread.

For example, considering the shape and length of the cog, it can be felt that the thin and long cog is sharper and has a large area of contact with the tissue, so the cog is easily caught in the tissue. Therefore, these cogs can be expressed to be anchored better and to have better anchoring strength than short and blunt-shaped cogs (Fig. 2.21).

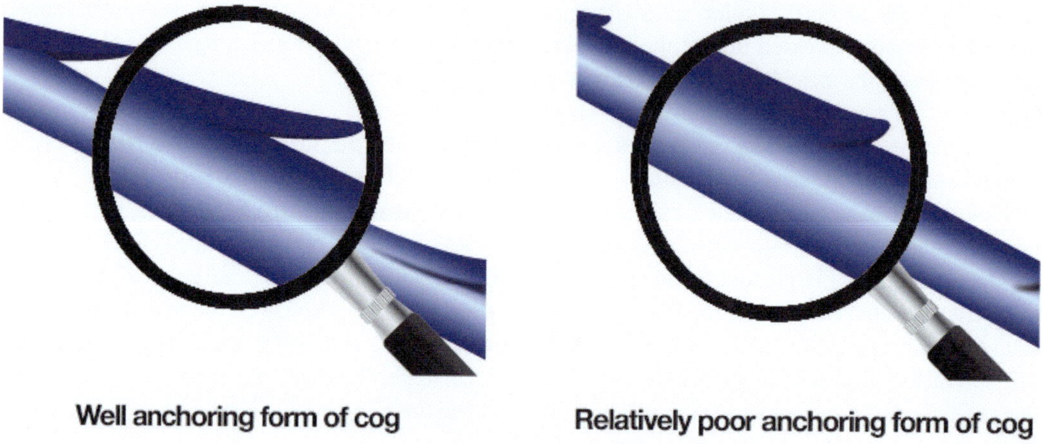

Fig. 2.21 Difference in anchoring strength according to the shape and size of cogs

However, once the cog is properly caught in the tissue, the holding strength, which indicates how well it will maintain the force that bites and pulls the tissue, may appear in reverse depending on the shape of the cog. Thin and long cogs are likely to weaken over time as the force opposite to the force being held by the tissue load and the movement of the face continues to act (Fig. 2.22).

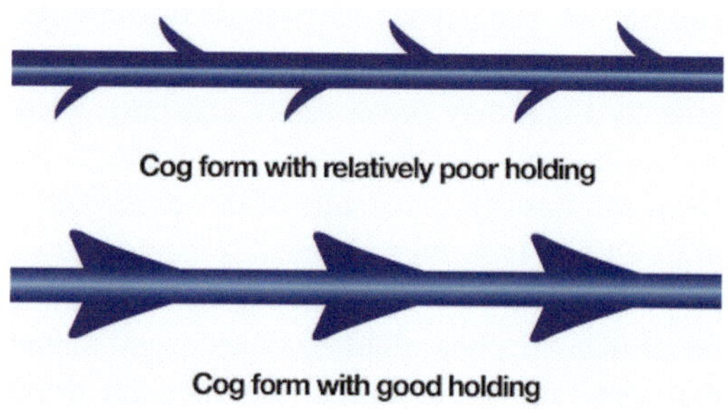

Fig. 2.22 Difference in holding strength according to the shape and size of cogs

Therefore, it is not desirable if the force is biased to either side. When inserting the cogged thread at first, it is good to anchor the tissue well, so that the force to bite and pull the tissue is easily felt. At the same time, after being caught in the tissue, the thread that holds the tissue as well as the force that acts as opposed to the pulling force does not loosen and maintains it as well as possible is a good cogged thread. However, it is not good to say that the cog of thread is unconditionally large and long because if the thread cog is too large and long, patients with thin skin may be touched on the outside, and the longer the cog, the larger the cannula used during the procedure. Therefore, it is good to check whether the cogged threads we use are threads that can play this role well and have an appropriate shape and size.

Another factor that may affect the anchoring and holding strength of the cog is the location of the cogs. In a single bidirectional cogged thread with the same other conditions, it can be said that in the twin-sided type where cogs are located on both sides of the thread, or the spiral-sided type where cogs are located surrounding the surface of the thread, tissue is more likely to get caught by the thread than in the single-sided type where cogs are located on one side of the thread. Even after the cog is caught in the tissue, when the cogs are located on various sides of the thread, stress that resists the force acting opposite to the pulling force of the cogs can be exerted in various parts of the thread, so the holding strength of the cog is also better (Fig. 2.23).

Another factor that can affect the anchoring and holding of cogged threads is the number of cogs. When all other conditions are the same, it can be seen that threads with a large number of cogs are easily caught in the tissue. In addition, after being caught, the probability of maintaining the pulling force increases. The number of cogs can be said to be important, especially in older

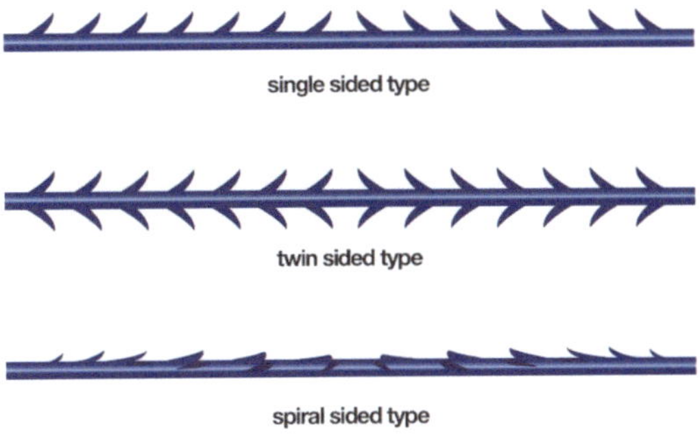

Fig. 2.23 Difference in anchoring and holding strengths according to the location of cogs in bidirectional cogged threads

patients with thin, weak skin and tissues and severe sagging. Patients whose skin tissue is relatively hard and elastic and does not droop much show good treatment results without using many cogged threads with strong pulling power. The reason is that the tissues that make up the skin and soft tissue are relatively tough and elastic, so the cogs are easily caught in the tissue. In addition, even after being caught, the pulling force of the cogs can withstand well without tearing. Therefore, in this case, the number of cogs can at least produce a better result. However, if the skin and soft tissue are made of relatively soft and loose tissue, more cogs must catch the tissue to show pulling force. Only then, the probability of holding on to some extent without loosening the pulling force after that can be increased.

For this reason, the long-length U- or V-shaped bidirectional cogged threads, which can serve as two lines due to the long length of even one thread, have a higher overall number of cogs before each shape or size of the cog, so it can show stronger anchoring and holding than short- or medium-length cogged threads.

Therefore, when all other conditions of the cogged threads used for the purpose of the procedure are similar, in order to pull loose tissues as strongly as possible, the cogs must be evenly located on various sides of the thread and the number of cogs are large. Otherwise, the number of cogged threads used should be increased to increase the total number of cogs that pull the tissue as a result.

2.5.4 Direction of Cogs

As described above, the cogged threads used for thread lifting can be largely divided into two types according to their shape and length. One is mainly used by bending a long thread, and the cogs on both left and right threads face one direction to bite and collect tissue in the middle of the thread, and the other is a short- or medium-length cogged thread type that can be designed in various directions. Since the direction of the cogs of the long cogged threads is basically determined, we will mainly talk about short- or medium-length cogged threads that may have different action mechanisms and treatment purposes depending on the direction of the cogs.

In the past, short- or medium-length cogged threads used unidirectional cogged threads with all the directions of the cogs facing one place, but these days, they are rarely used for lifting. It can be broadly divided into a single bidirectional cog type (usually referred to as a bidirectional type) in which both opposite cogs face the middle area depending on the direction of the cogs and a multidirectional cog type in which the direction of the cogs faces two or more places, not the center of the thread. The exception here is that the single bidirectional cogged threads used for the nasal shaping and contouring do not collect the skin of the nose in the middle, but pull the nose skin out from the middle to make the nose look longer, so it can be called reversed single bidirectional cogged thread. Multidirectional cog types can be further subdivided into double bidirectional, triple bidirectional, and multiple bidirectional types according to their form, but for ease of classification, all of the cogged threads facing more than one place are called multidirectional cog types (Fig. 2.24).

When comparing the characteristics of the two types of threads, the short- or medium-length bidirectional cogged thread designed to gather tissues in the middle while facing each other around the empty part in the middle has a good effect of raising tissues, but the tissue may gather in the middle to appear bulging.

In order to apply these features to benefit clinical practice, if you pull the side of the face by inserting a short- or medium-length I-shaped bidirectional cogged thread from top to bottom in patients with subzygomatic hollow, it is most ideal to hold an entry point near the hair line according to the length of the thread and insert the thread so that the middle part of the thread without cogs is located at the subzygomatic depression part under the zygomatic arch (Fig. 2.25).

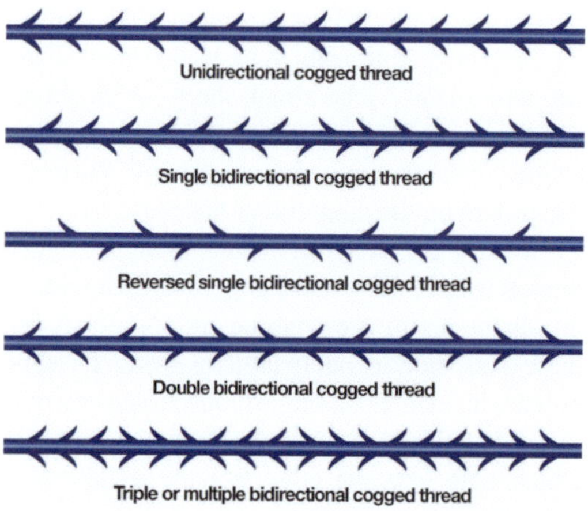

Fig. 2.24 Classification of short- or medium-length cogged threads according to the direction of cogs

During this procedure, the stretched and bulging parts of the lower face are pulled on the cogs and flattened, and the area under the zygomatic arch improves the depressed shape as the tissue is concentrated, and the overall facial shape is also improved. It should be noted that if the center of the thread is placed below the depressed area, the area may bulge and the depressed part may appear to be recessed in the shape of an uneven shape. On the contrary, if the center of the thread is located in the zygomatic arch area, the side cheekbones may appear to protrude, so it is important to position them accurately.

However, like the early models of the short- or medium-length bidirectional cogged thread, if the number of both cogs are the same around the middle part, the upper part of the protrusion bites the tough tissue of the temple, and the lower part of the cogs holds the relatively loose cheek tissue weak. In particular, in patients with relatively long faces, when the middle part of the cogs is placed directly under the zygomatic arch to soften the shape of the side of the face, the length of the thread placed on the lower cheek is shortened, resulting in a relatively insufficient number of cogs and weak strength level. As explained in

Fig. 2.25 Position the noncogged middle part of the thread on the subzygomatic depression

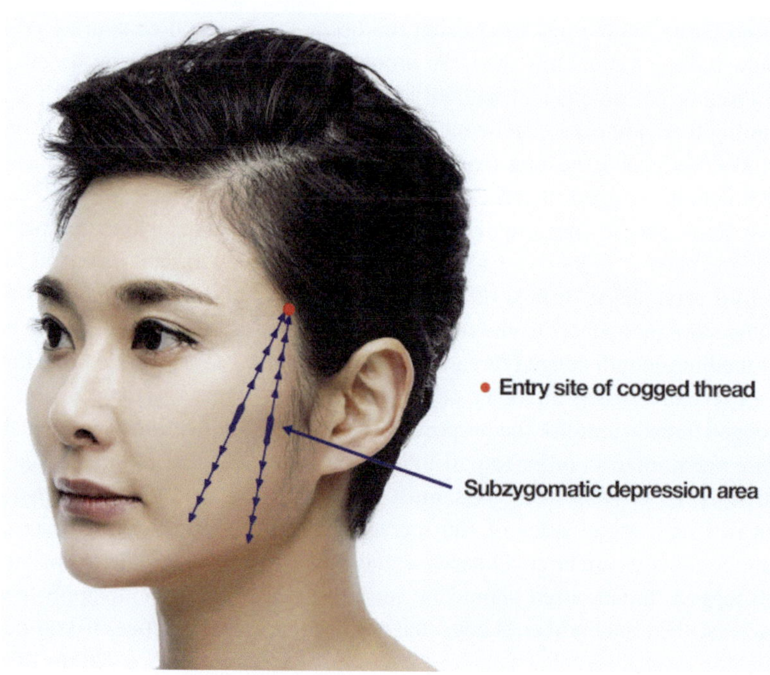

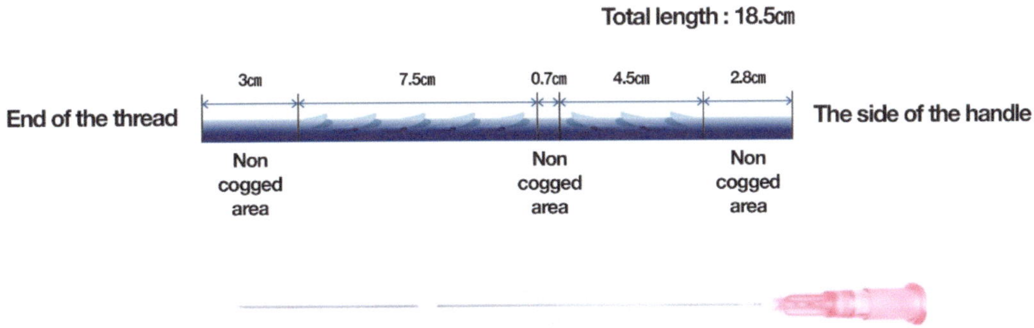

Fig. 2.26 Existing modified single bidirectional cogged thread (i-THREAD Cog L-cannula, HEALUX)

the number of cogs, the number of cogs pulling the lower loose tissue must be relatively large to achieve the effect of pulling the loose tissue. So, in some companies, when creating short- or medium-length bidirectional cogged threads that are inserted from the head to the bottom of the face, the numbers of both cogs based on the center of the thread are not the same. Short- or medium-length bidirectional cogged threads with improved direction of cogs are produced to increase the number of cogs placed on the lower loose area and reduce the number of cogs on the handle side to sufficiently create a lifting effect of loose tissues (Fig. 2.26).

Unlike ordinary bidirectional cogged threads, which collect and pull tissue only in the middle of the thread, multidirectional cogged threads cause cogs to bite and hold the tissue in several places. Therefore, it can be said that the traction power, or lifting ability, that is, to bite the tissue and strongly gather and pull it only in the middle is poor. However, as is the trend these days, when the patient is lying down, the tip of the chin is raised, head down, and the cogged thread is inserted for fixation, the ability of multidirectional cogged threads to fix the tissue evenly as a whole so that is, the holding strength is better. Therefore, it is suitable for producing a natural lifting effect overall in patients with less sagging. These days, many combination treatments can maximize the advantages of the two types of cogged threads that first collect and pull tissues with bidirectional cogged threads and then use multidirectional cogged threads to keep pulled tissues in place.

2.5.5 Insertion Depth of Threads According to the Toughness of Tissues

As mentioned earlier when explaining the anchoring and holding strength of the cogged thread, one of the treatment conditions that can affect the results of the cogged thread lifting is which tissue the cogs of the thread are caught in. In addition, depending on the condition of the patient's skin and tissue undergoing the procedure, the degree to which the anchoring and holding of the cogged thread appear varies. For example, even if the same cogged thread is used, when the tissue caught by the cogs is a tough tissue such as SMAS (superficial musculoaponeurotic system), the cogs of the thread show higher anchoring and holding than when the cogged thread enters the subcutaneous fat layer with little tissue resistance (Fig. 2.27).

The layer of tissues in which the threads are inserted is very important in terms of the lifting effect and reducing the side effects. Usually, the area around the head and ears is made of very tough, so it serves to hang the cogged thread so that the cogged thread biting the loose tissue at the bottom does not droop again. Therefore, the upper part of the cogged thread should find deep tissues such as the SMAS or around the SMAS and the cogged thread should be inserted into those tissues. The lower part of the cogged thread should be inserted so that the skin and subcutaneous fat layers that cause sagging are caught.

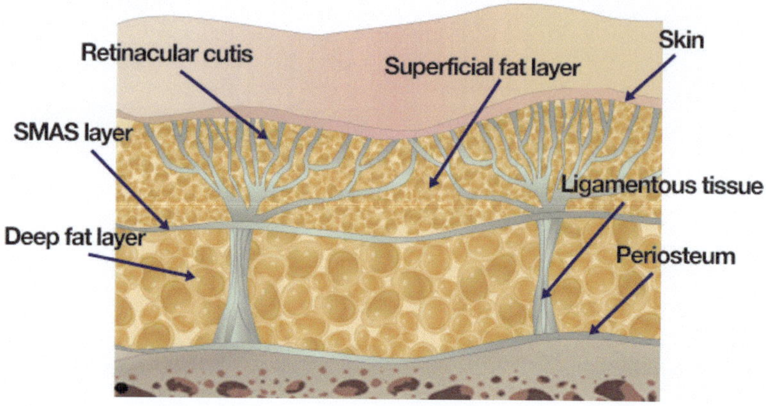

Fig. 2.27 Basic structure of facial skin and soft tissue

Even if it is the same subcutaneous fat layer, there are a lot of fibrous tissues that are formed when ligamentous tissues spread closer to the skin, therefore, as the thread is inserted closer to the skin, the thread gets a stronger anchoring and holding strength. When comparing the strength level, when the cogged thread enters the subcutaneous fat layer close to the skin, it shows a higher strength level compared to the middle of the subcutaneous fat layer. However, if the thread enters only the subcutaneous fat that is too close to the skin, the pulling force of the cog is not transmitted to the deep subcutaneous fat, and the force of the cog acts only on the subcutaneous fat connected to the skin. And, if the threads are inserted too superficially, a dimple could be formed on the surface, and the thread can be visible from the outside through the facial skin.

Generally, when using a thread thicker than 1-0, the risk of the formation of dimples increases as the thread is inserted into the subcutaneous layer near the skin. Therefore, it is desirable to insert a thread into the SMAS layer or the subcutaneous tissue around the SMAS tissue. Since there are fibrous septa in the fat layer as well, the thread may hold some amount of the tissues, but it wouldn't be as strong as the threads holding the tissue around the SMAS. Therefore, when using a thread with a thickness of 1-0, it is recommended to place the thread into the SMAS or around the SMAS to reduce the side effects and optimize the effects. When I have inserted threads into a fresh cadaver in the cadaver workshop many times in a similar manner to in practice, the thread was found to be inserted in the SMAS or around the SMAS. Also, in actual patients who had thread lifting procedures, it was found that the thread was inserted in the SMAS or around the SMAS, as I made confirmation by face lifting surgery later (Fig. 2.28).

2.5.6 Selection of Appropriate Lifting Vectors and Fixing Points According to Facial

2.5.6.1 Areas

When carefully examining the drooped facial tissues on the face, you may see that not all tissues are drooped, but the tissues around the tightly attached head and ears do not get sagged well, whereas tissues on cheeks, perioral region, or jawline that are not firmly attached to the inner structures, get easily drooped (Fig. 2.29).

Therefore, to maximize the effect and duration, it is necessary to focus on the loose tissue that is structurally easy to get drooped rather than just simply lifting the tissues forcibly. It is important to lift the loose tissues to be fixed to the tight tissues that are relatively maintained firm even with aging.

Therefore, it is important to find a fixing point with a tough tissue that does not move well and hang the loose tissue well so that the cogged thread does not fall again. There are tight tissues around the temple and ear that can hang cogged threads such as temporal fascia, temporal septum, zygomatic ligaments, Lore's fascia, and platysma auricular ligaments. Anatomically, if these tough tissues are well identified and used, the

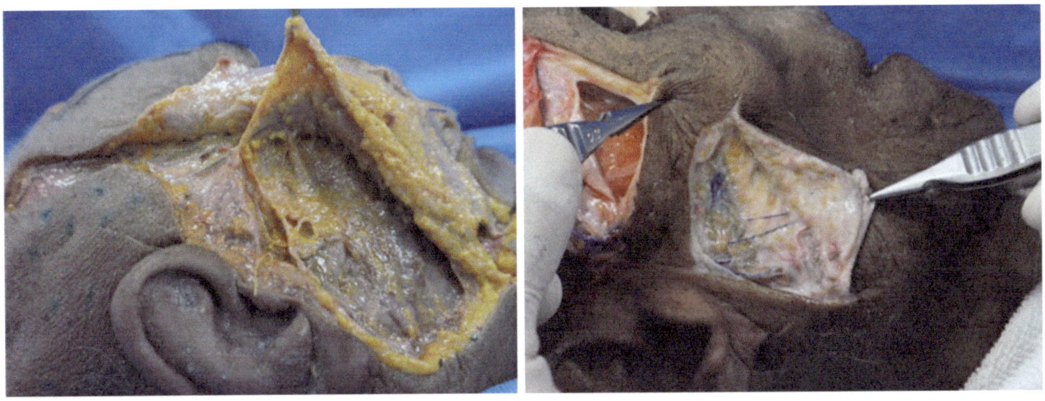

Fig. 2.28 Cogged threads inserted into SMAS or periSMAS plane

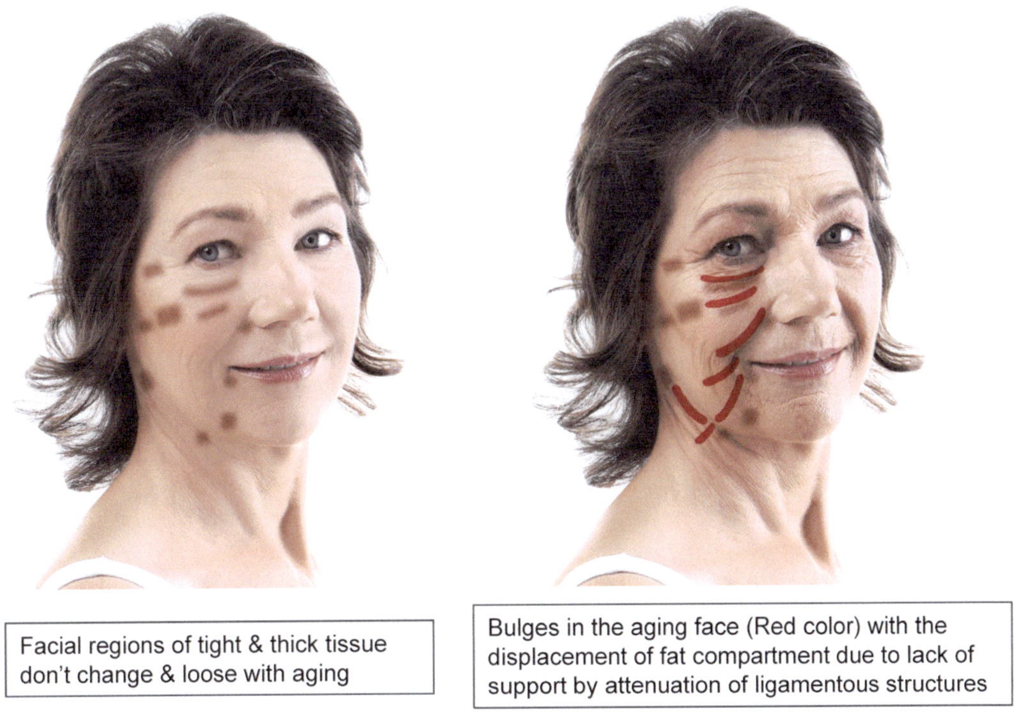

Fig. 2.29 Tight and thick tissue regions do not get loose with aging

effect and duration period of thread lifting can be improved.

In order to properly use the fixing point to hang the cogged threads biting these loose tissues, it is necessary to think about how to differently use the vector of the cogged threads and to which fixing point the thread should be hung according to the target area to be pulled and moved next (Fig. 2.30).

In the face lifting surgery, it used to be explained that pulling the skin and tissues of the mid-face and lower face unconditionally obliquely to the upper and the periauricular region. But the concept of pulling vertically gradually is now

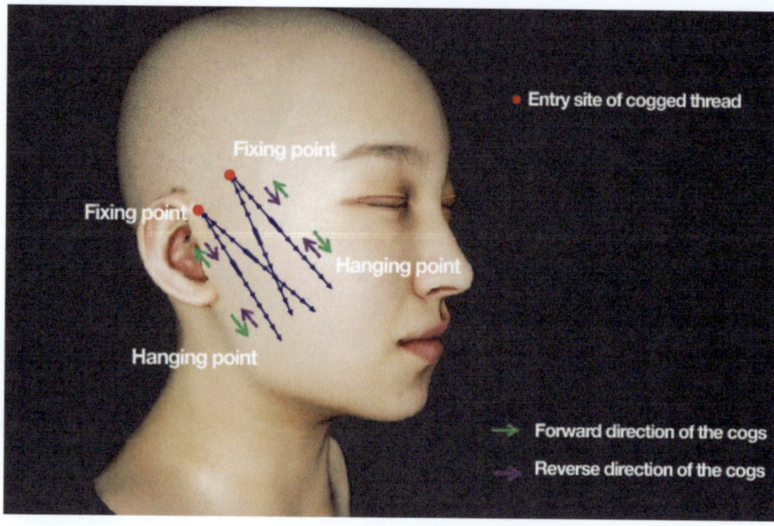

Fig. 2.30 Determination of lifting vector according to hanging and fixing points for bidirectional cogged thread lifting

being preferred. In the past, thread lifting was also preferred to be slightly oblique from the bottom to the top, but nowadays, vertical lifting is preferred. But, what we have to think about at this point is that even though gravity causes the tissue to sag down at right angles, pulling in only a vertical direction is not natural. When examining the direction of sagging of the facial tissues, wrinkles are formed according to the position and role of the strong ligaments that hold the skin and soft tissues, and it is believed that the insertion of the thread in the vertical direction to the wrinkles appearing can maximize the lifting effect.

For example, the soft tissues of the lateral cheek are droopy with aging vertical to the jawline, so pulling them vertically to the temporal region may seem most effective. On the other hand, since the vertical direction of jowling on the perioral tissues and the wrinkles on the nasolabial fold is toward the periauricular region, oblique lifting can be an effective method in this case. It is effective to lift and fix the tissues on jawline that droops out of the prejowl sulcus that are held by tough mandibular ligament by pulling to the tight tissue of the inferior temporal septum attached to the periauricular region, superior to the zygomatic arch. It would be the most ideal lifting vector to lift the tissues without disturbing the facial structures as much as possible vertically to the anatomical drooping direction (Fig. 2.31).

2.5.7 Difference Between Flap and String Methods

The thread lifting procedure was initially explained only as a concept of lifting the tissues with threading, but nowadays, the mechanism of the thread lifting effects can be divided into two aspects depending on the shape of the cogs and the purpose of the procedures.

The first mechanism is to lift a certain length of skin tissues in one direction, like a skin flap used in skin reconstruction surgery and the long-length U- or V-shaped thread lifting with single bidirectional cogs is a typical example of a lifting method that lifts skin tissues like a skin flap (Fig. 2.32).

Second, unlike the flap method, there is a string method in which thread cogs do not bite a certain area of skin and tissue and pull it in a certain direction, but mark a drooping skin and tissue and move it as if pulling a string in a target direction. If the skin and tissue to be pulled are wide, the number of points to be hung are bound to increase, but the direction in which each line is pulled can be designed in various ways depending on the shape of the patient's face or the aspect of drooping tissue (Fig. 2.32).

Although it is hard to say that a certain method is absolutely better than the other, it is advisable to use the two methods selectively depending on the patient's condition and the purpose of the procedure.

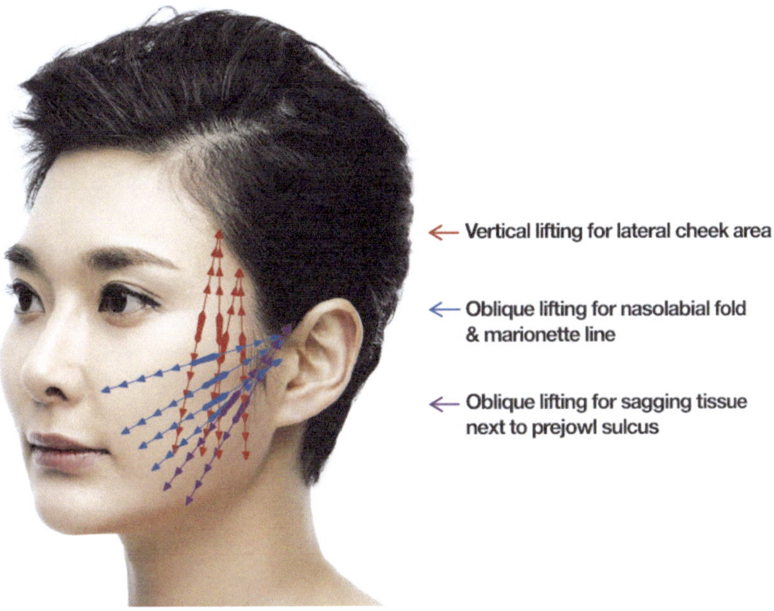

Fig. 2.31 Determination of lifting vector according to facial area for bidirectional cogged thread lifting

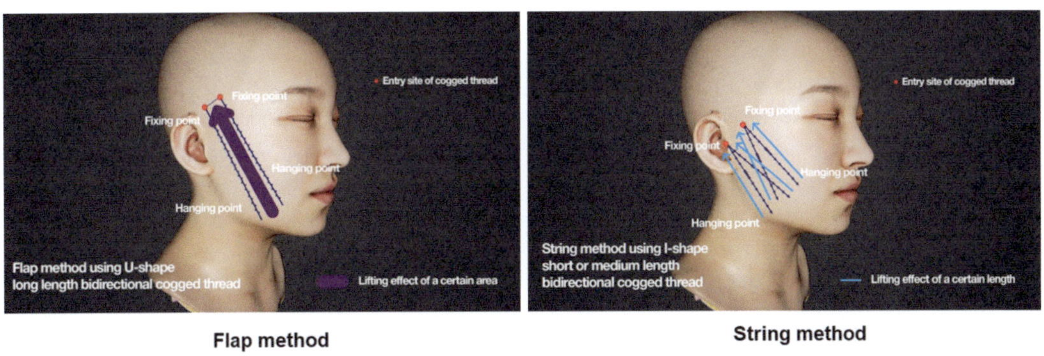

Fig. 2.32 Differences in the lifting effects of flap and string methods according to the type of cogged thread

The author personally prefers the string method using the short- or medium-length I-shaped cogged threads, which retains the lifted tissues on the site where the tissues are lifted naturally according to the facial tissue repositioning with changes of posture, more frequently rather than the flap-type of procedure that holds and lifts skin and soft tissues in one direction. When performing string-type cogged thread lifting, you can choose whether to use a bidirectional cogged thread that focuses on the traction that gathers tissues according to the patient's skin, soft tissue condition, and purpose of the procedure, or a multidirectional cogged thread that focuses on stress that holds moved tissues in place according to changes in posture. In some cases, the two types of cogged threads may be appropriately mixed and used.

No matter whether using the long U- or V-shaped cogged threads or short- or medium-length I-shaped cogged threads, the basic principle of flap-type thread lifting is based on the traction force that enables the cogs to catch and lift the tissues of forward direction with the cogs toward the opposite direction to the center by positioning the cogs in the opposite direction to the central part.

With these lifting methods, it may be felt as a lot of skin tightness at first, which makes the patients feel like having a strong lifting procedure. However, this method has the disadvantage of weakened tissue lifting effects due to rapidly decreased traction force when the tension of the central part of the thread, where the cogs don't exist and the strength is concentrated to maximize the traction force, gets weakened. In other words, due to the cogs positioned in one direction in order to gather the tissues, the strength is not evenly distributed to all of the cogs and therefore, once the tissue holding strength of the cogs in the central part of the threads is weakened, the anchoring strength that lifts the skin and soft tissues gets rapidly decreased.

We may feel our loose tissues on the cheek and jawline naturally leaning on the sites of firm tissues around the head and ears in the position of sitting back and then leaning back with our chin lifted slightly. The repositioning method of thread lifting developed for natural thread lifting procedures aims not to lift the lower facial tissues forcibly upwards, but rather to retain the leaned tissues on the spot even after the patients change their posture, sitting back again. It is important for this method, which seems ideal theoretically, to prevent the cogs from falling from the tissues they are holding after the patient changes the postures. Initially, it was difficult to manufacture cogs with sufficient tensile stress to hold out against the loads on the tissues. Also, due to the lack of strong tissue lifting effects in one direction unlike the flap method, this procedural method was only partially used. However, as the quality of the product and technique of cogs production improved, the lifting threads for repositioning methods have been increasingly produced, resulting in the recent production of string-type cogged threads that maximize the capability of the cogs by adjusting the shape, direction, and position of the cogs.

2.5.8 The Expiration Date of Absorbable Threads

Additionally, the period of time during which PDO thread, the most commonly used material for cogged threads, is absorbed and completely lost in the face should be considered. Practically, it is only possible to guess the changes in the inserted threads over time. It is commonly known that the lifting effect is not completely lost even after the thread is absorbed and gets loose, since the skin and tissues are regenerated due to collagenesis. However, further systematic studies are required to identify whether the lifting effects due to collagenesis last for some time even after the threads are absorbed and lost or, as some clinicians claim, the effects are only confined to histological findings, with clinical effects almost lost.

The quality of lifting threads from domestic manufacturers is generally verified due to domestic production conditions of lifting threads. Since there are only two factories in Korea producing the original threads, even giving consideration differences in length, shape and position, shape and a number of barbs of threads according to each manufacturer, the basic quality of any threads that are domestically manufactured can be guaranteed to some extent, whether it is designed from the production factory in the first place or not.

However, the manufacturers produce cogged threads through the process of processing PDO threads and making cogs on them, making the final product by putting the processed threads through a needle or deforming their shapes with sterilization and sealing afterward and since the hydrolysis starts immediately after unsealing, resulting in complete hydration of PDO threads after about 6–8 months, some clinician might experience, when using old threads that are unsealed for a long time ago, the threads snapping into pieces. Once the threads are unsealed, the efficacy of threads gets lost faster by being absorbed in the body more quickly. For this reason, even if the quality of products is similar, threads from the manufacturers whose manufacturing process is not thoroughly controlled are likely to have already been exposed to moisture in the air during the process of manufacturing, resulting in decreased maintenance duration of the thread as well as its efficacy.

3 Facial Anatomy for Thread Lifting

Contents

3.1 Layers of the Face

The face is composed of five layers similar to the scalp and they correspond with each other. However the face is different from the scalp in the fifth layer, as it contains masticatory muscles in some areas, not bone. Also, the layers are named differently in the temporal region (Fig. 3.1, Table 3.1).

S. M. Oh et al., *The Art and Science of Thread Lifting Based on Pinch Anatomy and Moving Plane*,
https://doi.org/10.1007/978-981-97-5516-5_3

Fig. 3.1 Layers of face. Diagram of coronal view

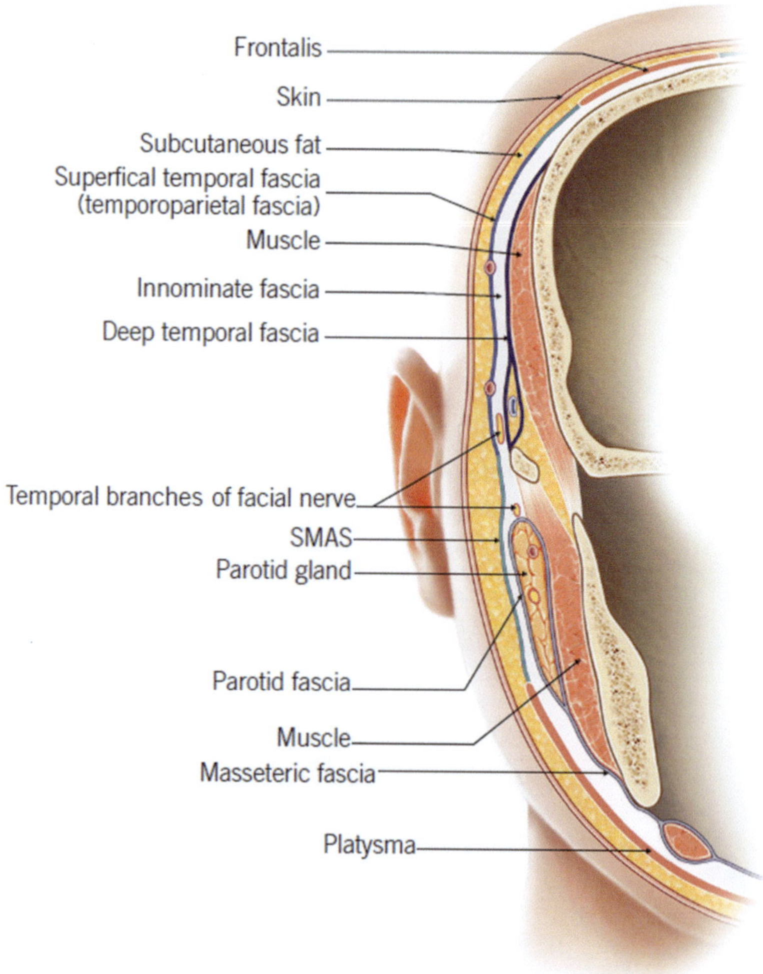

Table 3.1 Layers of face

Layers	Scalp	Face	Temple
1st	Skin	Skin	Skin
2nd	Subcutaneous tissue	Superficial fat	Subcutaneous tissue
3rd	Aponeurosis	Musculoaponeurotic layer	Superficial temporal fascia
4th	Loose connective tissue	Deep fat or spaces	Innominate fascia
5th	Periosteum	Deep fascia or periosteum	Deep temporal fascia

3.1.1 Skin

The skin thickness of the face was reported variously according to measurement methods. But in general, the thickness of the dermis is similar between Asians and Westerners, otherwise, the epidermis is thicker in Asians than in Westerners.

The total skin of males is about 20–25% thicker than females due to the difference in the dermal thickness, not the epidermis. Also, young ages have thicker skin than old ages. In addition, the person with a high BMI had a thicker skin than a low BMI. But the individual difference is the most important factor of skin thickness. The regional thickness of the skin on the face is shown in Fig. 3.2 and Table 3.2.

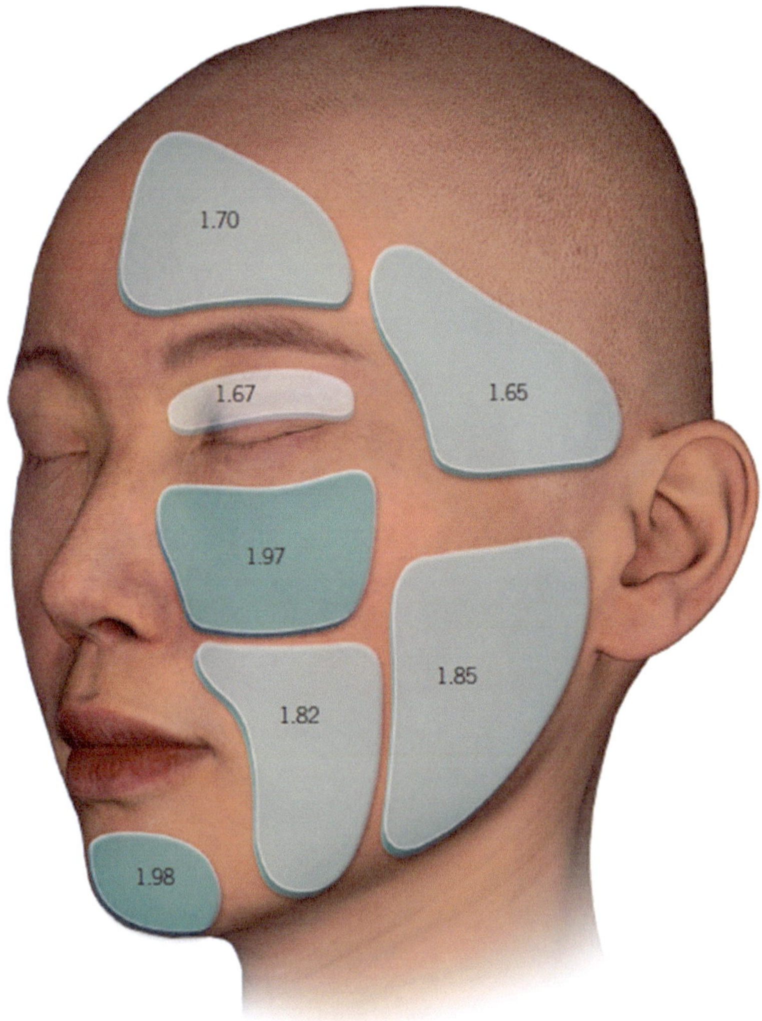

Fig. 3.2 Thickness of skin

Table 3.2 Thickness of skin

Region	Thickness (mm)
Forehead	1.70
Temple	1.65
Lateral cheek	1.85
Cheek	1.82
Malar	1.97
Chin	1.98
Eyelid	1.20

3.1.2 Subcutaneous Tissue (Fat)

The subcutaneous tissue (fat) is mainly composed of fat, and it is the same term as hypodermis. The subcutaneous fat is superficial to facial expression muscles, and it is known that it is divided into many compartments. But it is hard to be divided anatomically. This layer is a main drooping layer by aging (Fig. 3.3).

3.1.3 Facial Expression Muscle/ SMAS

The third layer is composed of facial expression (mimetic) muscles and aponeurosis continuous with these muscles. The medial face is mainly composed of muscles and the lateral face is mainly composed of fascia (aponeurosis) (Fig. 3.4). The aponeurosis is extended to lower

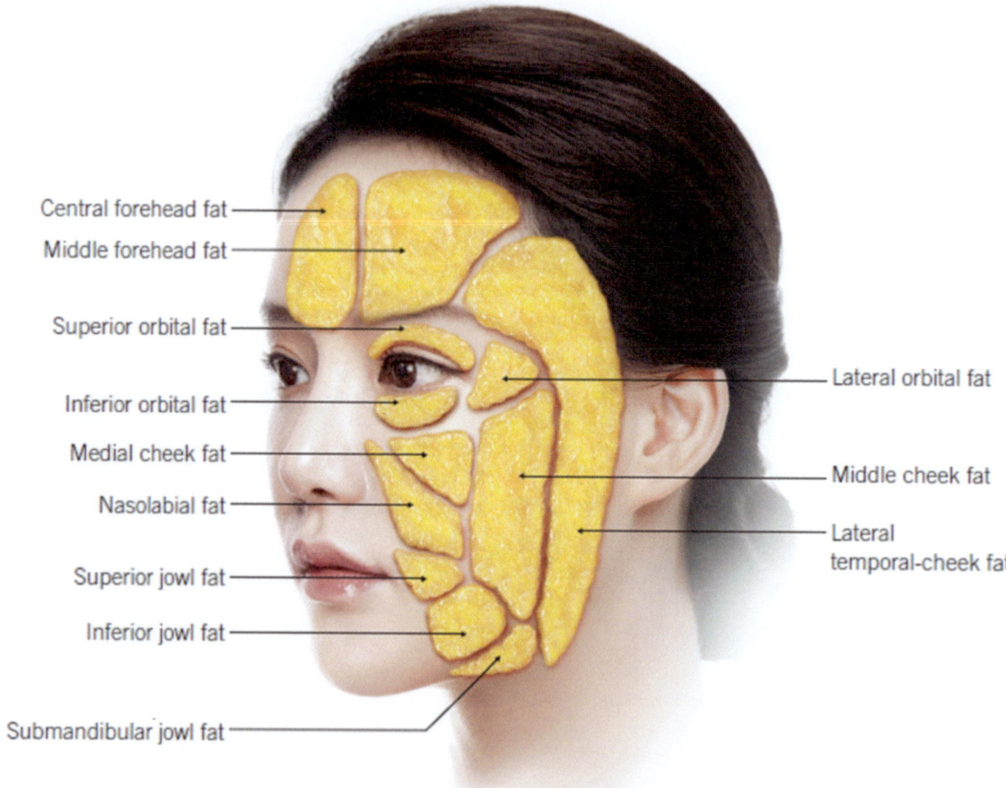

Fig. 3.3 Superficial fat compartments

platysma and upper frontalis muscle, but it has different names with reference to the zygomatic arch. The upper lateral part of the aponeurosis is named as superficial temporal fascia or temporoparietal fascia, and the lower part is named as superficial musculoaponeurotic system (SMAS).

3.1.4 Deep Fat or Spaces

The fourth layer of the face continues with the loose connective tissue layer of the scalp. This layer is inherently "loose," as the word itself suggests, so it either contains some fats or remains as potential empty space at intervals. Deep fat lies beneath the facial expression muscles or SMAS and is also divided into several compartments, similar to subcutaneous superficial fat (Fig. 3.5). However, deep fats are much more compartmentalized than superficial fat compartments.

Several spaces are located in this fourth layer of the face, depending on the region. The main trunk of the retaining ligament, connecting from the deep fascia or periosteum to the skin, is situated in this layer. In the temporal region, there is the innominate fascia, which appears to be more of a space than a sheet-like structure. This is because the fascia is very loose and easily separable.

3.1.5 Periosteum or Deep Fascia

The deepest fifth layer is the periosteum covering the bones of the face, but there are masticatory muscles in the temporal or mandibular region between deep fat and the periosteum. Therefore, the fifth layer in the temporal and lateral mandibular regions is composed of the deep fascia covering masticatory muscles. The deep tempo-

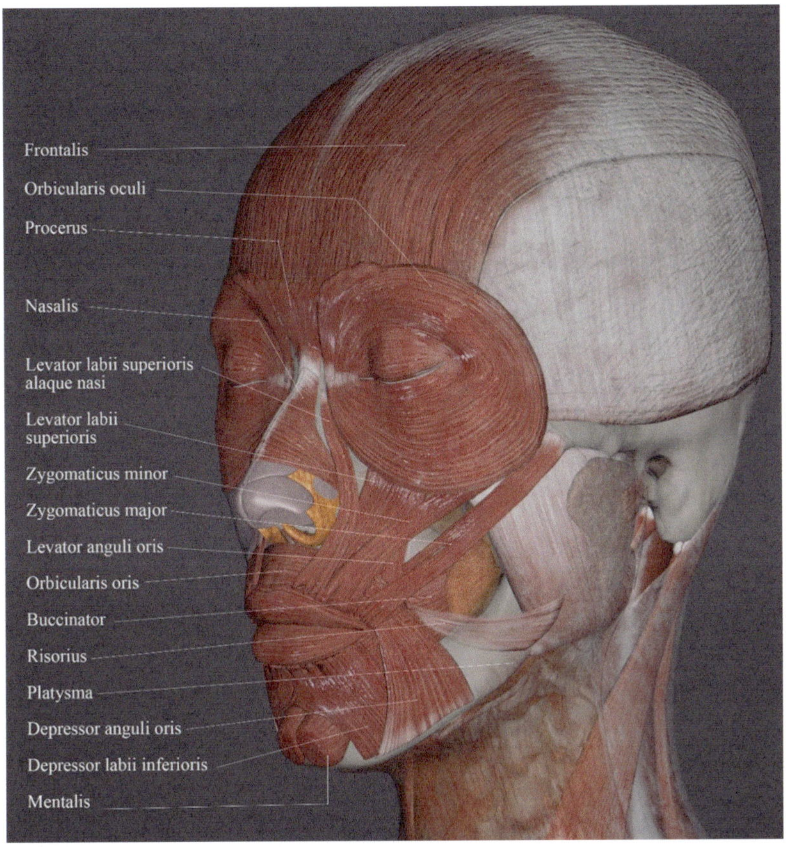

Fig. 3.4 Facial expression muscles

ral fascia investing temporalis muscle is separated into superficial and deep layers, and they are attached to the superior border and lateral surface of the zygomatic arch (Fig. 3.6).

The superficial temporal fat pad is a fat tissue in the space between the superficial and deep layers of the deep temporal fascia. The deep temporal fat pad extending from the buccal fat pad is a fat tissue between the deep layer of the deep temporal fascia and temporalis muscle.

The deep fascia below the zygomatic arch is named parotidomasseteric fascia, because it invests parotid gland as well as the masseter muscle. It is attached to the inferior border of the zygomatic arch. That is, the upper and lower SMAS, the third layer, are a continuous layer crossing the surface of the zygomatic arch, but deep fasciae, the fifth layer, are not a continuous layer between the upper and lower parts.

3.1.6 Moving Plane

The fourth layer of the face, which consists of deep fat or spaces, is similar to the fourth layer of the scalp, composed of loose connective tissue. The skin, subcutaneous tissue, and SMAS layers are relatively harder than the loose fourth layer, while the fifth layer of the periosteum or deep fascia is very hard and thick. Therefore, the superficial three layers move on the fifth layer via the loose fourth layer. We want to consider this fourth layer as a "moving plane."

The threads are commonly placed in the supraSMAS or subSMAS layer for face lifting. However, whether the threading is done in the supraSMAS or subSMAS layer, all three superficial layers are lifted by the thread on the periosteum or deep fascia.

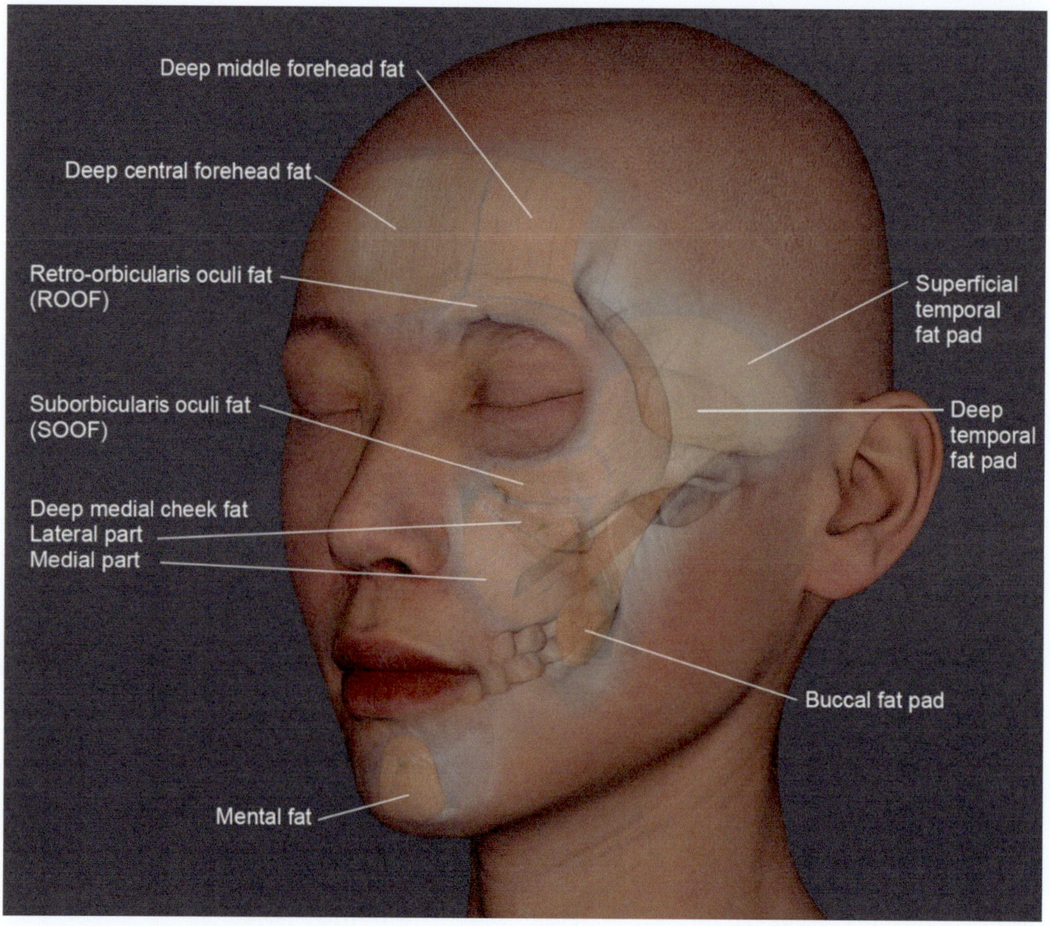

Fig. 3.5 Deep fat compartments

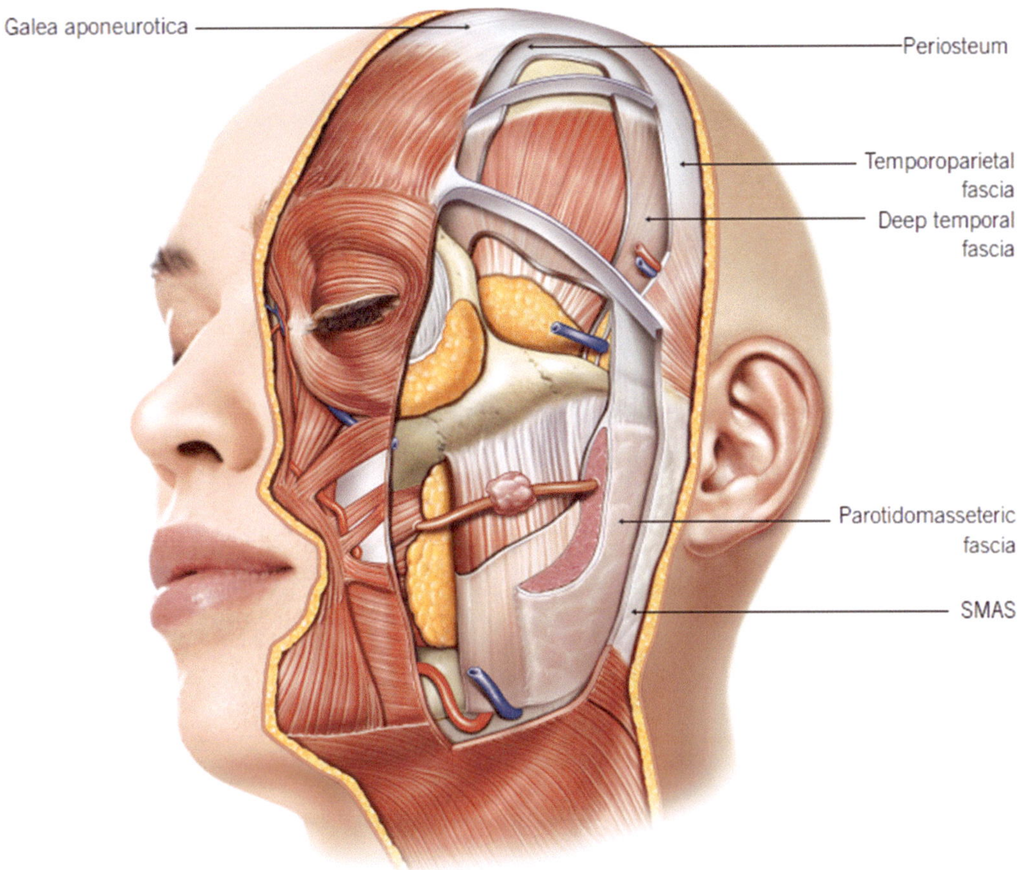

Fig. 3.6 Deep fascia of face

3.2 Anatomic Finding of Layers of the Face

After removing the skin and subcutaneous tissue, the third layer, the facial expression muscles/SMAS layer, was exposed (Fig. 3.7). The platysma, orbicularis oculi, and frontalis muscles and the aponeurosis that connect them can be seen. The thin muscle sheet (temporoparietalis muscle) is also shown in the temporal region.

Below the zygomatic arch, you can see an aponeurosis (or fascia) called the SMAS, and above the zygomatic arch, you can see the superficial temporal fascia or the temporoparietal fascia. This layer is the most important during lifting surgeries and procedures.

Figure 3.8 is a photo taken during the process of reflection of the SMAS forward. While the areas around the temporal and mandibular regions are relatively well reflected because of the easily separable fourth layer, it is not as easy to reflect in the middle portion near the ear due to Lore's fascia.

After reflection of the SMAS layer, the fourth layer was exposed (Fig. 3.9). Some deep fat tissue with loose areolar tissue on the parotidomasseteric fascia can be seen. The fourth layer of the temporal region, the innominate fascia, can be seen. Some thin temporal branches of the facial nerve were also seen.

In another cadaver, the deep temporal fascia above the zygomatic arch and masseteric

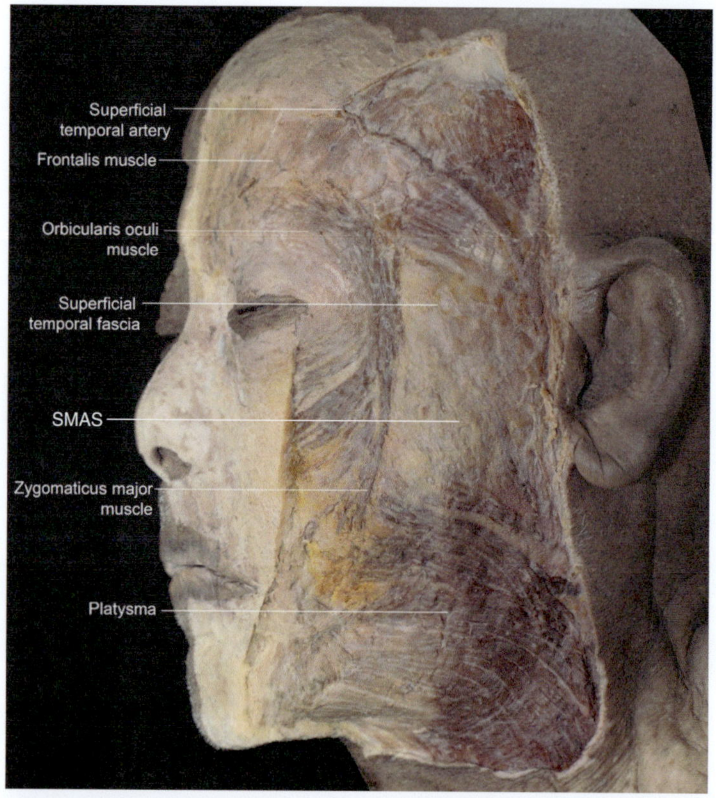

Fig. 3.7 Anatomic finding of SMAS

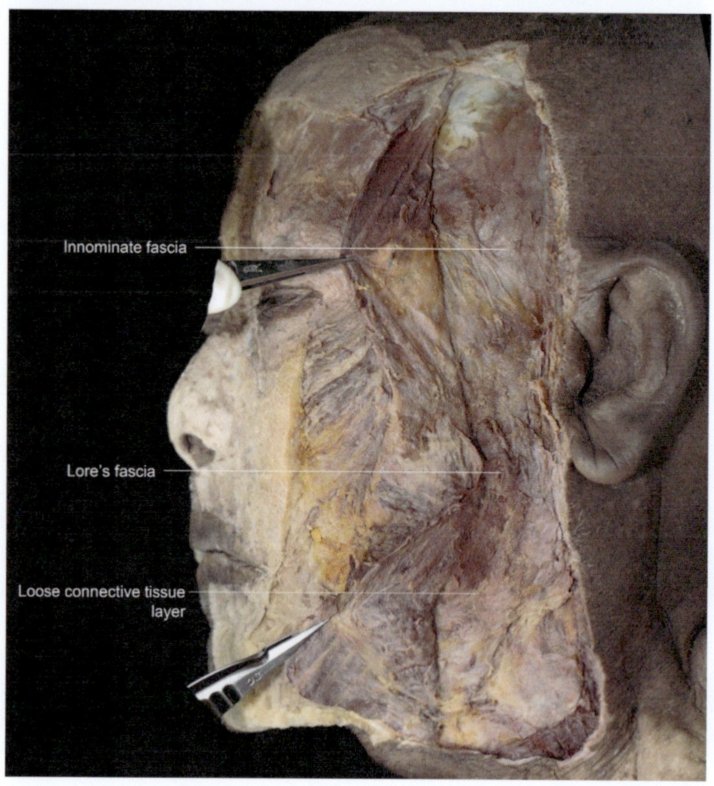

Fig. 3.8 On reflecting of SMAS

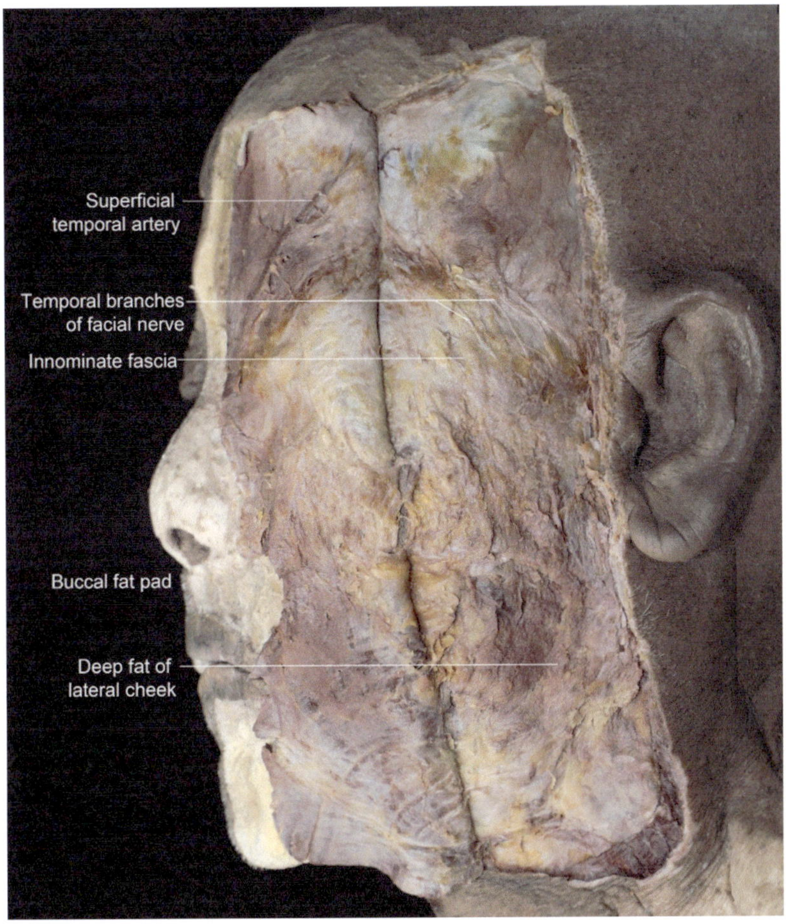

Fig. 3.9 Reflection of SMAS and superficial temporal fascia

fascia below the zygomatic arch are well revealed, which was thick when covering the masseter muscle (Fig. 3.10). A part of the parotid gland on the masseter muscle was also seen.

The parotidomasseteric fascia was removed to expose the parotid gland (Fig. 3.11). The branches of the facial nerve and parotid duct emerge from the anterior border of the parotid gland. The temporal branches of the facial nerve ascending to the forehead were also visible above the parotid gland.

This is a cadaveric photo and illustration showing the layers in the temporal region (Fig. 3.12). The superficial temporal artery is seen running through the superficial temporal fascia. The middle temporal vein runs through the superficial temporal fat pad, buried between the superficial and deep layers of the deep temporal fascia.

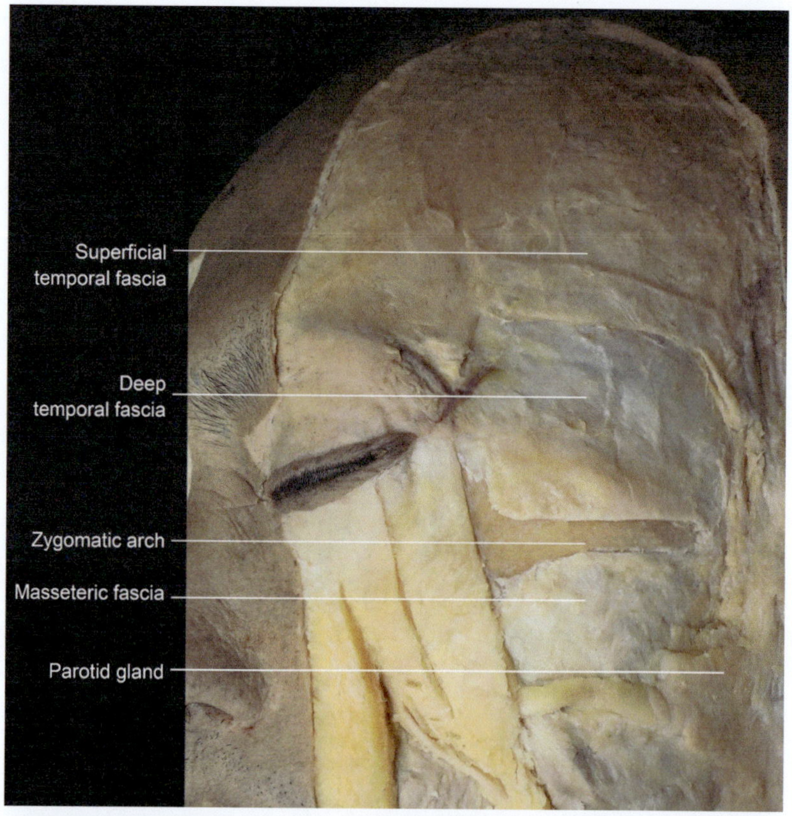

Fig. 3.10 Deep temporal fascia and masseteric fascia

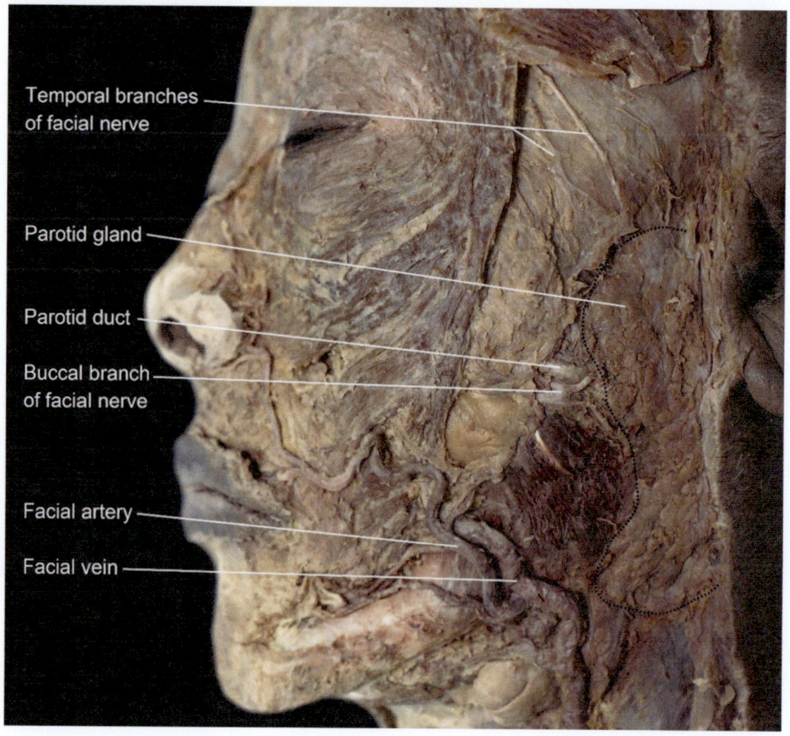

Fig. 3.11 The structures emerging from the parotid gland. Dot line is the border of the parotid gland

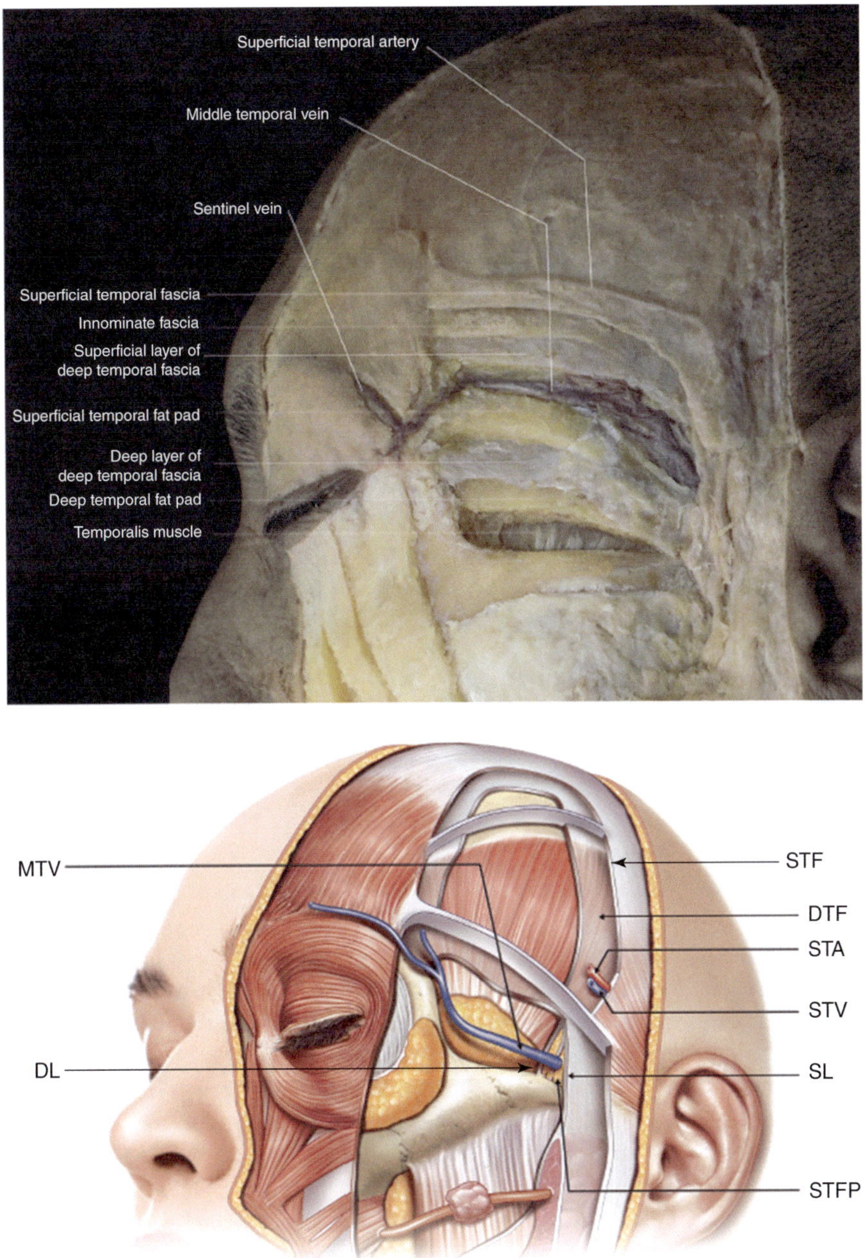

Fig. 3.12 Layers of the temporal region

3.3 Vessels of the Face

Thread lifting is less likely to cause vascular side effects such as intravascular injection of fillers. However, side effects associated with vascular injury by thread lifting include bruit, hematoma, swelling, and pain. Fortunately, such side effects are not common.

During thread lifting procedures, bleeding occurs more frequently than during filler procedures. This is because, in thread lifting, tissues need to be pulled upward, resulting in a longer

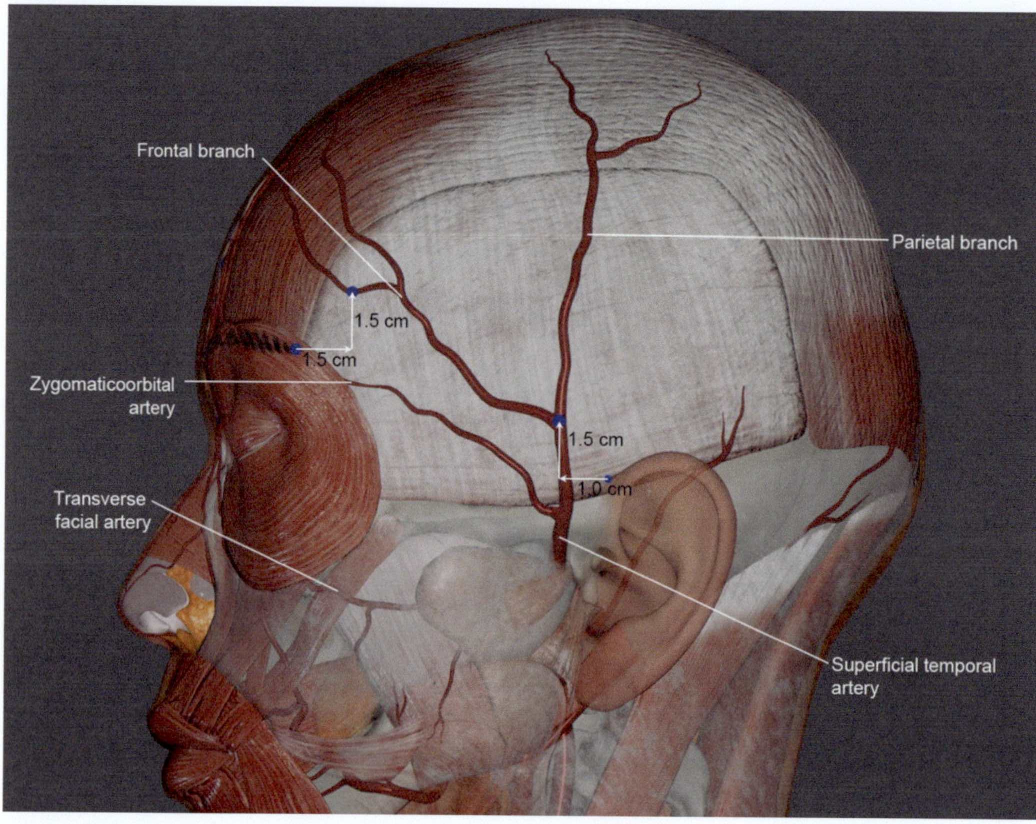

Fig. 3.13 Superficial temporal artery

path for the thread to travel and pass through some blood vessels along the way. While vascular injury can occur due to cannulas or needles, it can also happen due to the cogs on the threads in the case of cog threads. Special attention should be paid to the injury of the superficial temporal artery, the zygomatico-orbital artery, the transverse facial artery, and the middle temporal vein during thread lifting.

3.3.1 Superficial Temporal Artery

The superficial temporal artery, as the terminal branch of the external carotid artery, bifurcates into the frontal branch and parietal branch at approximately 10 mm in front and 15 mm above the superior root of the auricle, respectively. While they are sometimes referred to as the anterior and posterior branches, these terms are not precise. The frontal branch courses diagonally forward before reaching the forehead, then ascends upwards. It travels along the surface of the frontalis muscle, entering at a point approximately 15 mm above and 15 mm lateral to the outermost point of the eyebrow (Fig. 3.13). The parietal branch ascends almost straight toward the vertex.

The superficial temporal artery travels enveloped by the superficial temporal fascia. However, due to its relatively large diameter (1.5–2.7 mm), although it is enveloped by the superficial temporal fascia, it often protrudes through the skin or subcutaneous tissue, making its course visible from the skin surface (Fig. 3.14).

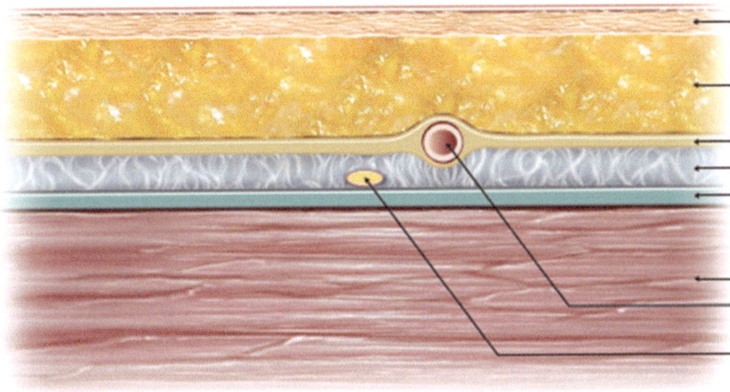

Fig. 3.14 Superficial temporal artery in layers

After emerging from the parotid gland as the terminal branch of the external carotid artery and passing upwards beyond the parotid gland, the superficial temporal artery remains enveloped by the parotid fascia, the fifth layer deep fascia, before gradually emerging above the zygomatic arch and eventually becoming enveloped by the third layer superficial temporal fascia.

3.3.2 Zygomatico-Orbital Artery

The zygomatico-orbital artery is a branch of the superficial temporal artery and is present in 23% of individuals. This artery generally originates from the trunk of the superficial temporal artery, but sometimes it originates from the proximal part of the frontal branch of the superficial temporal artery (Fig. 3.13). The diameter of the artery is about 1.0 mm from its origin.

The zygomatico-orbital artery is enveloped by superficial temporal fascia like the superficial temporal artery because the zygomatico-orbital artery is a branch of the superficial temporal artery (Fig. 3.14). The zygomatico-orbital artery runs parallel or slightly obliquely to the superior border of the zygomatic arch toward the lateral end of the eyebrow, so the cannula probably crosses the artery during thread lifting with their positional relationship.

3.3.3 Transverse Facial Artery

The transverse facial artery is an artery from the superficial temporal artery before that vessel leaves the parotid gland. The artery runs across the lateral face as its name between the parotid duct and the inferior border of the zygomatic arch. It supplies the middle area of the lateral face including the parotid gland and duct.

The transverse facial artery originates from the superficial temporal artery in the parotid gland, so its main trunk is covered by parotid fascia just like the superficial temporal artery (Fig. 3.14). The diameter of the artery is about 1.0 mm from its origin. The transverse facial artery was present almost always (96%) differently from the zygomatico-orbital artery. There is generally a transverse facial artery, but sometimes two arteries are present.

3.3.4 Middle Temporal Vein

Middle temporal vein is a very important vein in the temporal region. The vein is buried in a superficial temporal fat pad between superficial and deep layers of deep temporal fascia, it drains into superficial temporal vein posteriorly. Middle temporal vein runs parallelly above the zygomatic arch at a distance 2–3 cm (Fig. 3.15). The vein is a relatively large vein with a mean diameter of 2 mm.

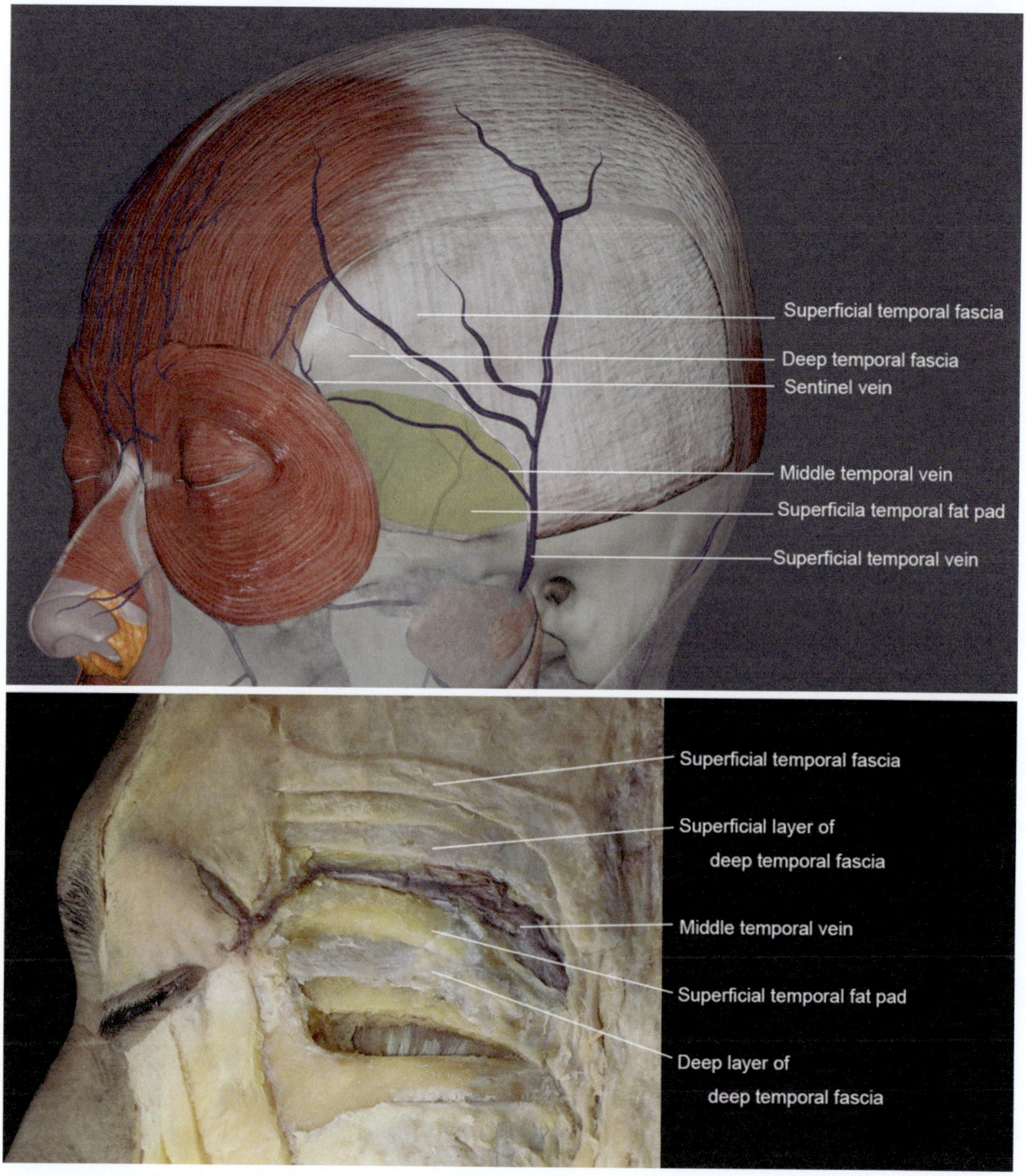

Fig. 3.15 Middle temporal vein

3.4 Nerves of the Face

3.4.1 Facial Nerve

The nerve of the face is mainly composed of the trigeminal nerve as a sensory nerve and the facial nerve as a motor nerve. The more important nerve during thread lifting is the facial nerve innervating facial expression muscles. The temporal, zygomatic, buccal, marginal mandibular, and cervical branches of the facial nerve exit from the parotid gland and travel beneath the SMAS (Fig. 3.16). The branches of the facial nerve are covered by deep fascia, parotidomasseteric fascia, just after exiting from the parotid gland.

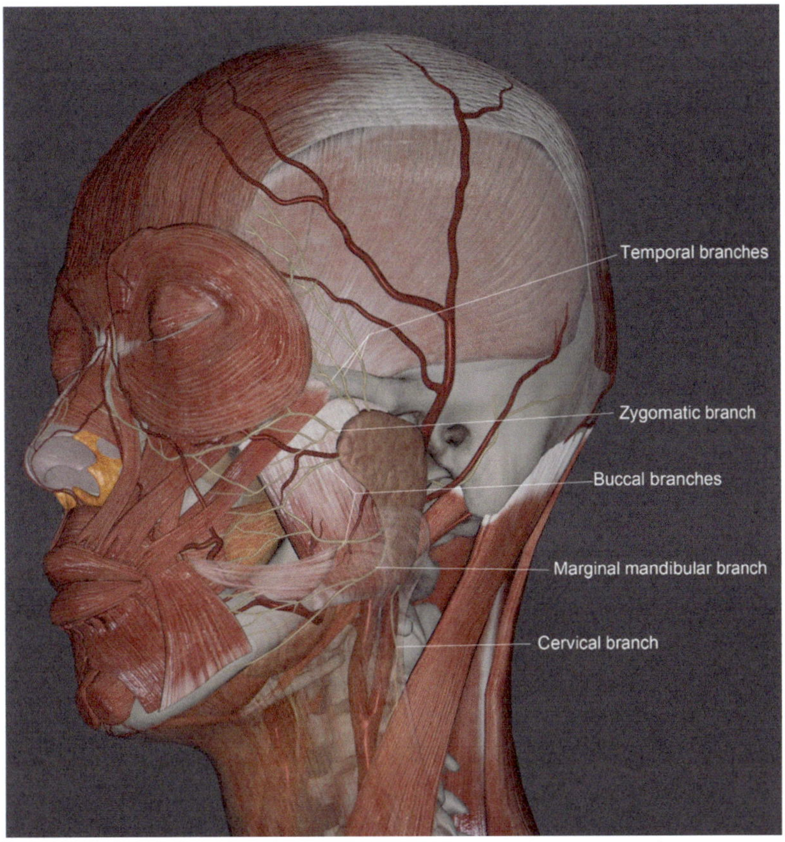

Fig. 3.16 The branches of the facial nerve

The temporal branch of the facial nerve is an important branch during thread lifting. The temporal branch pierces the deep fascia known as the parotidomasseteric fascia and exits the parotid gland covered by SMAS. It then travels across the zygomatic arch to reach the innominate fascia (4th layer in the temporal region) and runs at a height of 1.5–3.0 cm above the zygomatic arch.

There are multiple temporal branches of the facial nerve, which is located within a danger triangle connecting the tragus, hairline, and lateral end of the eyebrow (Fig. 3.17, blue triangle). In addition, there is another reference line to explain the course of the temporal branch. The average course of the temporal branch of the facial nerve follows Pitanguy's line, which connects a point 0.5 cm below the tragus to a point 1.5 cm from the lateral end of the eyebrow (Fig. 3.17, dot line). The temporal branch of the facial nerve crosses the middle third of the zygomatic arch (Fig. 3.17, green square). Therefore, we must be

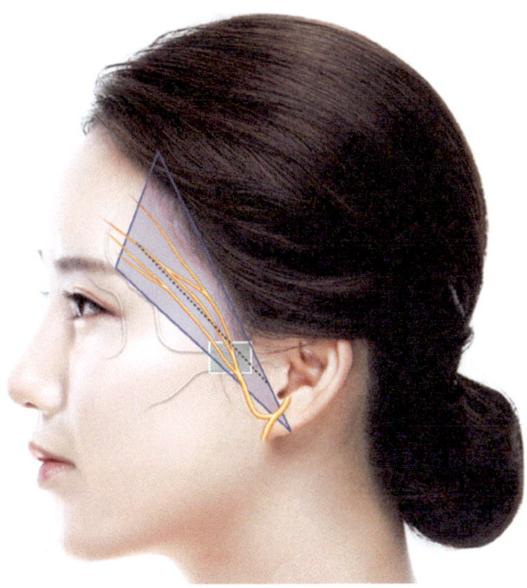

Fig. 3.17 Topography of the temporal branch of the facial nerve. Blue triangle: dangerous triangle. Dot line: Pitanguy's line. Green square: crossing area with zygomatic arch

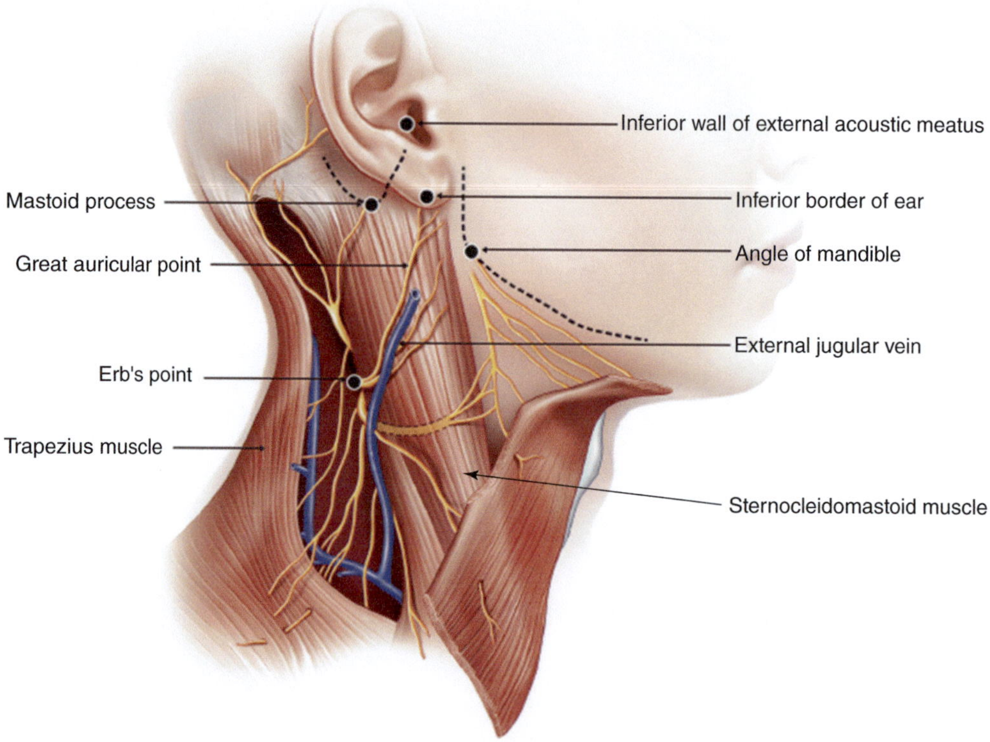

Fig. 3.18 Greater auricular nerve

very careful when the cannula passes through the zygomatic arch during thread lifting.

3.4.2 Great Auricular Nerve

The great auricular nerve is a cervical sensory nerve branch that originates from CN2–3. The great auricular nerve exits at the nerve point of the neck (Erb's point) with the other three cervical sensory nerves, which are located approximately in the center of the posterior border of the sternocleidomastoid muscle. This nerve runs between the sternocleidomastoid muscle and the platysma in its ascending course. It ascends to the lobule of the auricle, posterior to the external jugular vein, and then divides into two branches. The anterior branch supplies the skin around the anterior surface of the lobule, the angle of the mandible, and the parotid area, while the posterior branch supplies the skin around the posterior surface of the lobule and the mastoid area (Fig. 3.18). The great auricular nerve can be inadvertently crossed by a thread during a lower face lift procedure because this nerve is relatively thick and lies superficially.

3.5 Retaining Ligaments of the Face

The retaining ligaments are strong and deeply rooted fibrous attachments that originate from either the periosteum or the deep fascia. They traverse through various facial layers perpendicu-

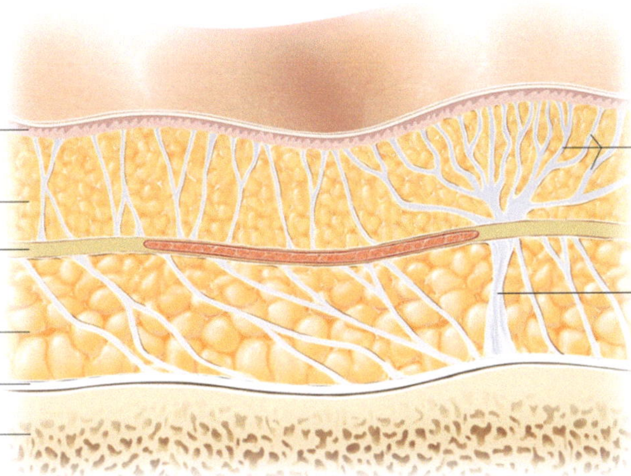

Fig. 3.19 Retaining ligament

larly and firmly attach to the dermis. Acting as strong hanging points, these ligaments play a crucial role in retaining and stabilizing the skin, superficial fascia, and SMAS in specific anatomic locations, ensuring a well-defined facial structure (Fig. 3.19).

Anatomically, a ligament is a fibrous connective tissue that attaches bone to bone and usually serves to hold structures together and keep them stable. Therefore, the retaining ligament is not an actual ligament anatomically.

Each retaining ligament resembles the shape of a tree and is well-known. The portions attaching to deeper structures, such as the periosteum or deep fascia, are relatively thicker, while those closer to the SMAS branch into smaller branches. These branches progressively become thinner and finer as they attach to the dermis, ultimately playing a role in supporting the entire layer of facial soft tissue. However, these retaining ligaments are not uniformly firm throughout the entire face. While they may be firm in certain facial areas as depicted in the illustration below, in most cases, this fourth layer is loose, allowing the superficial three layers of the face to slide over it.

Remarkably, the superficial projections of the retaining ligaments into the subcutaneous layer (known as retinacula cutis) are believed to play a role in the formation of septa that partition this layer into discrete fat compartments within the face. This theory is substantiated by the finding that specific boundaries of subcutaneous septa correspond with the positions of deeply embedded retaining ligaments. Therefore, the deep-seated retaining ligaments and the subcutaneous fibrous septa harmoniously form adhesive areas, effectively dividing the facial fat compartments and aiding in maintaining the overall shape of the facial key structures.

The important retaining ligaments during thread lifting are as follows (Fig. 3.20).

1. Zygomatic ligament
2. Zygomatic cutaneous ligaments
3. Masseteric ligaments
4. Mandibular ligament

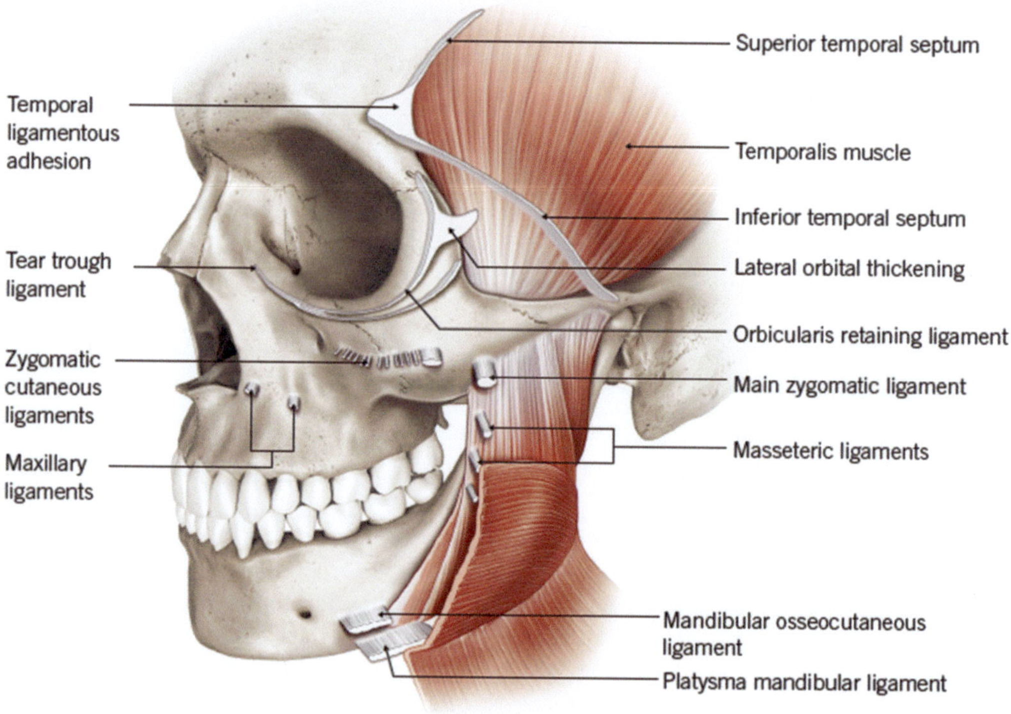

Fig. 3.20 Notable retaining ligament

3.6 Fat Compartments of the Face

The location of the retaining ligaments overlaps with some of the boundaries of the superficial fat compartments of the face. The temporal portion of the lateral temporal-cheek fat compartment is bounded superiorly by the superior temporal septum and inferiorly by the inferior temporal septum. The lateral orbital compartment is sandwiched between the inferior temporal septum superiorly and the superior cheek septum inferiorly. The deeply located zygomatic ligaments overlap with the more superficial superior cheek septum, separating the lateral orbital compartment from the middle cheek fat compartment (Fig. 3.21). The masseteric cutaneous ligaments overlap with the septum, separating the middle and medial cheek fat compartments. The mandibular septum separates both the superior and inferior jowl fat compartments superiorly from the submandibular jowl fat compartment inferiorly.

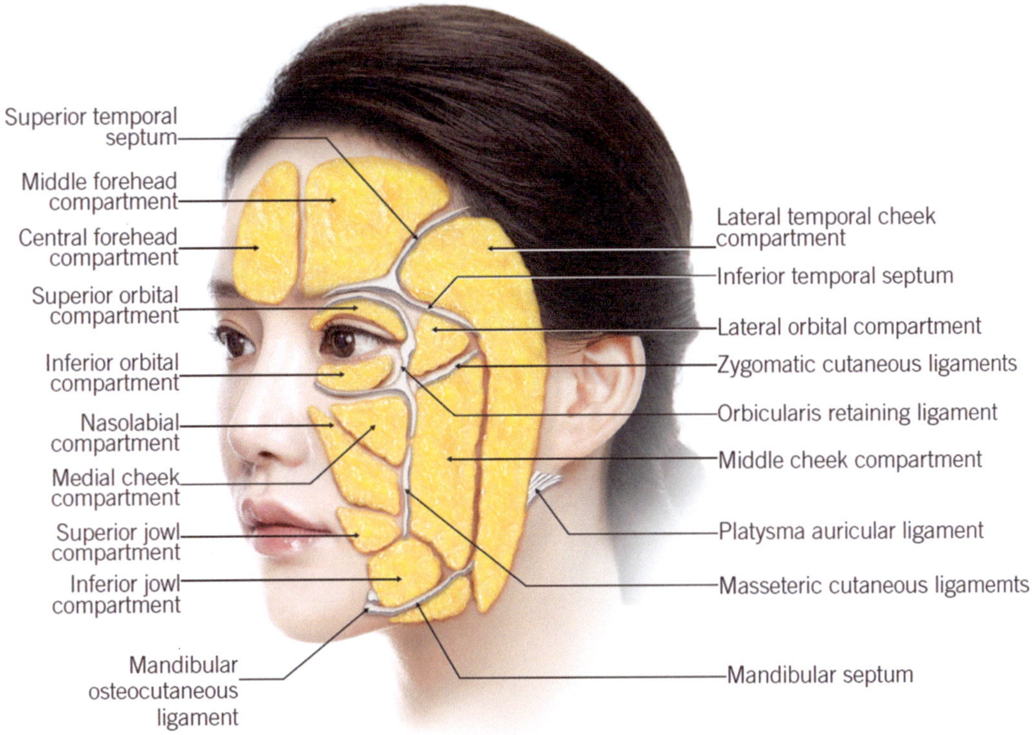

Fig. 3.21 Superficial fat compartments and retaining ligaments

3.7 Space of the Face

The spaces of the face lie in the fourth layer of the face under SMAS. The spaces have an importance not in thread lifting but in facial volumization. Almost all spaces of the face are occupied with deep fat tissue (Fig. 3.22).

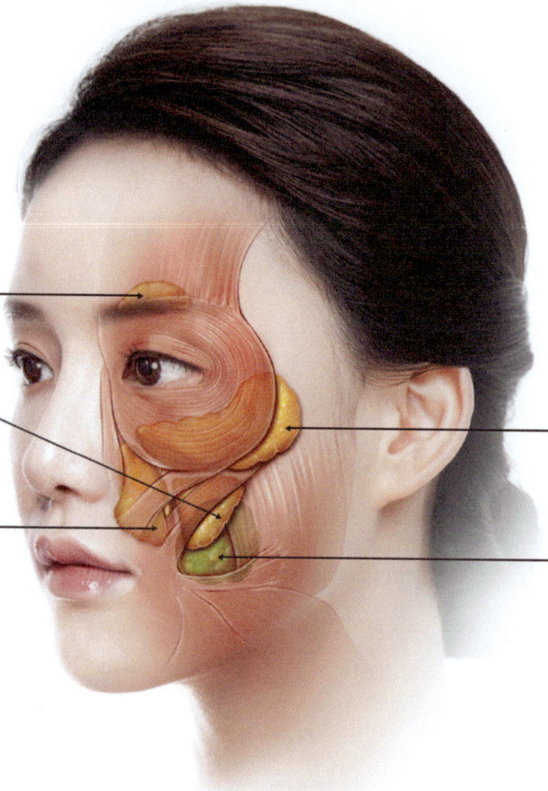

Fig. 3.22 Spaces of the face

3.8 Parotid and Submandibular Glands

The parotid gland is a major salivary gland on either side of the lateral face. The anterior part of the parotid gland is relatively thin and the posterior part is thick because the posterior part folds the posterior border of the mandibular ramus (Fig. 3.23). The thick parotid fascia covers the gland and it continues to masseteric fascia anteriorly. So, the combined parotidomasseteric fascia is commonly used in the clinical field.

The parotid duct exits from the anterior border of the parotid gland, runs anteriorly on the masseter muscle, and enters oral cavity piercing the buccinator muscle. The parotid duct is about 5 cm in length and 3 mm in caliber. The parotid duct is an important structure in thread lifting due to its large size easily be injured (Fig. 3.10). The transverse facial artery and facial nerve branches are closely located around the duct. These structures including the parotid duct were covered by masseteric fascia under SMAS (Fig. 3.23).

Submandibular gland is also a major salivary gland inside the body of the mandible and it is smaller than the parotid gland (Fig. 3.23). Submandibular gland is something oval and the most of the gland is not visible and palpable. But the concave inferior surface can be palpable on the internal side of the inferior border of the mandible. A large or descended gland by aging can be visible and more palpable below the inferior border of the mandible.

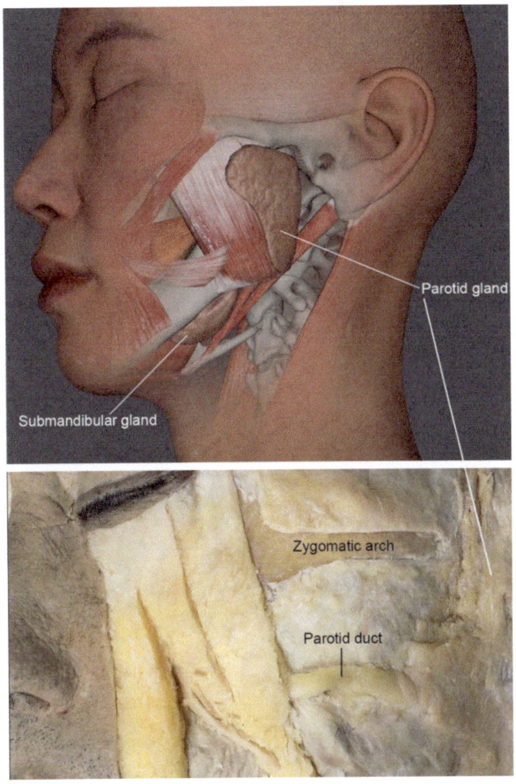

Fig. 3.23 Parotid and submandibular glands

3.9 Fibrous Connective Tissue of the Face

The deep fasciae in the fifth layer of the face cover masticatory muscles such as the masseter and temporalis muscles. They can be used as fixing structures during thread lifting because they are relatively thick and immobile.

The deep temporal fascia covers the temporalis muscle, the superior part of the fascia is one layer, while the inferior part is divided into two layers, the superficial and deep layers (Fig. 3.12). These two layers are attached to the superior border and lateral surface of the zygomatic arch. The middle temporal vein and superficial temporal fat pad are located between these two layers. The deep temporal fascia is commonly used as a fixing structure during cogged thread insertion in the temporal area due to its thickness and strength.

The deep fascia below the zygomatic arch is distinct from the deep temporal fascia. The masseter muscle originates from the inferior border of the zygomatic arch, and the parotid gland lies on the masseter muscle. Therefore, the posterior part of the deep fascia below the zygomatic arch is referred to as the parotid fascia, while the anterior part is called the masseteric fascia. However, the posterior parotid fascia continues and joins with the anterior masseteric fascia. These two fasciae are often considered as a single structure known as the parotidomasseteric fascia, which is also thick and strong like the deep temporal fascia.

There are many clinically important septa, adhesions, and thickened areas on the face in addition to the retaining ligaments. These structures are fundamentally similar to retaining ligaments but are named differently based on their morphology and location. The superior and inferior temporal septa are narrow bands of fusion between the superficial and deep temporal fasciae. They are named septa due to their morphological features, rather than being referred to as ligaments or fasciae. They serve as boundaries separating the superior part of the lateral temporal-cheek fat compartment from the frontal and orbital fat compartments (Fig. 3.21).

Pinch Anatomy for Thread Lifting

4

Contents

4.1 Definition of Pinch Anatomy

The facial structure seen in cadaveric photographs or illustrations is a natural appearance without any manipulation such as pinching or pulling. On the other hand, the appearance changed after a procedure or when tissue is pulled during the procedure is slightly different from the original appearance. This difference can be observed not only externally but also within the tissue itself.

In general, practitioners sometimes perform procedures with the skin in a pinched state for ease of procedure, but it is not clear what changes occur beneath the skin in this state. Therefore, the new state of anatomy that changes when tissue is lifted or pulled is called "Pinch anatomy," and research has been conducted based on it. Figure 4.1 is the logo of pinch anatomy.

S. M. Oh et al., *The Art and Science of Thread Lifting Based on Pinch Anatomy and Moving Plane*,
https://doi.org/10.1007/978-981-97-5516-5_4

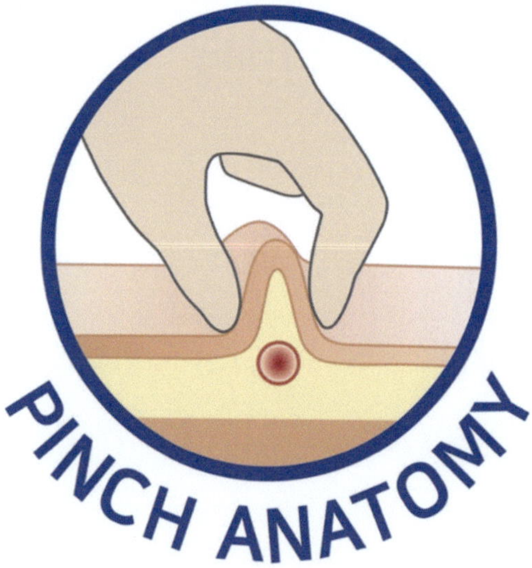

Fig. 4.1 Logo of pinch anatomy

4.2 Importance of Pinch Anatomy

During the thread lifting procedure, the practitioner should be careful of nerve and blood vessel injury. Especially if the cannula containing the threads is a sharp needle type, there is a risk of bleeding or nerve injury. Thread lifting is a petit procedure, not a surgical one. The advantages of petit procedures are that they have fewer side effects, faster recovery, and shorter procedure time. Therefore, minimizing the risk of bleeding and nerve injury during the procedure maximizes the value of thread lifting.

Knowing the main nerves and blood vessels and which layer they pass through based on facial anatomy is fundamental to thread lifting. As a result, knowledge of pinch anatomy can help produce safer and more effective results.

Practitioners often manipulate tissues in a pinch state to facilitate the procedure. At this point, the internal anatomic structure changes. If we can clearly understand the changes in anatomy in the pinched state and proceed with thread lifting based on this knowledge, we can avoid blood vessel and nerve injury.

Considering the depth and course of main blood vessels and nerves, it is essential to know which layer is being pulled up during the pinch maneuver, and whether blood vessels and nerves are being pulled up or not. Assuming they are being pulled up, the thread should be passed through the deeper layer for safety, and if not, it should be passed through the relatively more superficial layer.

4.3 Method of Studying Pinch Anatomy

4.3.1 Methods

After marking the hairline on a fresh cadaver, the hair was shaved, blue dots were marked along to hairline, and red stickers were placed on significant areas for the thread lift procedure (Fig. 4.2). Soft pinching was performed on each area, and excision was made on the lower side of the lifted skin (Fig. 4.3).

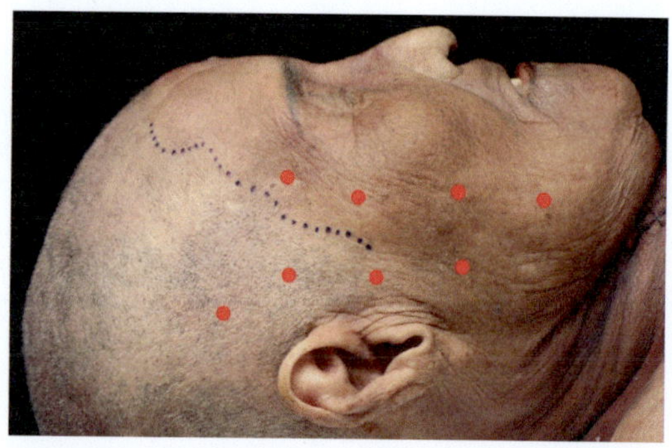

Fig. 4.2 Points for pinch

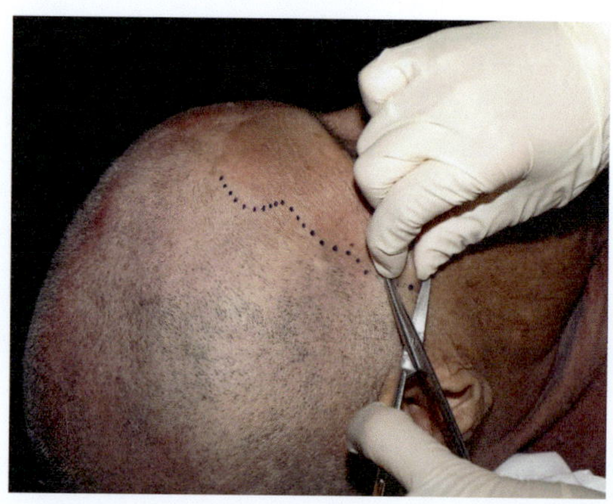

Fig. 4.3 Cut after pinch

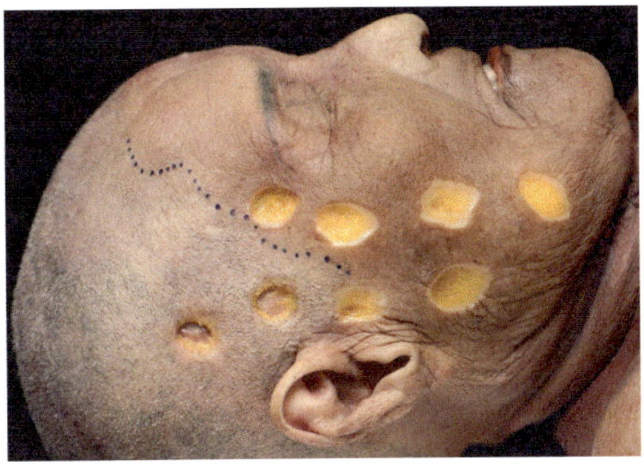

Fig. 4.4 Results after cut

It is thought that the cutting after pinching was done slightly deeper than the actual layer of cannula insertion. After the skin excision, the exposed area was observed with the naked eye to determine which layer had been removed by the pinch and excision. The excised tissue samples were processed and Masson's trichrome was stained for histologic examination.

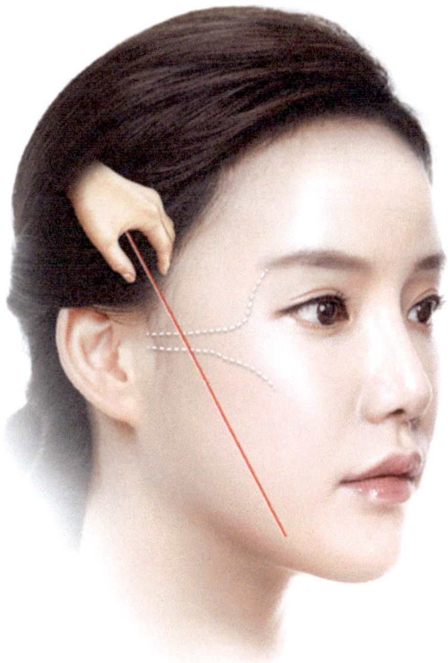

Fig. 4.5 Pinch of posterior temple

4.3.2 Overall Results

In the temporal area posterior to the hairline, the subcutaneous fat layer was cleanly removed and the superficial temporal fascia and the superficial temporal artery that protruded to the surface of this layer were not injured. In all other areas, almost subcutaneous fat remained. In some areas where some muscle was visible with rare subcutaneous fat (lateral orbital area), but histologically, the muscle was not injured (Fig. 4.4). That is, the muscles were not pulled up enough to be cut by pinching.

4.4 Pinch Anatomy for Each Part of the Face

4.4.1 Posterior Temple

It is very important to determine how deep to insert thread during long thread lifting. This is because the temporal fascial layer provides much stronger fixing points than the subcutaneous fat layer. It is necessary to understand how the temporal fasciae are pulled up during pinch manipulation because it is impossible to visually confirm which layer is pulled up. This is why the fixing procedure itself is a blind procedure.

When making a fixing point on the temporal region, it is important not to injure the superficial temporal artery that is enveloped in the superficial temporal fascia. Understanding how the vessels and fasciae in this region move during pinch manipulation can also help reduce the risk of vascular injury (Fig. 4.5).

4.4.1.1 Gross Anatomic Finding: Posterior Temple (Fig. 4.6)

- After the pinch, the subcutaneous fat layer was removed by excision and exposed to the superficial temporal fascia. No injury was visible to the superficial temporal fascia.
- Indirectly, it can be seen that only the subcutaneous fat layer was pulled up by the pinch. This demonstrates that the fascial layer is not easily pulled up during the pinch.

- Since there is almost no difference in the amount of skin and subcutaneous fat layer that was removed, it can be inferred that separation occurred between the subcutaneous fat layer and the fascia due to the pinch.

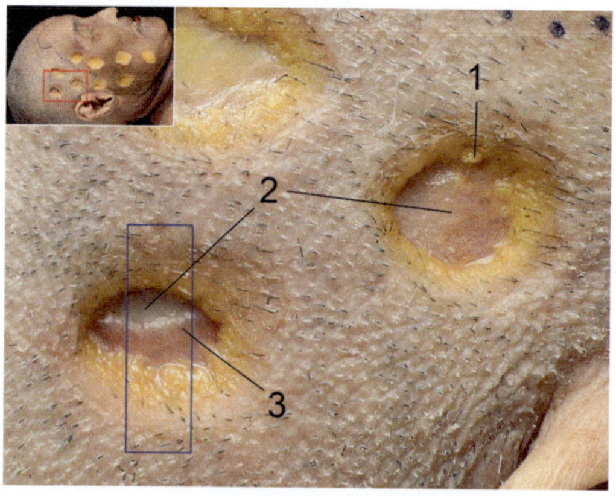

Fig. 4.6 Anatomic finding of posterior temple. (1) Subcutaneous fat, (2) superficial temporal fascia, (3) superficial temporal artery

- Although the superficial temporal artery is enveloped in the superficial temporal fascia, it protrudes through the subcutaneous fat layer due to its large caliber. The fact that the superficial temporal artery was not injured despite the removal of the same level of fat layer also demonstrates that separation occurred between the subcutaneous fat layer and the superficial temporal fascia due to the pinch.

4.4.1.2 Histologic Finding: General Pinching in Posterior Temple (Fig. 4.7)

- This is a histologic image to confirm the blue rectangular area of Fig. 4.6 from the pinched and excised remaining portion of the posterior temple.
- There is not much fat in the subcutaneous tissue of the posterior part of the hairline.

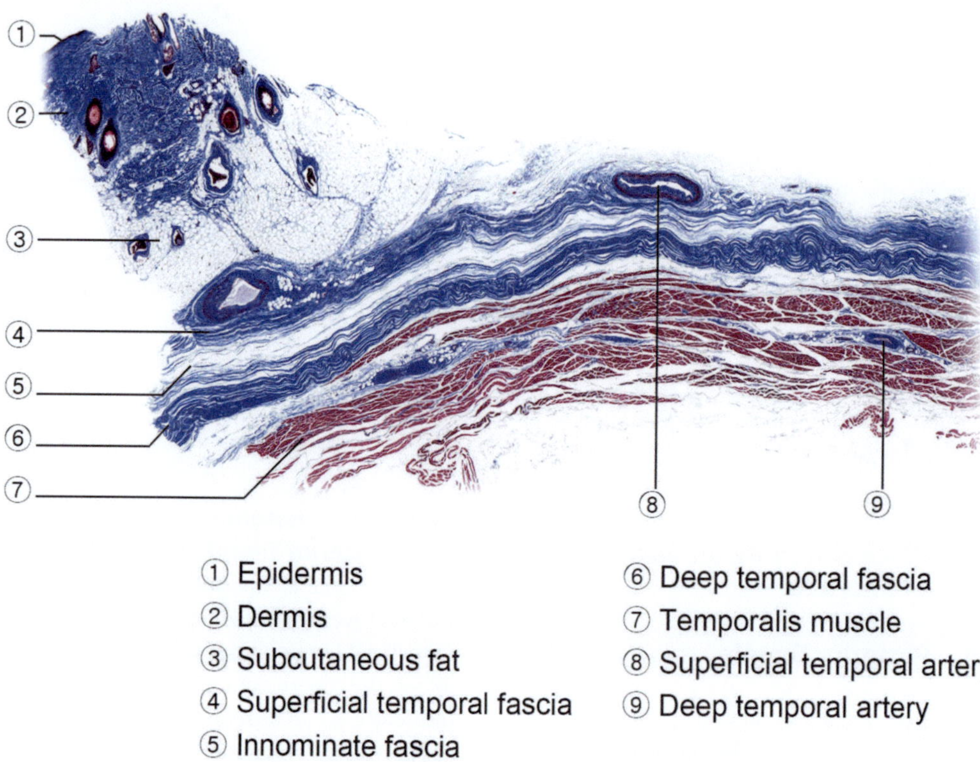

Fig. 4.7 Histologic finding of posterior temple

- As seen in the gross anatomic findings, after pinching, almost all of the subcutaneous fat has been excised.
- The superficial temporal fascia was not injured even after pinching and excision, thus the branches of the superficial temporal artery and branches of the facial nerve were not injured.
- It can be observed that the superficial temporal artery is enveloped in the superficial temporal fascia.

4.4.1.3 Gross Anatomic Finding: Comparison of General Pinching and Thick Pinching in Posterior Temple (Fig. 4.8)

- A thicker pinching and excision were applied above the area of general pinching commonly employed in thread lifting. This was done to determine whether the superficial temporal fascia was pulled up by the thick pinching.
- When a gentle or general pinching and excision were performed, only the subcutaneous fat was removed, and neither the superficial temporal fascia nor the superficial temporal artery was injured.
- However, when a stronger or thicker pinch was applied and tissue was dissected, along with the skin and subcutaneous tissue, some portions of the superficial temporal fascia and innominate fascia were removed, exposing the deep temporal fascia. However, the deep temporal fascia itself remained not injured.
- In the excised area at the lower right, pinching was performed in an area devoid of branches of the superficial temporal artery, making it impossible to confirm injury to the artery. However, if there were arterial branches in this area, there is a high likelihood they would have been injured.
- This demonstrates that the layers involved in pinching can vary depending on the technique used, including the width and intensity of the pinch.

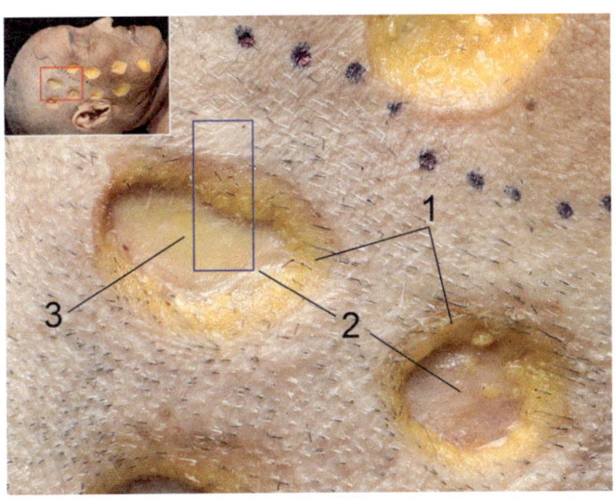

Fig. 4.8 Anatomic finding of general pinching (right bottom) and thick pinching (left top) in the posterior temple. (1) Subcutaneous fat, (2) superficial temporal fascia, (3) deep temporal fascia

4.4.1.4 Histologic Finding: Thick Pinching in the Posterior Temple (Fig. 4.9)

- This is a histologic image from the remaining portion of the thickly pinched and excised area at the posterior temporal region, aimed at identifying the blue rectangular area of Fig. 4.8.
- In cases where thick pinching was applied, as opposed to the general pinching shown in Fig. 4.7, both the superficial temporal fascia and the innominate fascia were pulled up together and excised.
- However, the very thick deep temporal fascia remained not injured. This suggests that when pinching is performed thicker, the innominate fascia widens, without causing injury to the thick deep temporal fascia.

4.4.2 Anterior Temple

This area is bordered by the lateral orbital rim, zygomatic arch, and hairline (Fig. 4.10). It is anatomically important as the temporal branch of the facial nerve and the frontal branch of the superficial temporal artery pass through this area. The temporal branches of the facial nerve in this region run deeper than the superficial temporal fascia.

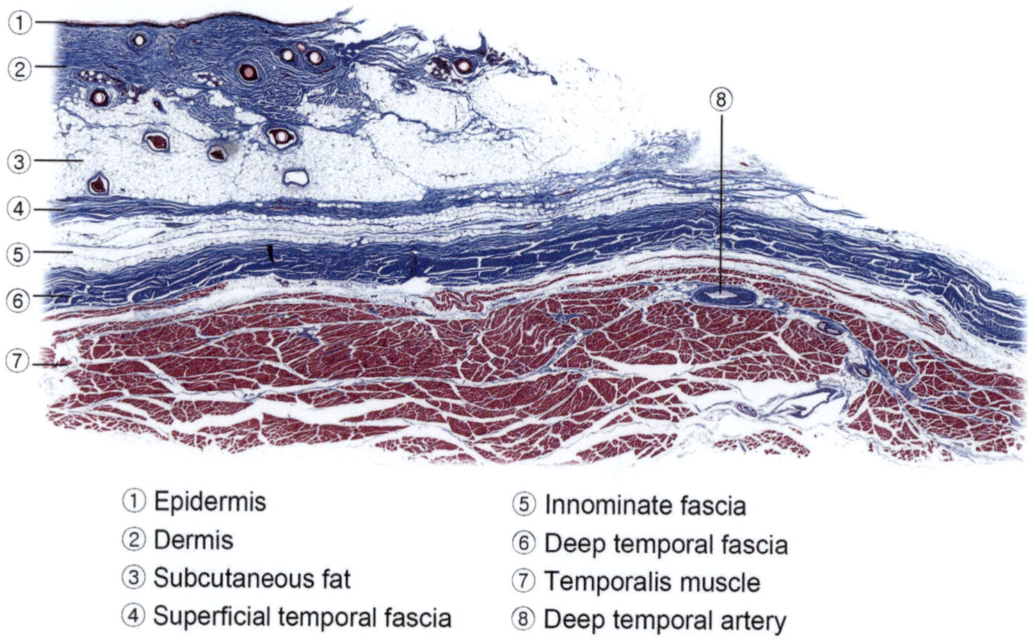

Fig. 4.9 Histologic finding of general pinching and thick pinching in the posterior temple

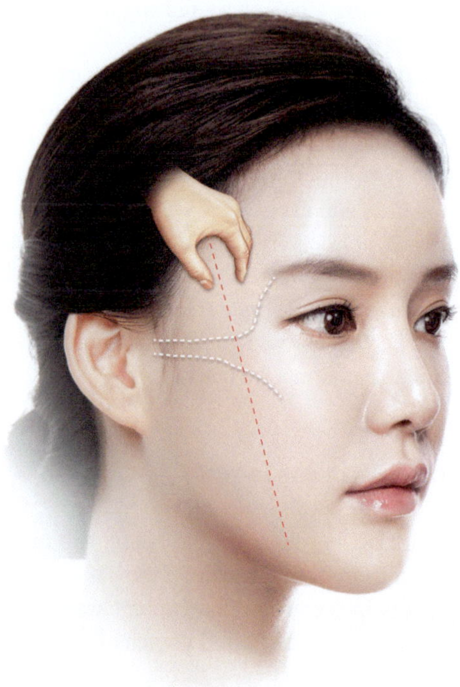

Fig. 4.10 Pinch of anterior temple

4.4.2.1 Gross Anatomic Finding: Anterior Temple (Fig. 4.11)

- As a result of pinching and incising the lower part of the anterior temple, only some subcutaneous fat along with the skin was removed.
- Visually, it was evident that some subcutaneous fat remained even upon gross inspection, and the superficial temporal fascia located deeper than this, along with the orbicularis oculi muscle in front of it, remained not injured.
- Therefore, it can be inferred that neither the superficial temporal artery, which runs enveloped by the superficial temporal fascia, nor the temporal branch of the facial nerve, which runs deeper, was injured.

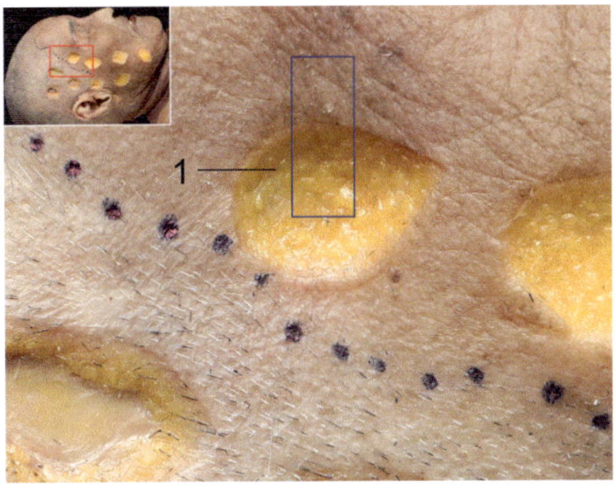

Fig. 4.11 Anatomic finding of the anterior temple. (1) Subcutaneous fat

4.4.2.2 Histologic Finding: Anterior Temple (Fig. 4.12)

- This is a histologic image from the remaining portion after pinching and excision of the anterior temporal region, aimed at identifying the blue rectangular area of Fig. 4.11.
- The skin and some subcutaneous fat were excised together, while some subcutaneous fat remained.
- The orbicularis oculi muscle beneath the subcutaneous fat was not injured.
- The temporal branch of the facial nerve, which runs deeper than the anterior orbicularis oculi muscle and the posterior superficial temporal fascia, as well as the zygomatico-orbital artery, remained not injured.

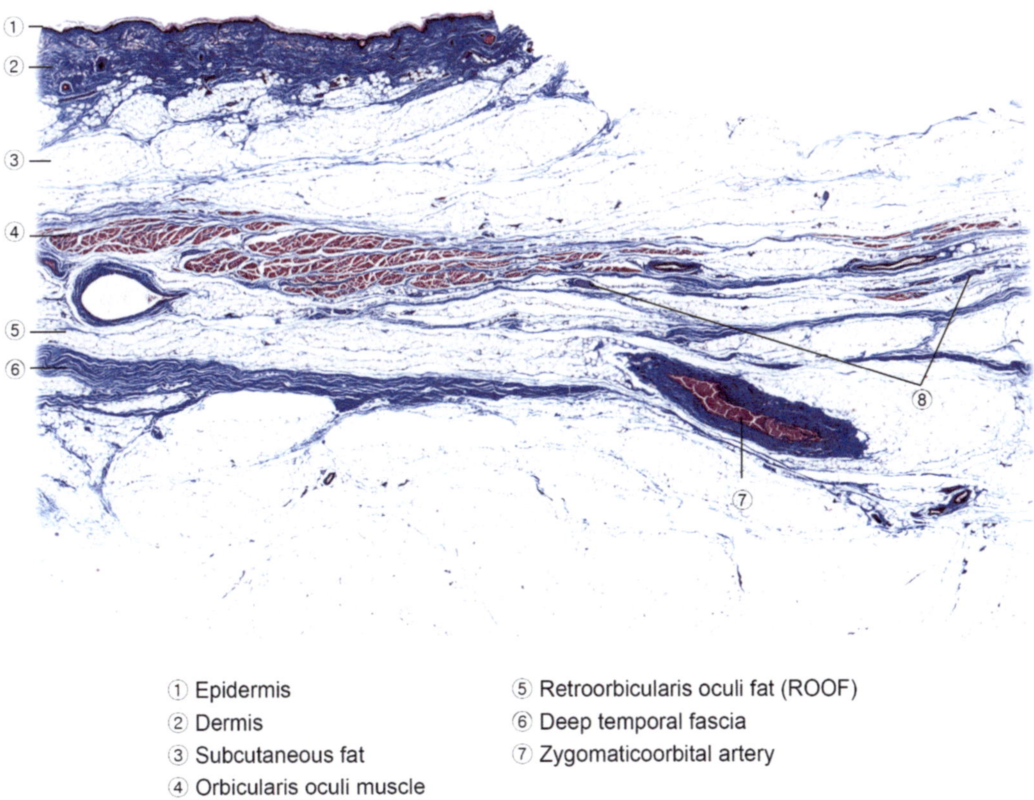

Fig. 4.12 Histologic finding of anterior temple

4.4.3 Zygomatic Arch

The zygomatic arch region is of significant interest regarding changes due to pinching, as there is a high concern for potential injury to the facial nerve (Fig. 4.13). In the zygomatic arch region, the temporal branch of the facial nerve runs deep within the superficial temporal fascia, making it crucial to understand which fascial layers are pulled up during pinching. Additionally, in the zygomatic arch region, the branches of the facial nerve are still largely undivided into smaller branches and exist as major trunks, thus nerve injury in this area could lead to much more serious consequences.

As depicted in the diagram below (Fig. 4.14), in the zygomatic arch region, the facial nerve ascends through the "loose" innominate fascia situated deep within the SMAS from a superficial position of the zygomatic arch, penetrating it as it progresses toward the temporal region. Typically, when using the temporal region as a

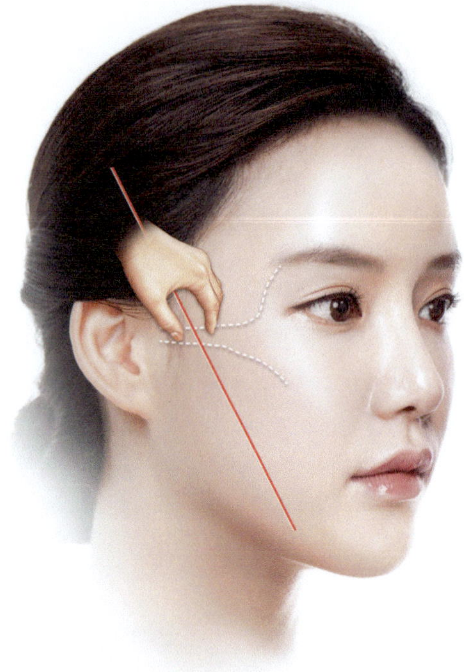

Fig. 4.13 Pinch of the zygomatic arch area

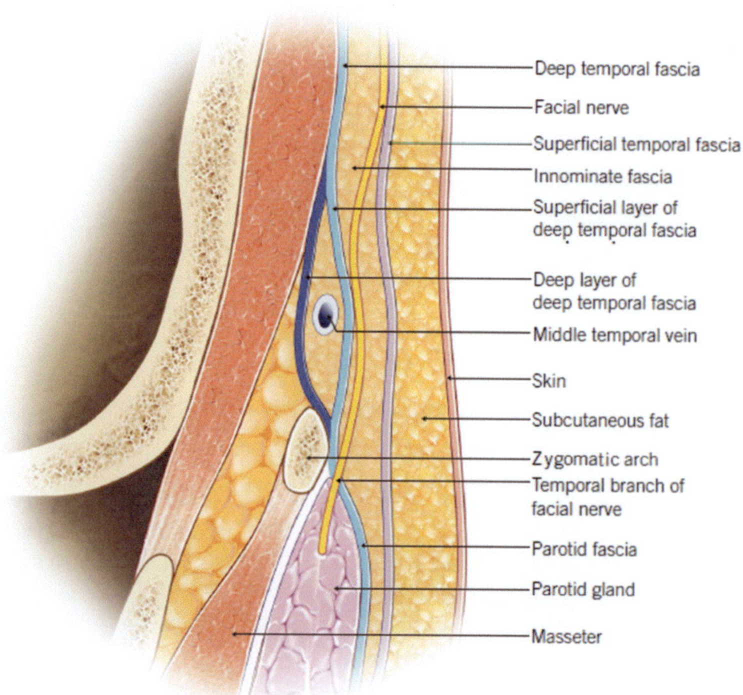

Fig. 4.14 Temporal branch of the facial nerve in the zygomatic arch area

fixing point for thread lifting procedures, the cannula passes through the surface of the zygomatic arch and descends toward the lower cheek. Here, the facial nerve passes deeper than the superficial temporal fascia, which is part of the SMAS above the zygomatic arch. Therefore, there is no need to worry about injuring the facial nerve after the subcutaneous fat layer has been loosened through pinching. However, if the cannula scrapes the surface of the zygomatic arch during descent, it can potentially injure the temporal branch of the facial nerve, so caution is advised.

4.4.3.1 Gross Anatomic Finding: Zygomatic Arch (Fig. 4.15)

- Following pinching and excision of both the anterior and posterior portions of the zygomatic region, only some subcutaneous fat along with the skin was removed, leaving behind some subcutaneous fat.
- Gross examination revealed the presence of subcutaneous fat, and it was observed that the SMAS, situated deeper than the fat, remained intact and not injured.
- Therefore, it can be inferred that the temporal branch of the facial nerve, which runs deeper than the SMAS, was not injured.

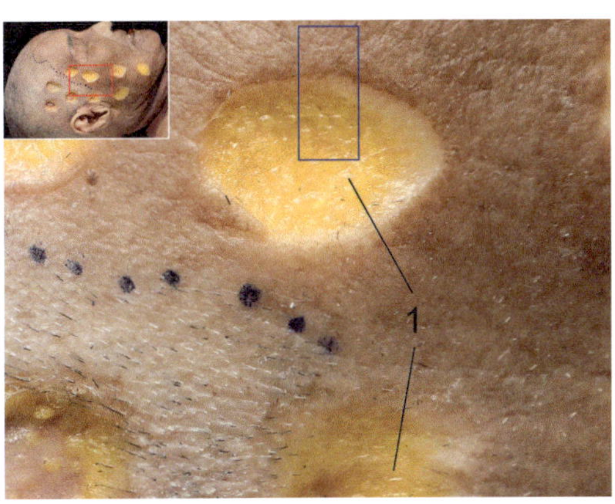

Fig. 4.15 Anatomic finding of the zygomatic arch area. (1) Subcutaneous fat

4.4.3.2 Histologic Finding: Zygomatic Arch (Fig. 4.16)

- This is a histologic image from the remaining portion after pinching and excision of the zygomatic region, aimed at identifying the blue rectangular area of Fig. 4.15.
- The skin and some subcutaneous fats were excised together, while some subcutaneous fat remained.
- The orbicularis oculi muscle, located deeper than the subcutaneous fat, remained not injured.
- The temporal branch of the facial nerve, which runs deeper than the orbicularis oculi muscle, was not injured.
- The subcutaneous fat appears to be slightly thicker compared to that of the temporal region.

4.4.4 Subzygomatic Area

Subzygomatic area is generally hollowed. It is a region with abundant fibrous tissue and relatively strong adhesion (Fig. 4.17). Therefore, when placing cog threads in this area, they can withstand the pulling force well and achieve good lifting results. However, for the same reason, if the characteristics of this area are not clearly understood during thread lifting, side effects such as hollowing may occur easily. Therefore, it is essential to create an optimal procedure based on various skills and design know-how, including pinch manipulation.

4.4.4.1 Gross Anatomic Finding: Subzygomatic Area (Fig. 4.18)

- The subzygomatic area contains a certain amount of subcutaneous fat, so after pinching and excision, only some subcutaneous fat was removed along with the skin.
- Some subcutaneous fat remained, and it can be inferred that the SMAS, situated deeper than the fat, was not injured.
- Therefore, it can be inferred that the parotid gland, located deeper than the SMAS, was also not injured.

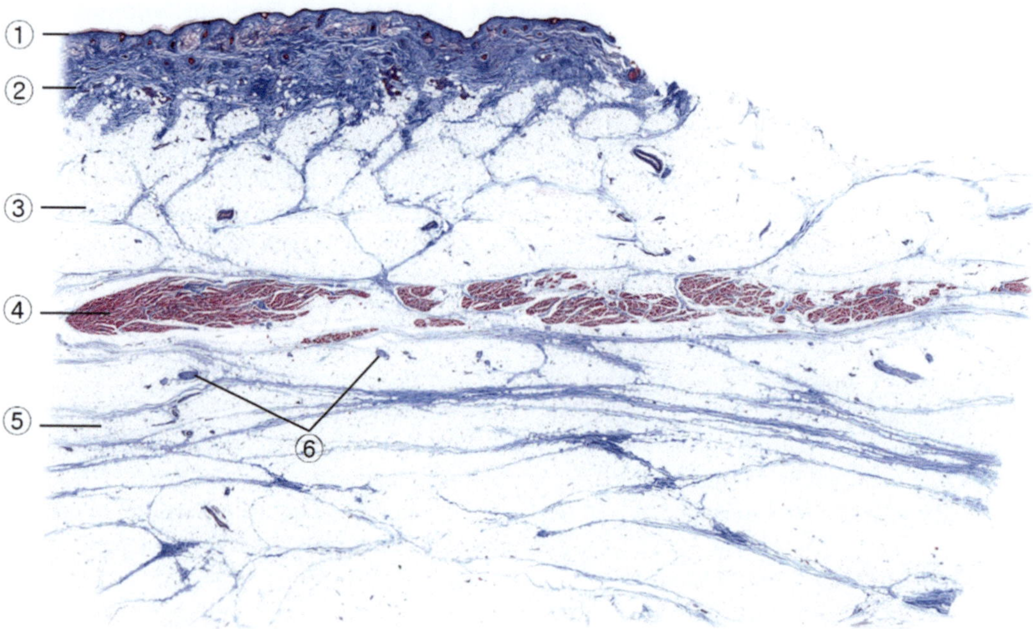

① Epidermis
② Dermis
③ Subcutaneous fat
④ Orbicularis oculi muscle
⑤ Suborbicularis oculi fat (SOOF)
⑥ Temporal branch of facial nerve

Fig. 4.16 Histologic finding of the zygomatic arch area

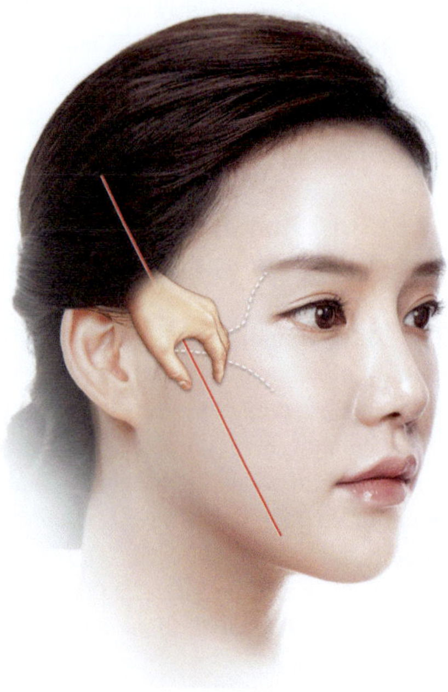

Fig. 4.17 Pinch of subzygomatic area

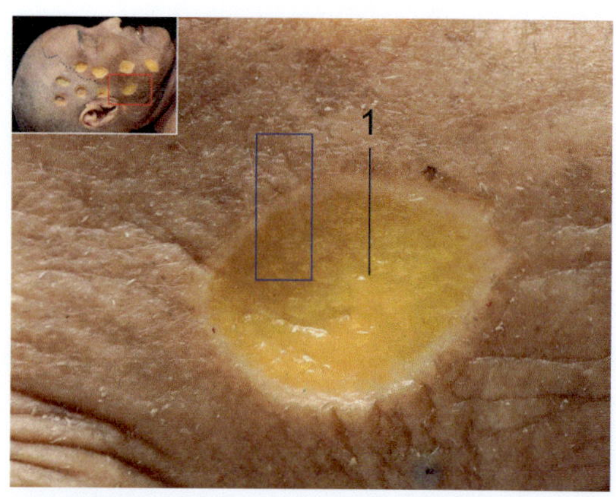

Fig. 4.18 Anatomic finding of the subzygomatic arch area. (1) Subcutaneous fat

4.4.4.2 Histologic Finding: Subzygomatic Area (Fig. 4.19)

- This is a histologic image from the remaining portion after pinching and excision of the subzygomatic area, aimed at identifying the blue rectangular area of Fig. 4.18.
- While the skin and some subcutaneous fats were removed, the SMAS remained not injured.
- The relatively large branches of the facial nerve regarded as zygomatic branches, situated deeper than the SMAS, were not injured.
- The subcutaneous fat appears to be thicker in the upper portion.

4.4.5 Lateral Cheek

During pinch maneuvers before thread insertion, it may occur that only the subcutaneous fat layer is being pulled up, but in thin individuals, it is important to adjust the depth of the procedure carefully. The practitioner should aim to lightly pinch and then proceed cannula by puncturing the lifted tissue.

In this area, caution must be taken to avoid injury to the parotid gland, parotid duct, branches of the facial nerve, transverse facial artery, and other structures (Fig. 4.20). After leaving the gland, these structures travel deeper than the SMAS. It is important to identify the layer pulled up by the pinch maneuver and insert the appropriate layer before performing the lifting procedure.

It is important to be cautious about facial nerve injury in the lower cheek area. The branches of the facial nerve travel within the parotid gland and then proceed deeper than the SMAS and deeper than the parotidomassteric fascia, after leaving the gland. It is crucial to identify which layer is being pulled up by the pinch maneuver and to determine in advance the thread into the appropriate layer for the lifting procedure.

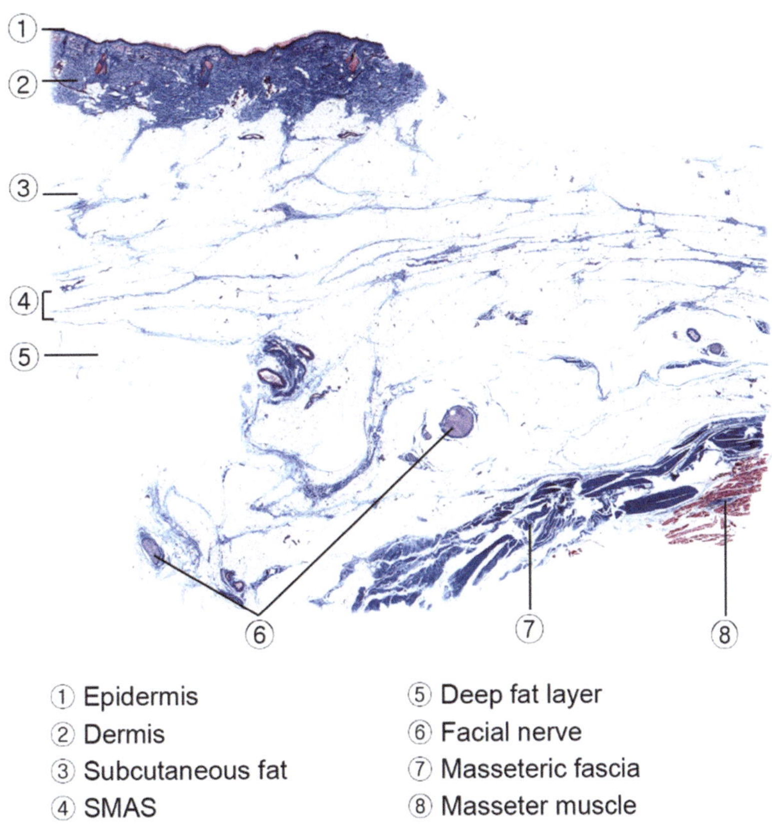

Fig. 4.19 Histologic finding of the subzygomatic arch area

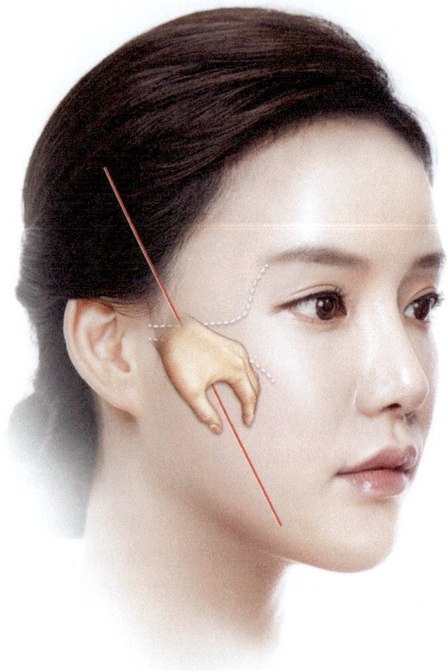

Fig. 4.20 Pinch of lateral cheek

4.4.5.1 Gross Anatomic Finding: Lateral Cheek (Fig. 4.21)

- Following pinching and excision, only some subcutaneous fat was removed along with the skin, leaving behind some subcutaneous fat.
- It was evident upon gross examination that some subcutaneous fat remained, thus it can be inferred that the SMAS, situated deeper than the fat, was not injured.
- Therefore, it can be inferred that the parotid gland, located deeper than the SMAS, was also not injured.

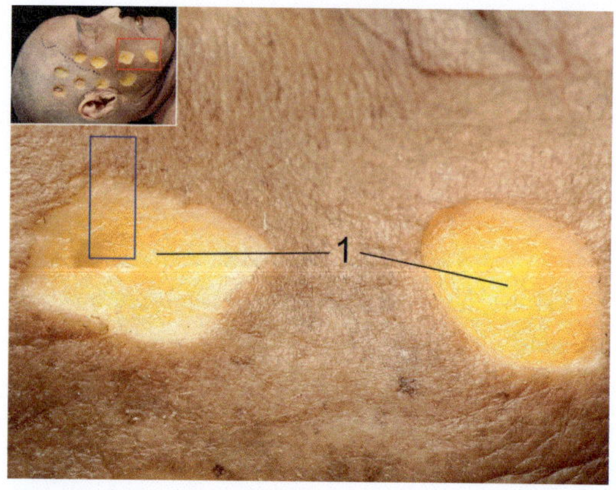

Fig. 4.21 Anatomic finding of the lateral cheek. (1) Subcutaneous fat

- Furthermore, it can be inferred that the buccal branch of the facial nerve, which runs deeper than the parotidomasseteric fascia, was also not injured.

4.4.5.2 Histologic Finding: Lateral Cheek (Fig. 4.22)

- This is a histologic image from the remaining portion after pinching and excision of the cheek area, aimed at identifying the blue rectangular area of Fig. 4.21.
- Only some subcutaneous fat was removed along with the skin.
- It can be observed that the subcutaneous fat is significantly thicker compared to other areas.
- Deep within the thick subcutaneous fat, the SMAS is visible.
- Located deeper than the SMAS, a bundle of facial nerves is visible, which can be inferred to be the buccal branch based on its location.

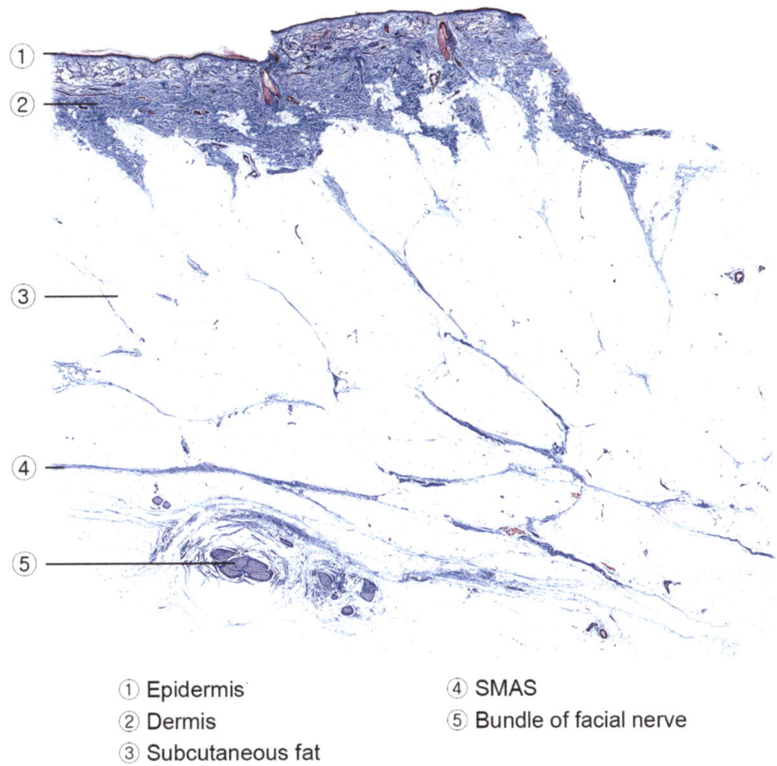

Fig. 4.22 Histologic finding of lateral cheek

4.5 Summary of Pinch Anatomy

4.5.1 Important Area for Pinch Anatomy

The significance of pinch anatomy is that it can help with performing safe procedures. In particular, it can help prevent vascular injury in the temporal region and prevent nerve injury in the zygomatic arch area. This is related to the movement of the nerves and blood vessels that are surrounded by connective tissue in each area when the pinch maneuver is performed.

4.5.1.1 Posterior Temple

Pinch anatomy in the temporal region reveals several important facts. When the temporal region was pinched and excised, it showed a similar appearance to Fig. 3.7. Particularly in the area where the superficial temporal artery is located, the fat around the artery can be seen being cut away. In other words, the fat layer at the depth of the artery is injured, but the artery itself is not injured. This can be illustrated as shown in Figs. 4.23, 4.24, and 4.25.

When pinching the temporal region, the subcutaneous fat layer widens, and the deeper portion of the fat layer becomes loosened, creating space between it and the superficial temporal fascia, which can be cut. Therefore, the superficial temporal artery, which is enveloped by the superficial temporal fascia, remains not injured.

Consequently, when pinching with moderate force for thread lifting procedure, there is minimal risk of vascular damage, providing reassurance for proceeding with the procedure.

We observed interesting findings when we pinched the posterior temple more deeply and then excised the tissue. As we pinched the area more deeply or thicker, we could see that the superficial temporal fascia was also cut (Fig. 4.26).

While thread lifting, fixing the thread to the fascia of the temporal region is the most effective lifting method, it is technically challenging. Moreover, as it involves blind procedures within

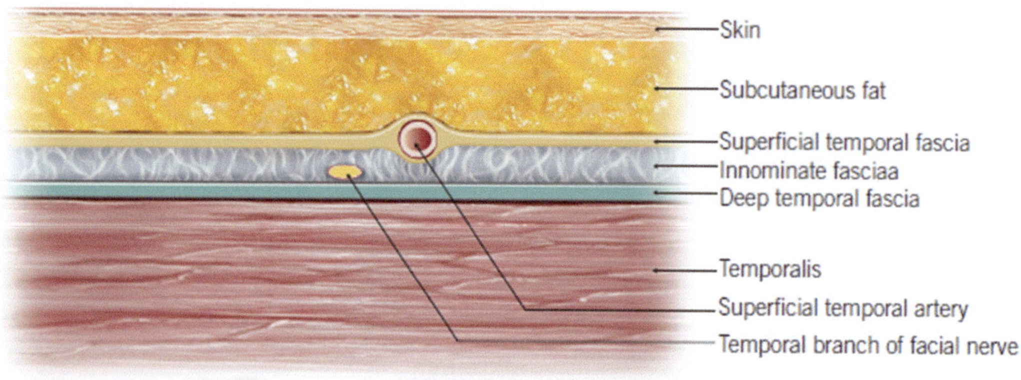

Fig. 4.23 Superficial temporal artery in temporal layers

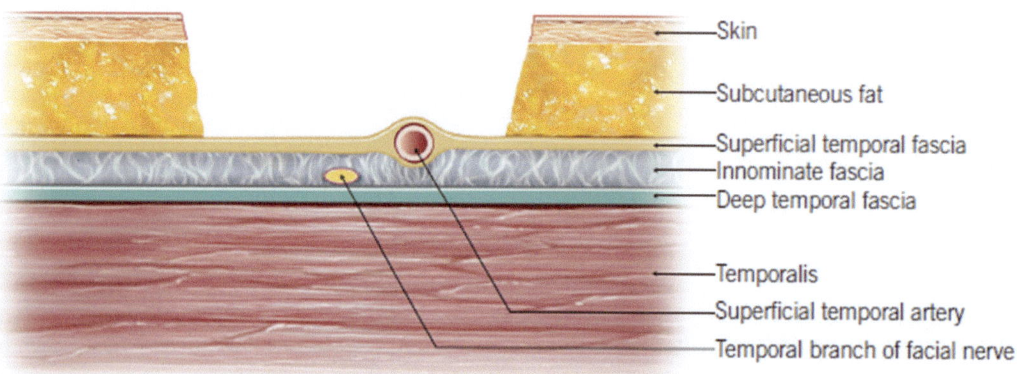

Fig. 4.24 Temporal layers after pinch and excision

the skin, it is not possible to directly confirm whether the fixing is actually caught in the superficial temporal fascia (tagging) or extends deeper to the temporalis muscle merely through visual inspection. The fixing must certainly catch onto the fascia to create a firmer fixing point. However, it is difficult to ascertain during the procedure whether the fixing has indeed caught onto the fascia.

When summarizing the findings of the pinch biopsy in the temporal region, the following conclusions can be drawn:

1. When performing a pinch, a specific layer of the tissue becomes loose and is pulled up.
   (a) When generally pinched, the layer between subcutaneous fat and the superficial temporal fascia becomes loose.
   (b) When thickly pinched, the innominate fascia (just like a space between the superficial temporal fascia and the deep temporal fascia rather than a fascia) becomes looser.
2. When generally pinched, the superficial temporal artery is not significantly pulled up as it is enveloped within the superficial temporal fascia.
3. When pinching while avoiding vascular areas and tagging, envisioning an imaginary line drawn over the presumed location where the temporalis muscle resides, and performing the procedure with the sensation that the tagging needle passes through the area where this line exists, enables the sutures to catch onto either the superficial or deep temporal fascia.

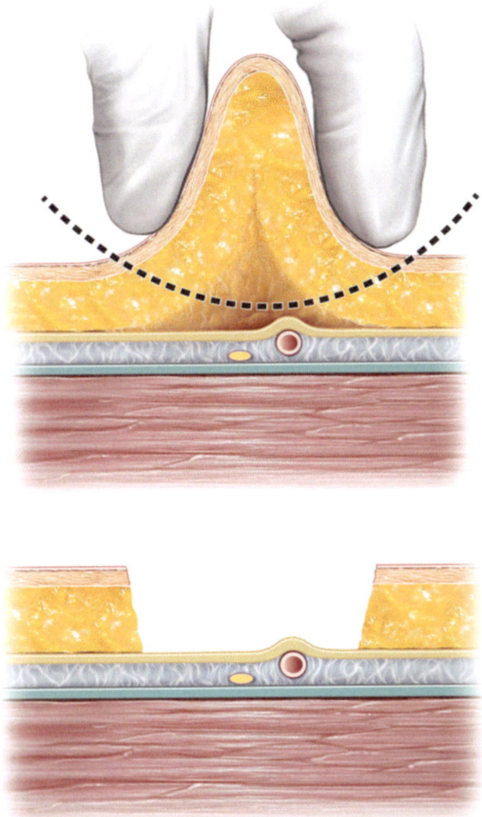

Fig. 4.25 Temporal layers changed during general pinching (top) and after excision (bottom)

4.5.1.2 Zygomatic Arch

The temporal branch of the facial nerve traverses across the midsection of the zygomatic arch. When this branch is injured during facial lifting surgery, it can lead to paralysis of the frontalis muscle, resulting in a side effect where the eyebrows are drooped.During thread lifting as well, caution must be exercised when the threads pass through the zygomatic arch. The temporal branch of the facial nerve travels deeper than the superficial temporal fascia, so even when pinching, it does not get caught. This is illustrated in the diagram below (Fig. 4.27). Since the superficial temporal fascia does not be

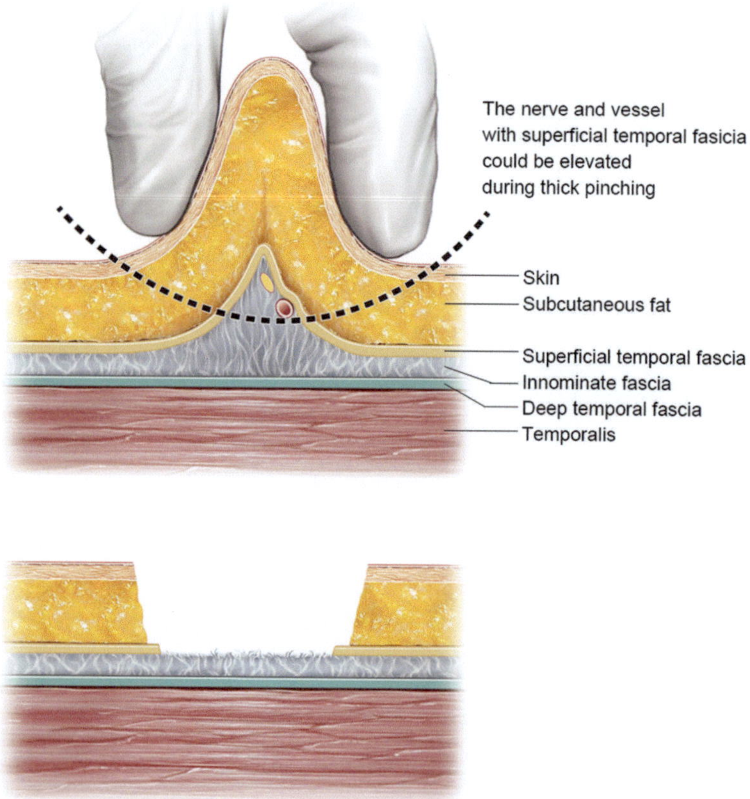

Fig. 4.26 Temporal layers changed during thick pinching (top) and after excision (bottom)

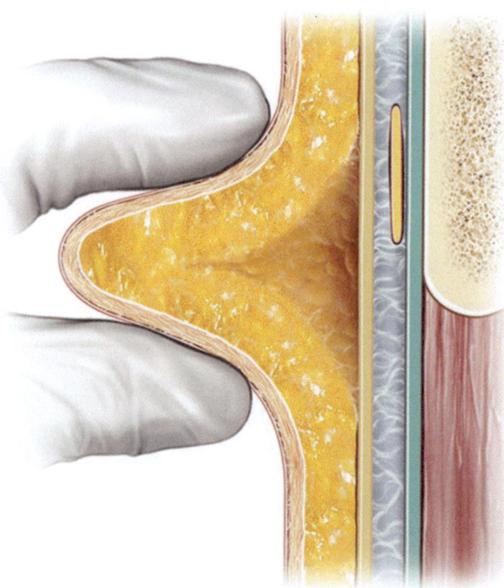

Fig. 4.27 Pinch of the zygomatic arch area

pulled up during general pinching, it is safe to perform the procedure with a sensation of traversing the subcutaneous layer when advancing the cannula. If the cannula descends along the zygomatic arch like scratching, it can injure the temporal branch.

Areas where pinch manipulation is useful
1. Posterior temple (a) Reduces the risk of injuring the superficial temporal vessels during fixing or puncture (b) Allows for appropriate depth of initial progression to prevent vascular injury 2. Zygomatic arch (a) Reduces the risk of facial nerve injury (b) During pinch, the branches of the facial nerve located deeper in the SMAS/superficial temporal fascia will not be pulled up

5 PDO Thread Lifting

Contents

5.1 Beginning of PDO Monofilament Thread Lifting

The theory that the thick cogged threads penetrating the loose fat tissue under the skin make the tissue firmer by giving mechanical stimuli to the tissue through signaling is well explained in *Mechanical signaling through connective tissue: A mechanism of therapeutic effect of acupuncture* by Dr. Langevin HM, a study that established academic theories on the effects of acupuncture. Usually, stimulating underlying soft tissue by using techniques of rotating or winding up the needle when acupuncturing may not only relieve the pain by tissue remodeling through the mechanotransduction pathway but also contract the skin and soft tissue of the treated site, improving the quality of the skin and firming the tissues. Assuming that these effects can be reproduced with thin absorbable threads instead of needles, it could be seen that embedding therapy, using chromic catgut, which was initially performed at the oriental medicine, has provided the basis for the absorbable monofilament thread lifting (Fig. 5.1).

However, it should be considered that the tissue contraction effect, hypothesized by Dr. Langevin as being induced by physical stimuli during acupuncture, is most substantially found when stimulating the sub-SMAS loose areolar layer, rather than stimulating the skin or subcutaneous tissue, when dividing the layers of middle third of the face, into the skin, subcutaneous tissue, SMAS, deep fat layer, and facial muscle layer. The subcutaneous fat of the face can be divided into superficial fat tissue firmly held by vertically oriented fibrous septa above the SMAS and deep fibroadipose connective tissue with obliquely oriented fibrous septa which may hold the tissue more loosely under the SMAS. Mechanical and physical stimulation on the sub-SMAS loose tissue may lead to activation

S. M. Oh et al., *The Art and Science of Thread Lifting Based on Pinch Anatomy and Moving Plane*,
https://doi.org/10.1007/978-981-97-5516-5_5

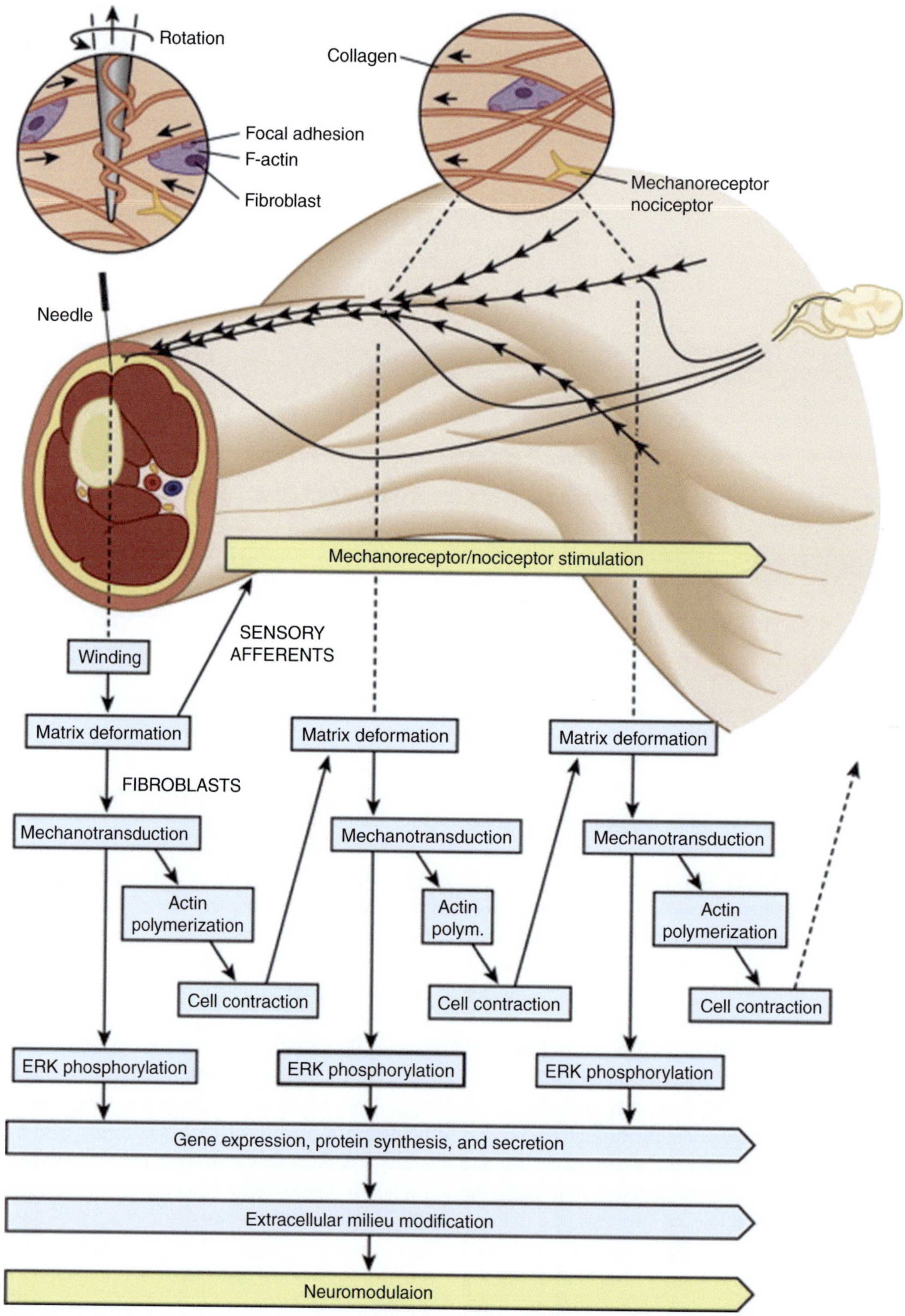

Fig. 5.1 Mechanical stimulation of sub-SMAS loose areolar layer. Change of cytoskeleton of fibroblast. Mechanical signaling through connective tissue: a mechanism for the therapeutic effect of acupuncture. Langevin HM, Churchill DL, Cipolla MJ. FASEB J 15: 2275–2282, 2001

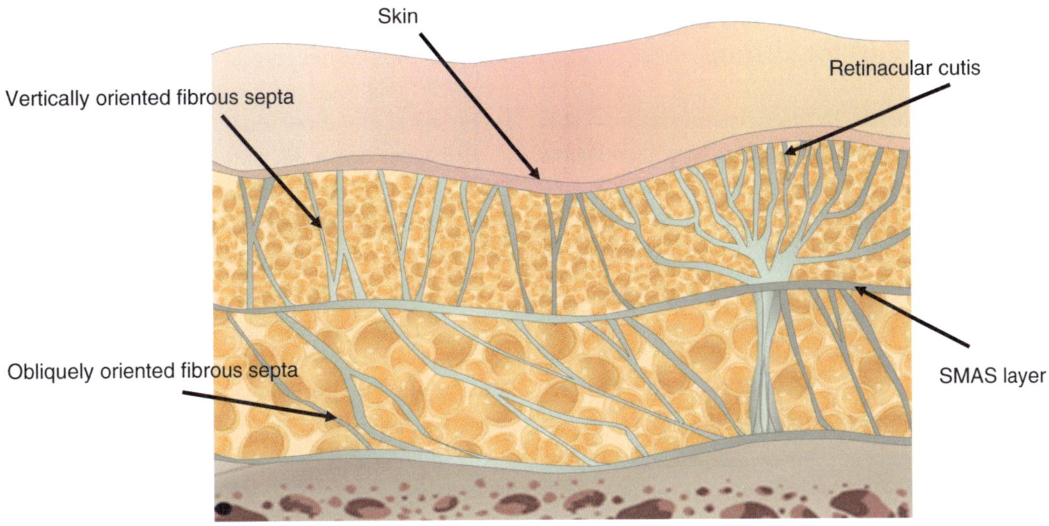

Fig. 5.2 Difference of the fibrous septa between superficial and deep fat layer

and proliferation of fibroblasts by immediate cell contraction due to changes in the cytoskeleton of fibroblasts and tissue remodeling to adapt to these changes (Fig. 5.2).

Based on these theories, some believe that stimulating subcutaneous soft tissues induces changes in subcutaneous white adipose tissue (sWAT), not neocollagenesis, resulting in the expansion of mature adipocyte along with activation and proliferation of adipose-derived stem cells (ADSC) and thereby, ultimately inducing volumizing effect and tissue tightening in the long term by hyperplasia and hypertrophy of ADSC and mature adipocytes.

In addition, combination therapy using fillers, toxins, injection therapies, liposuctions, fat grafts, or various energy-based devices such as laser, ultrasound, and high frequency is currently popularly performed procedure, rather than singly using lifting threads. The reason for the usage of these combination procedures is that the purpose of the minimally invasive procedure is not simply confined to pulling, raising, or lowering a certain part of the face but rather aims to create an attractive appearance that matches each person. The attractive face that matches each person can be formed by a combination of various procedures with various materials providing a harmonious ratio and morphological facial appearance, rather than a sharp nose, prominent forehead, V-line jaws, and protruding apple cheek.

Also, as the types of short monofilament threads equipped with needles are varied, further advanced from maximizing the existing effects with an increase in the contact surface between the thread and tissue by rolling up the threads on the needle or putting two lines of threads on the needle, threads with cylindrical mesh and forms of brooms, springs, or braids became available.

These threads are increasingly utilized due to their characteristics of mimicking the effects of fillers as well as tightening the skin to revive and firm the sunken tissues due to wrinkles. They also play a role as porous scaffold strengthening adhesion after insertion and thereby, inducing target-specific outcomes with various cells that are involved in fibrosis and regeneration, settling on the porous structure.

These threads are called volumizing threads that can create volume effects by separately dividing them, their utilization is increasing these days, which is explained separately in the volumizing multifilament PDO thread lifting.

5.2 Beginning of PDO Cogged Threads for Lifting

In the early 2010s, domestic manufacturers that had produced absorbable monofilament and short and thin straight-formed cog threads came to produce U-shaped absorbable lifting barbed threads, such as EZ Lift, a thick PDO thread with various cogs, and they gained great attention as threads for actual lifting purpose.

As various types of threads with different manufacturing methods were produced by different manufacturers, lifting procedures using the U-shaped long-length PDO cogged threads had become a general trend for some time. The author also used to mainly use thick and absorbable U- or V-shaped long-length cogged threads from a domestic manufacturer for lifting procedures. However, the threads still had a limitation for various applications due to the inconvenience of fixing threads to the temporal region in order to pull the lower third part of the face upward. In the meantime, many products with cogs of different thicknesses, directions, and locations, advanced from the basic bidirectional type cogged threads were released. At the same time, the preexisting I-shaped short- or medium-length cogged threads, which had been evaluated to be relatively inferior to U- or V-shaped long-length cogged threads in lifting effects, were newly released with significant improvements in lifting effects. Especially, the cause of adverse effects such as protrusion of threads or rugged skin due to concentrated loads were identified with clinical outcomes using bidirectional type threads. The N-Cog threads, multiple bidirectional type, which were uniquely designed to distribute the load evenly throughout the cogs of threads are the representative example.

Until recently, despite its various applications due to its simplicity and convenience in that it can be equipped with a cannula without the need for other apparatuses, the I-shaped short- or medium-length cogged threads have been considered to be confined to have skin tightening effect or tissue repositioning effect rather than significantly lifting the lower parts of face due to its less satisfying lifting outcomes.

However, these I-shaped cogged threads are released in various types with cogs of more advanced shape and position with various lengths, thicknesses, and directions.

Advanced from the initial method of making cogs on the threads, simply cutting out of the thread with a knife and making short cogs like fish scales, press cutting methods using a hydraulic cutter were currently used, resulting in various products with different types of cogs, which are longer, more angular or firmly standing like cobra head available. Threads manufactured with molding techniques are currently popular. Threads made by injection molding method, which can be represented by threads with rose thorn-shaped cogs, are produced by the process of heating and absorbable plastic materials into fluids and injecting them into a mold cavity, where they harden to the configuration of the cavity. However, due to the domestic production conditions, the domestic lifting cogged threads are produced by the process of attaching the cogs preproduced by injection molding method on the threads with heating rather than producing threads equipped with cogs at once, which induce a decline in the tensile strength, which means the force to withstand the tensile force, which is the force to pull the threads.

In the press molding method making up for these drawbacks, threads are produced by injecting materials such as thermoplastic resin into the press molding machine, pressed and heated to form a certain shape. With this method, the cogs are usually made as wedge forms like arrowhead, and the tensile strength of threads is substantially preserved. However, as explained in the previous tensile strength experiment, friction energy is generated by the force pressed by the machine during the manufacturing process, and the original thread is inevitably deformed as heat is generated, which is less than the injection molding method, but the tensile strength is weakened. The product that minimizes this can be said to be a good product.

Threads with reversed trapezoid-shaped cogs are currently available, which maximize the contact surface of threads with tissues by changing the shape of threads produced by the press molding method (Fig. 5.3).

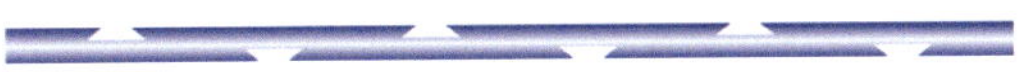

Fig. 5.3 Reversed trapezoidal PDO cogged thread

Threads made by molding methods are commonly promoted to be better than other threads made by preexisting methods with several versions of generation. Some threads have stronger tensile strength once they are inserted; however, they initially hold tissues less effectively than threads made by press-cutting method. Since a thread with less effective anchoring and holding effects in the first place has less lifting effects even though it has strong tensile strength, it is desirable to select lifting threads with reasonable price, which may serve the purpose of each procedure after testing and comparing various types of threads.

To sum up, lifting threads made by various advanced processing techniques have come to have cogs that have better abilities to hold and fix the tissues when compared to that of the threads of past generations. Therefore, rather than unconditionally using a certain type of cogged thread, it is desirable to choose a lifting cogged thread that meets the purpose of each procedure after using the product directly and comparing the effects.

5.3 Action Mechanism of PDO Thread Lifting

It seems that the concept of the action mechanisms of the absorbable lifting threads has been established to some extent, and in the aspects of the efficacy of the procedure, it can be divided into visible effects shown immediately after the procedure and invisible effects, subdivided into the biochemical part and the physical part.

As is commonly known, collagen regeneration caused by tissue reaction which occurs in the process of absorption of the inserted absorbable thread, takes up the largest portion of invisible biochemical effects. In particular, threads inserted superficially in the skin may promote collagen, elastin, and blood vessel regeneration, thereby improving the quality of the skin and restoring the thickness of the dermal tissue. Also, the thread inserted into the skin may induce lipolysis of the tightly adherent adipose tissue, causing loosening of the adipose tissue and continuous stimulation of the subcutaneous fat to promote the decomposition of the fat, thereby reducing the volume of the treated site and simultaneously increasing the collagen regeneration, with tightening effects expected on the site. Some also believe that, based on the principles of oriental medicine on acupuncture, the inserted threads may improve cellulites and relax the surrounding muscles by stimulating blood circulation and metabolism, relieving the pain caused by muscle contraction and tension, and reducing muscle size.

Table 5.1 Factors that control direction and force during skin and tissue tightening using absorbable monofilament threads

1. Direction and position of threads according to site
2. Number of threads (more threads increase tensile force)
3. Length of threads (more lengths increase tensile force)
4. Insertion depth of threads (more depth increases tensile force)
5. Width between inserted threads (narrow width increases tensile force)
6. Overlapping of inserted threads (closer overlapping of threads increases tensile force)

In addition to artificially twisting the threads when inserting or manufacturing the threads in twisted forms in the first place to maximize the lifting effects, threads with different thickness and length in different number, depth, and direction were used for each facial part to differentiate the tensile forces applied to each thread, adding physical effects to the basic biochemical effects of the absorbable monofilament threads. The author assumes this effect as a procedural manual to maximize the tightening of skin and soft tissue rather than actual lifting effects (Table 5.1).

The physical effects are mainly attributed to the improvement in the quality of skin that is induced in the process of skin regeneration that is physically damaged by needle pricking in all procedures, not necessarily lifting, and tissue contraction caused by the thread inserted in the subcutaneous tissue stimulating the soft tissue.

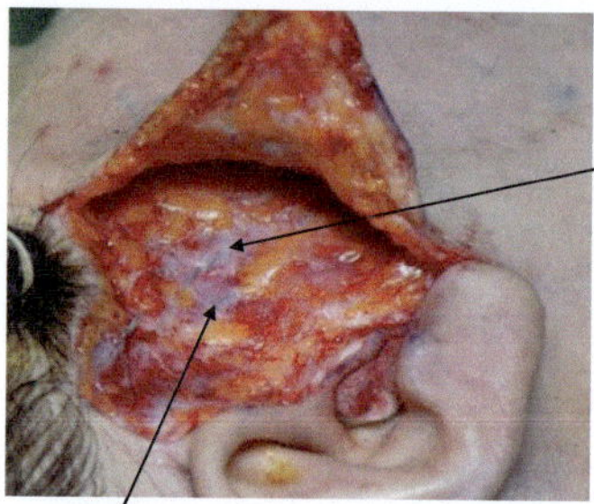

Fig. 5.4 Fibrosis of tissue around the thread after insertion of the cogged thread into the face

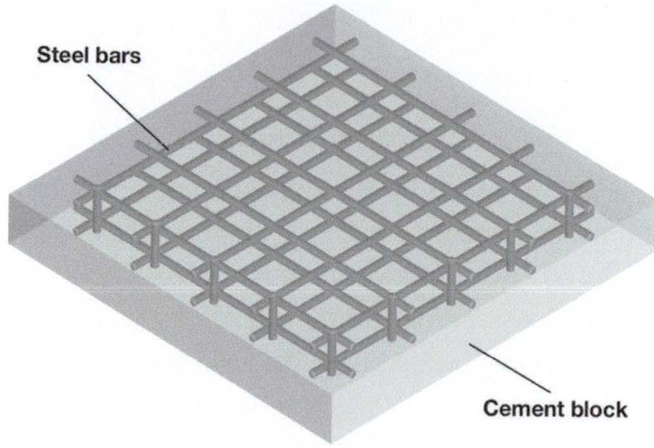

Fig. 5.5 Steel bars contained in cement blocks to create a reinforcement effect

Skin and tissue are constantly damaged physically in the process of penetrating skin with thread insertion and its passaging under the skin, which leads to the fibrosis of the cellular tissue that could be seen in the wound healing process after trauma or surgery. Therefore, internal splinting effects which firmly support from inside, are shown in skin and tissues where thread lifting is performed since fibrosis like a scar from the wound healing process is induced by the physical stimuli until the thread is absorbed (Fig. 5.4).

Tissues that have been firmed by the physical stimuli get to lose the effects, as scar tissue softens and fibrosis gets lost gradually over time. In the filler procedure, better results can be expected with less volume if retreated before the filler is completely absorbed. Likewise, if the thread lifting procedure is performed before the effect of the former procedure is completely lost, the lifting effect and its duration can be maximized even with less effort.

The healing process of the physical damage caused by the needle of absorbable monofilament thread pricking skin and penetrating tissue is mostly attributed to the biochemical effects induced by the regeneration of tissues, rather than the direct procedural effect. However, with improvements in the quality of absorbable cogged threads containing actual lifting effects, the main effects of the procedure are not just confined to collagen regeneration but also induced by soft tissue repositioning, which moves the softer tissues toward the side of firmer tissues, and internal splinting, which is caused by the multiple thick threads, not fibrosis of the surrounding tissues, constantly stimulating and putting strains on soft tissues under the skin and resultantly, resulting in tissue contraction.

5.3.1 Reinforcement Effect

One of the most basic effects of thread insertions is a supportive effect. This effect can be slightly shown in all thread lifting procedures, regardless of whether it is thin PDO thread with no cogs or thick cogged thread, absorbable or nonabsorbable. It is easy to understand the effect of putting the reinforcing steel bars in between, for example, rather than just putting the concrete into the frame when constructing a building (Fig. 5.5).

When the threads are inserted parallel to the skin, the tensile strength acting in parallel and the force against compressive force become stronger and if several strands of threads are inserted in cross stripes pattern, the supportive effects may be superimposed (Fig. 5.6).

Even though it is difficult to accurately quantify these effects, the supportive effects induced by the multiple strands of threads inserted in the tissues may relieve the bulging tendency of fat tissues due to the process of aging and the uneven skin surface could be kept soft and smooth. However, this relieving effect can be retained stronger when the threads are retained unabsorbed and may somewhat get gradually weaker after the threads are absorbed. In the case of absorbed threads, the more and wider the fibrous tissue generated by the reaction between the threads and surrounding tissues, the greater the support effect and the longer the duration period.

5.3.2 Scaffold Effect

If the threads remain in the tissue and serve as scaffolds, inducing a volume effect, this can be explained differently with preexisting known lifting or supporting effects of threads. There have been many attempts to create such scaffold effects in the past and it used to be expected that volume effects in forms of scaffold can be found by twisting the threads forming a whirlpool. Unfortunately, it is found that there is no difference between using a simple PDO thread and using the twisted PDO threads because the twisted form is not maintained once the thread is inserted into tissues (Fig. 5.7).

It is of course possible to insert thick threads to give a volume and scaffold effect, but the thick thread can be outlined on the surface and hard, which can cause discomfort to patients and cannot be inserted shallowly for the depressed area.

Recently, multifilament PDO threads that compensate for these shortcomings have been released and are increasingly widely used, and the PDO volumizing threads mentioned above are threads developed to maximize this scaffold effect.

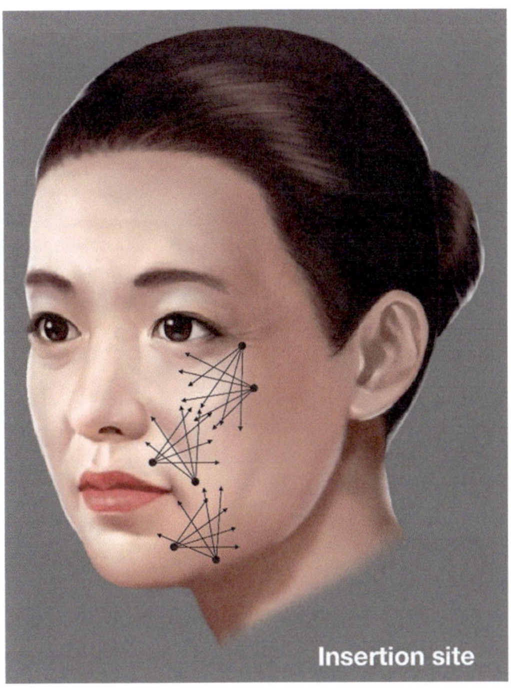

Fig. 5.6 Noncogged threads inserted in a grid pattern for supporting skin and soft tissue

5.3.3 Indirect Block Effect of Cutaneous Insertion Sites of Facial Muscles

There are various facial muscles and the movement of the muscles is transmitted to the skin making facial expressions and wrinkles. If the threads are inserted into the muscle in parallel with the muscle fibers, it may not have a significant effect on the transmission of muscle movement to the skin, but if the threads are inserted in vertical direction to the muscle fiber, which is parallel with the contraction direction of the muscle, the movement of skins will be found relatively less. In other words, in the case of crow's feet, nasolabial folds, or marionette lines, even with the insertion of thin and short PDO threads in the vertical direction to the direction of the wrinkles, these threads can prevent the movement of the muscles transmitted to the skin and thereby, reducing the wrinkles shown in the face (Fig. 5.8).

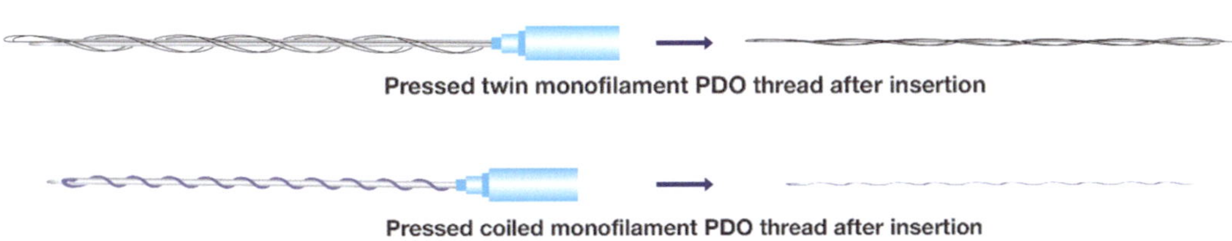

Fig. 5.7 Initial PDO volumizing monothreads pressed after insertion into the face

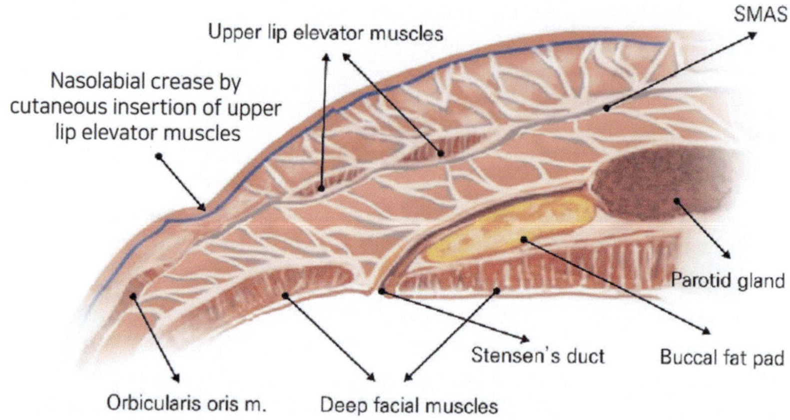

Fig. 5.8 Indirect block of cutaneous insertion sites of upper lip elevator muscles

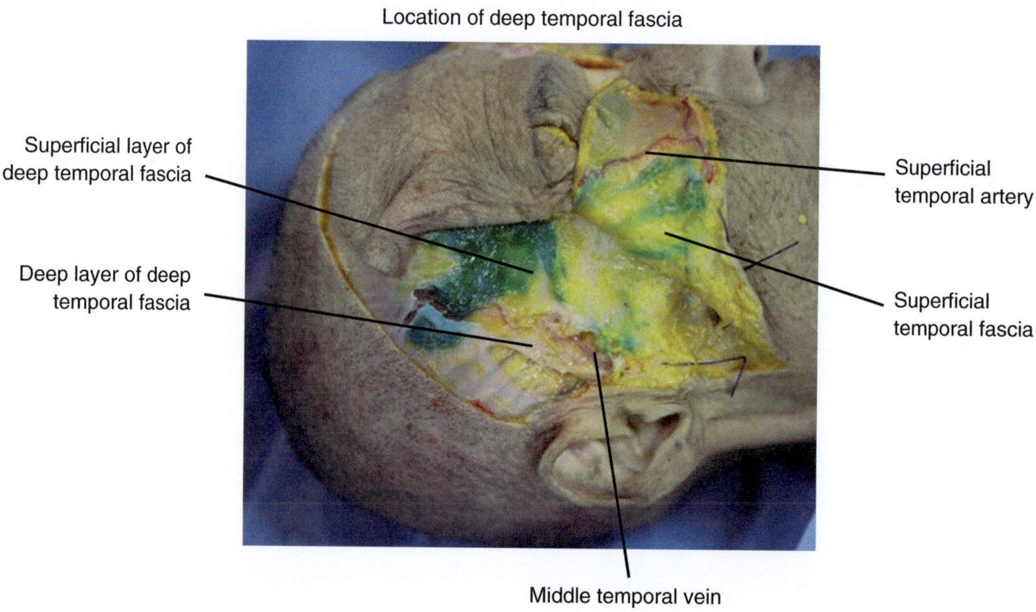

Fig. 5.9 Location of deep temporal fascia

5.3.4 Lifting Effect

The lifting effects among the effects of thread lifting mean the effects that genuinely lift the drooped tissue by gravity upwards. Strictly speaking, the supportive effect or scaffold effect discussed above is more like a tightening effect rather than a lifting effect. In order for the threads to have an actual lifting effect, a structure that may hold the tissues such as a cog is necessary. The point at which the cog of the thread is caught in the fixed area of our face is called the fixing point, and the point at which it is caught in the loose soft tissue that is not fixed is called the hanging point. In order to improve the results of the cogged thread lifting, a fixed point that is not easily affected by facial expression or aging is essential. The most commonly used site is the deep temporal fascia (DTF) of the temple area (Fig. 5.9).

The most commonly used method for making a firm fixation in this site is to make a slight incision in the temporal region and remove the overlying tissues to find the DTF and make a knot in that area to securely fix it and insert a thread with a cog in the mobile tissues on the lower part. Another method is to use a U-shaped long thread

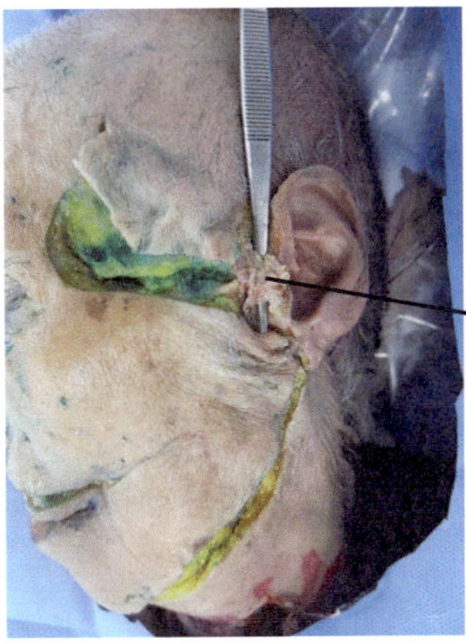

Fig. 5.10 Location of Lore's (tympanoparotid) fascia

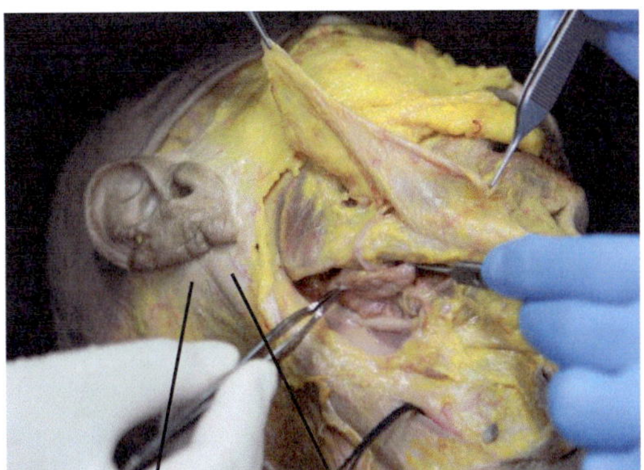

Fig. 5.11 Location of mastoid fascia

to put the middle noncogged part of the thread without a skin incision but with a hook or a large needle on the deep fascia and insert the remaining cogged threads into the tissue of the lower part of the face. The latter method has the advantage of not making a skin incision and the procedure time is short, thereby being simple and widely used.

In addition to the temple area, fixing point areas that are often used include mastoid fascia (Fig. 5.10) or Lore's fascia (Fig. 5.11) behind or in front of the ear. These two areas are not areas that can be cut because they are covered by hair-like DTF, but they can be used as fixing points for the cogged threads. These are the areas where the drooping jowl around the mouth, the sagging

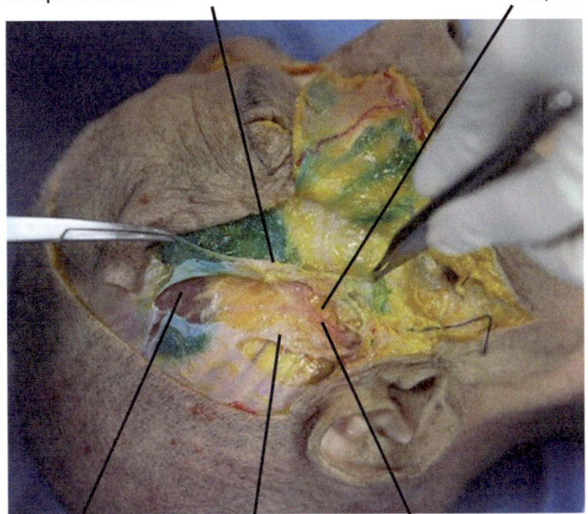

Fig. 5.12 Location of temporalis muscle

skin, or soft tissue around the chin or neck can be hung with thread cogs and pulled to fix them.

This U- or V-shaped long-length cogged thread lifting is usually more dramatic and lasts longer than the I-shaped cogged thread lifting because it lifts the tissue with a strong fixing point. However, because the underlying tissue moves all the way to the anchor point, it may initially feel a little overly performed and the cheek protrusion may last for 2–4 weeks. In addition, when the thread enters the scalp at the temporal region, it is troublesome to avoid the site of hair. If the thread passes through the DTF and the temporalis muscle, it may cause a headache (Fig. 5.12). In addition, when the DTF is hooked but the thread is too superficially inserted, excessive tension is applied to the subcutaneous fat area, which may cause alopecia with a rare chance.

The relatively short I-shaped cogged threads do not insert threads into the temple when pulling the lower cheek region, so it can be performed more easily. Depending on the patient's condition and the purpose of the procedure, it is necessary to decide whether to use a bidirectional cogged thread or a multidirectional cogged thread.

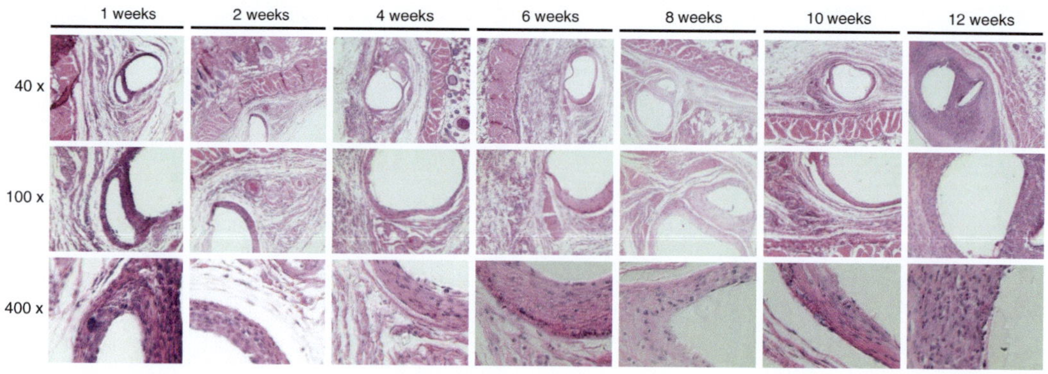

Fig. 5.13 Histological changes from 1 to 12 weeks after thread insertion into skin tissue of rat (H&E staining)

Bidirectional cogged thread can have a few more cogs on one side or the same number of cogs on both sides. When using bidirectional cogged thread, it is especially important to make sure that there is a fixing point in the upper part of the face, if the fixing point is not made in a tissue that is hard enough, not only the lower tissue can be lifted upwards, but the upper tissue may be lifted downwards. Therefore, it is recommended to fix the upper cogs to firmer tissues. Also, since the bidirectional cogged thread has the effect of gathering the lower tissue toward the central part of the thread, it is necessary to confirm in advance where the center of the thread will be located when designing the procedure. I-shaped cogged thread is usually easier to use than U- or V-shaped long-cogged thread because it does not require the hole inside the face through which the needle is pulled out and is simple to perform. Also, the outcome of the procedure is relatively natural, with less protruded cheeks after the procedure and the postprocedural adaptation period is relatively short. However, the duration period of thread lifting is relatively shorter and its effect can be less significant when compared to that of U- or V-shaped long cogged thread.

5.3.5 Histological Effect

When a thread is inserted into human tissue, a tissue reaction occurs around the thread. Even though the specific reaction could be different according to the thread type, in the case of the most commonly used type of threads, the PDO (polydioxanone) thread, lymphocyte, histiocyte, and eosinophil are gathered around the inserted threads, ultimately leading to fibrosis. The degree of fibrosis can be determined by the amount of myofibroblast or the thickness of the capsules formed around the thread. The histological changes around the PDO thread that occur over time after insertion of the PDO thread were observed through animal experiments (Fig. 5.13).

We can explain in more detail the tissue changes observed in animal experiments regarding the injection of absorbable PDO threads. PDO, a component of the threads, has been used as a suture material for a long time and is a substance with proven safety. It lasts longer than Dexon and Vicryl, is completely absorbed, and disappears from the body after 6 months. Therefore, it has been used for suturing areas where tension is required for a long time. Additionally, PDO threads have a smooth surface and can be made in monofilament form, which reduces the risk of latent infections that can be caused by bacteria settling on the surface of the thread. Hence, its safety and durability as a suture material are recognized. Generally, PDO is known to cause changes in the dermis, and as some studies have shown, it is effective in improving pores and fine wrinkles. It is particularly known to increase the thickness of the dermal papillae, achieved through a mechanism that promotes the formation of collagen in the dermal matrix.

Yoon et al, detailed the tissue changes after subcutaneous injection of PDO threads in a pig. The authors inserted PDO threads into porcine

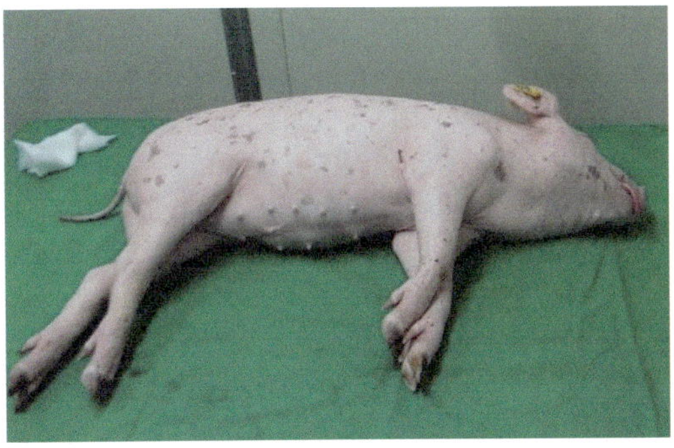

Fig. 5.14 The pigs used in the experiment

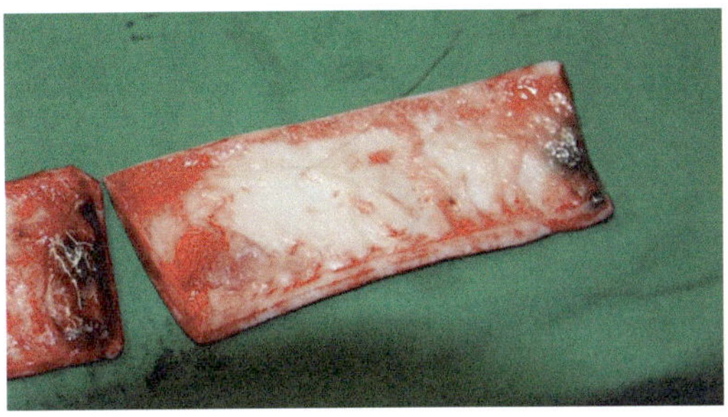

Fig. 5.15 Collected tissue

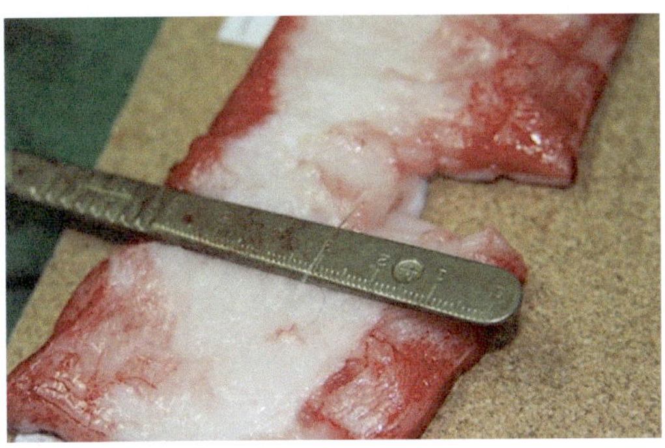

Fig. 5.16 PDO thread found within the tissue

subcutaneous tissues and tracked changes by collecting tissue samples after 1 month, 3 months, and 12 months (Figs. 5.14, 5.15, and 5.16).

The detailed changes in tissue after the insertion of PDO threads are as follows:

1. Many PMN cells, including eosinophils, gather around the area where the thread is inserted, forming granulation tissue. Within the granulation tissue, newly formed collagenous connective tissue is abundantly observed.
2. The newly formed collagenous connective tissue merges with the existing surrounding fibrous connective tissue (merging effect). Due to the merging effect, the inflammatory response process progresses around the inserted thread, and the cell signaling that occurs during the formation of granulation tissue spreads like a wave to the surrounding tissue, initiating mechanotransduction
3. Fibroblasts and myofibroblasts are seen within the granulation tissue formed around the thread. Myofibroblasts are closely related to wound contraction during the wound healing process and play a crucial role in making the treated area elastic and firm after skin regeneration procedures.
4. When comparing the area of capillaries in experimental and control groups, the thickness of capillaries was observed to be larger in the group injected with PDO threads. A high number of eosinophils were also observed, indicating a phenomenon that promotes fibrosis during the wound-healing process.
5. Denaturation of adipocytes due to the formation of granulation tissue was observed only around the area where the thread was inserted, with no changes in adipocytes away from the granulation tissue.

These changes can be summarized over time as follows:

At 1 month postprocedure, inflammation around the injection site, activation of myofibroblasts, and fat cell denaturation were observed.

At 3 months postprocedure, inflammation around the injection site had disappeared, and thick fibrous tissue had formed around the thread. The fat cell denaturation persisted.

At 6 months postprocedure, the thread was found to be broken, and the formed fibrous tissue had thinned. Fat cell denaturation was still present, and due to the merging effect with surrounding tissue, it was observed that fibrous tissues were interconnected.

Among the various tissue changes observed, the following five points can be considered significant in the context of thread lifting procedures (Fig. 5.17).

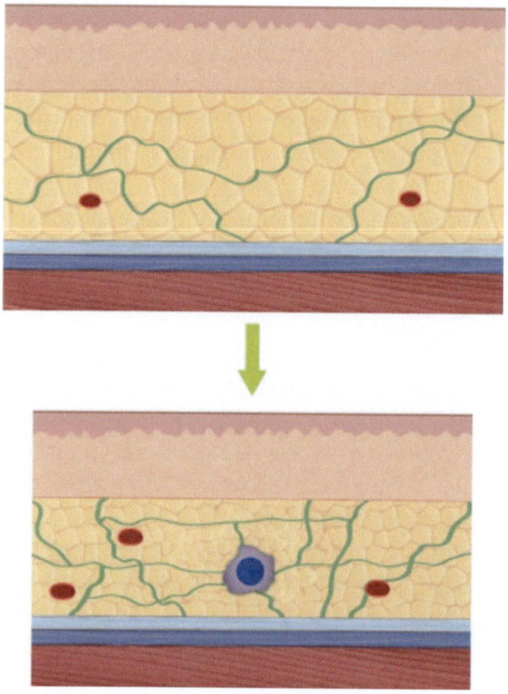

Fig. 5.17 Tissue change after PDO thread insertion

1. Formation of new connective tissue
2. Connection with existing connective tissue
3. Tissue contraction by myofibroblasts
4. Neovascularization of capillaries
5. Denaturation of adipocytes

The principle that the effect lasts even after the lifting threads are completely absorbed can be explained by the histologically formed capsules. However, a clinician should not unquestioningly depend on the effects of these capsules around threads. In fact, we can observe that the capsule formed around is way thinner than our expectations by performing facelift surgery on a patient who had a thread lifting procedure before the inserted threads were completely lost. Histological studies have shown that the thickness of capsules around the prolene with thickness of USP size 2-0 is 0.05–0.07 mm. In addition, the histological observation experiment using the PDO thread shows that the capsule thickness is difficult to exceed 0.2 mm. Actually, the capsules observed in patients with facelift surgery were almost invisible during dissection, and it would be difficult to expect the actual lifting effects from this kind of effect, but rather somewhat effective for the tightening, as described above.

Most lifting thread manufacturers insist that the histological effect of thread may retain the lifting effect for one or two years even after the threads are completely absorbed. However, considering the actual patient feedback and the thickness of the capsules found, it should be noted that the tissue effects may not be as significant as general expectation after the threads are completely lost. However, in fact, the patient's feedback felt in the clinical trial varies greatly depending on the type of product, the doctor who performed the procedure, the patient's age, and the condition of the skin tissue. Therefore, it is important to know that receiving a thread lifting procedure does not necessarily show a significant histological effect, and that the thickness of the capsule actually generated after the procedure can vary widely depending on various factors.

Recent Advances in Thread Lifting

6

Contents

S. M. Oh et al., *The Art and Science of Thread Lifting Based on Pinch Anatomy and Moving Plane*,
https://doi.org/10.1007/978-981-97-5516-5_6

6.1 Definition of Moving Plane

6.1.1 Understanding Facial Layer and Moving Plane

Facial lifting essentially achieves its final shape through the movement of the skin. Without the skin moving, the movement or change in position of the tissues beneath the face would not result in a perceivable lifting effect.

Previously, there was much debate about the ideal layer for thread placement in thread lifting treatments, with varying views among clinicians and anatomists. While it might appear safer to place threads in the subcutaneous fat layer, which has fewer nerves and vessels, doing so can still cause issues such as dimpling or noticeable threads, particularly with a thin subcutaneous fat layer or shallow thread insertion.

Yet, understanding the optimal depth for thread insertion to enhance the lifting effect might be more crucial than focusing solely on insertion depth to avoid complications. A procedure with few complications but ineffective is futile. Thus, it is best to first grasp scientifically how to boost the procedure's effectiveness and then address reducing complications, which is a sensible clinical strategy.

When considering all lifting procedures, not just thread lifting, the starting point of understanding a lifting procedure begins with knowing which layer of the skin and soft tissues moves during the treatment. Whether performing a direct lifting procedure on the face or simulating facial lifting with hands, the authors want to define the moving layer of the face as the "moving plane." The goal of all procedures under the banner of lifting is ultimately to move tissues effectively around this moving plane and maintain their position for an extended period.

In other words, understanding which layer of which part of the face is the moving plane, and then, figuring out how to conduct the procedure so that the tissues move along this moving plane and are well secured is the essence of understanding lifting procedures.

Typically, discussions about lifting procedures invariably include the SMAS layer. It is well-known that lifting effects are achieved by contracting or pulling this fascial layer that envelops the face. However, there appears to be a lack of proper discussion on why pulling the SMAS layer results in a lifted appearance of the face.

When simulating a lifting procedure by moving the forehead skin upwards while keeping the ultrasound probe fixed on the forehead, it is observable which layer of the forehead is moving. The layer of loose areolar tissue that lies above the periosteum and below the frontalis muscle is the one that shifts (Fig. 6.1).

Generally, the layers of the face vary depending on the region (Table 6.1).

When synthesizing ultrasonographic findings with anatomical observations, the following interpretation is possible:

Generally, when moving various parts of the face, including the forehead area, the actual mov-

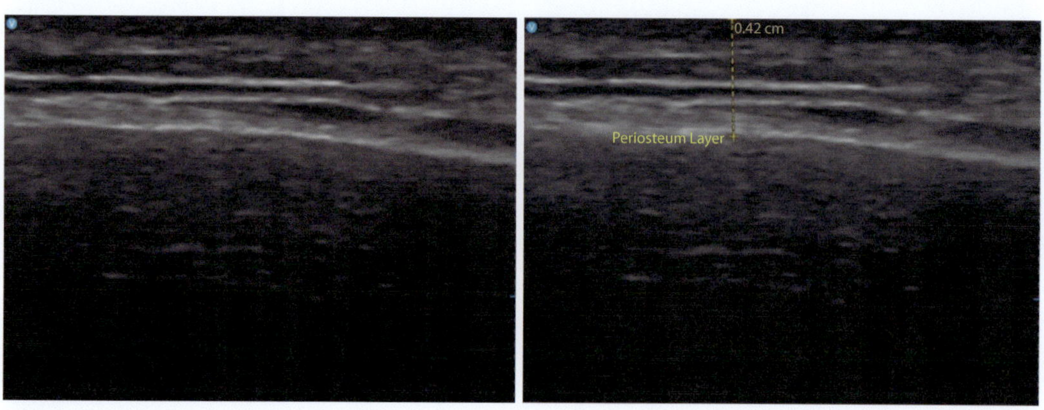

Fig. 6.1 Sonographic finding of the forehead

Table 6.1 Layers of each part of the face

Region	SCALP	Temple	Lateral cheek	cheek	Infraorbital area	Nose	Neck
Layer 1	Skin	Skin	Skin	Skin	Skin	Skin	Skin
Layer 2	Connective tissue	Subcutaneous fat	Subcutaneous fat	Subcutaneous fat	Subcutaneous fat	Superficial fatty layer	Subcutaneous fat
Layer 3	Frontalis muscle	Superficial temporal fascia	SMAS	Facial expression muscle	Orbicularis oculi muscle	Fibromuscular layer	Platysma muscle
Layer 4	Loose areolar tissue	Innominate fascia	Platysma auricular fascia	Buccal fat or deep medial cheek fat	SOOF and pre-periosteal fat	Deep fatty layer	Deep fat
Layer 5	Periosteum	Deep temporal fascia	Parotid-masseteric fascia	Periosteum	Periosteum	Perichondrium	Investing layer of cervical fascia

ing part is layer 4, which is the deep fat layer or the loose connective tissue layer. (Of course, there are exceptions.) This is because layers 1, 2, and 3 are tightly bound together. In other words, the reason why layer 1, the skin layer, layer 2, the subcutaneous fat layer or connective tissue layer, and layer 3, the SMAS, fascia, or muscle layer, move together as a unit is that they are relatively more firmly connected than layer 4.

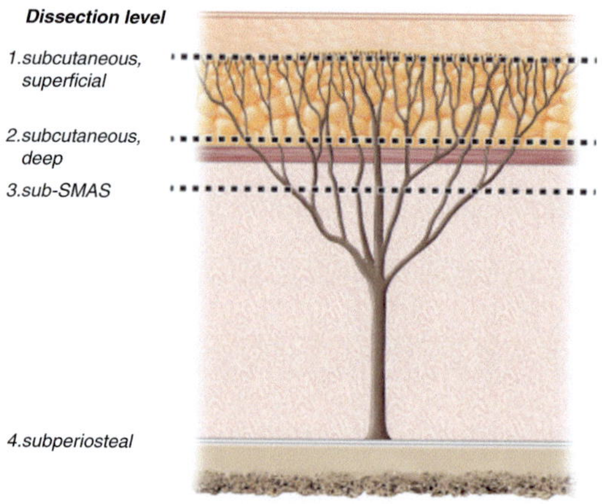

Fig. 6.2 Schematic diagram of the facial retaining ligaments

This is well represented in the schematic diagram of the facial retaining ligaments (Fig. 6.2).

The retaining ligaments in the subcutaneous fat are closely spaced, short, and stiff. In contrast, the ligaments in the deeper layers are more spaced out, slanted, and flexible. This means that the fourth layer, made of a looser connective tissue, serves as the moving layer during procedures.

Therefore, the skin layer, subcutaneous fat layer, and SMAS layer move as a single unit. When the layer corresponding to layer 3 is pulled through thread lifting or lifting surgery, the skin moves along with it, producing the lifting effect. In contrast, layer 4, being the moving plane, does not move with the SMAS when it is pulled.

It is necessary to conceptualize lifting with the understanding that layers 1, 2, and 3 act as a single unit, and generally, the moving plane is typically layer 4. However, this is not an absolute rule. As indicated by area b in the above figure, in some facial areas, layer 2 can be more movable than layer 4. Understanding which layer is the primary moving plane for each area of the face can lead to insights on how to design and perform thread lifting effectively for each specific region (Fig. 6.3).

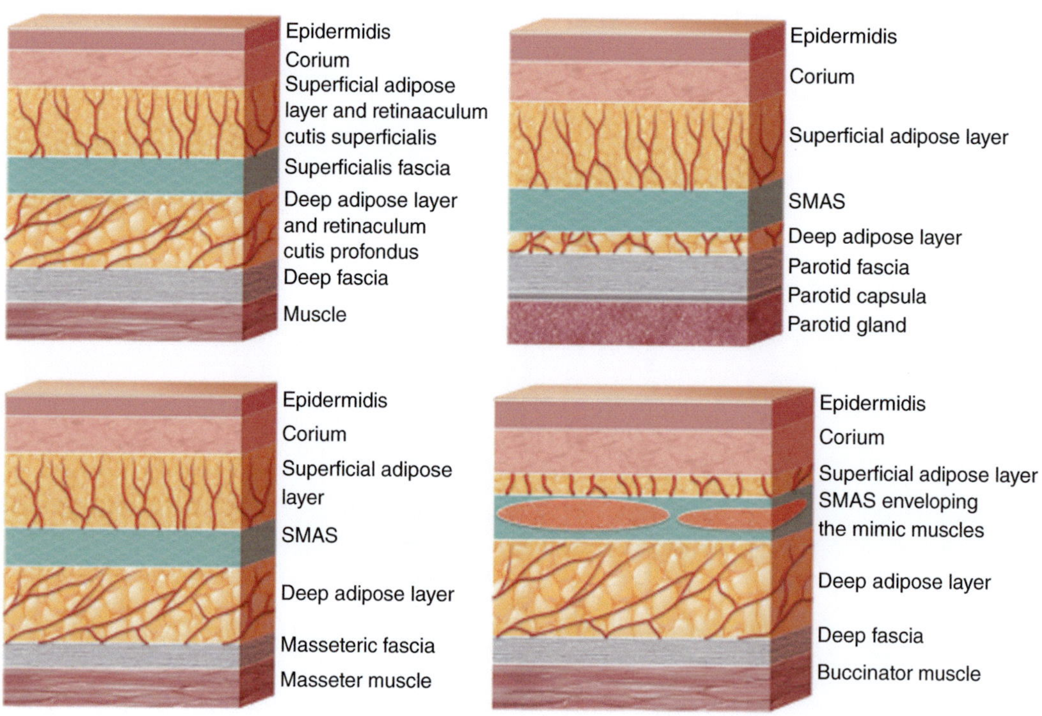

Fig. 6.3 Differences in the distribution of subcutaneous connective tissue by facial area

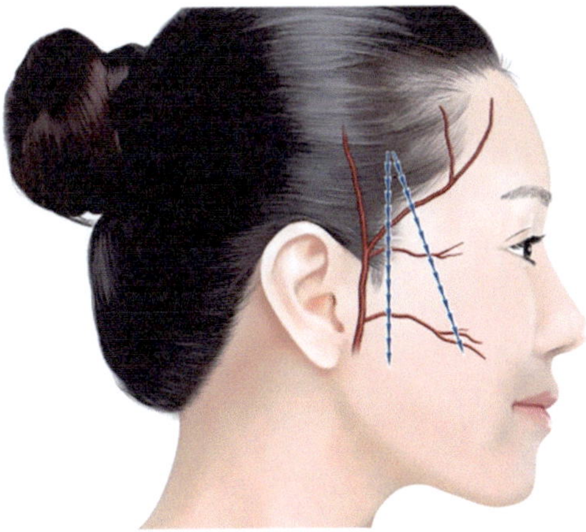

Fig. 6.4 Major blood vessels that require caution when performing the thread lifting

From the perspective of the safety of thread lifting procedures, injecting the thread into layer 2 is safer than into layer 4. In the facial areas where thread lifting is performed, the major blood vessels and nerves generally reside in the deeper layers (Figs. 6.4, 6.5, 6.6).

However, the frequency of serious complications in the actual clinical practice of thread lifting is low. This is because the tissues of the face are not rigid but flexible. In other words, even if blood vessels or nerves are encountered during thread lifting procedures using cannulas, they do not cause significant damage.

This can be partly explained by the difference in tensile strength between tissues. For example, considering blood vessels, the tensile strength of the vessel wall is greater than that of the subcutaneous fat layer. Therefore, when threading a thread through a blunt cannula and injecting it gently, the cannula passes through the fat layer smoothly, reducing the risk of vascular damage.

Through the manipulation of pinch and press techniques and the gentle injection of blunt cannulas, it can be inferred that the risk of vascular damage is reduced due to the difference in elasticity between blood vessels and the subcutaneous fat layer. While there is no direct comparison study, there is indirect evidence that can be considered.

Balazs et al. obtained transversal and longitudinal samples from the coronary vein of pig and measured the tensile strength of each (Table 6.2).

Meanwhile, Denise et al. measured the tensile strength of human adipose tissue. The purpose of the study was to compare the tensile strength of adipose tissue between healthy individuals and those with metabolic syndrome, which is unrelated to thread lifting research. However, it is possible to infer from the study results (Table 6.3).

One should interpret with the comparison between pig coronary vein and human subcutaneous adipose tissue in mind.

Considering the measured tensile strengths:

$$1\,\text{MPa} = 10^{6}\,\text{N} / \text{mm}^{2}$$

$$1\,\text{mN} / \text{mm}^{2} = 1000\,\text{N} / \text{m}^{2}$$

Therefore, with only the average values, let us estimate approximate ranges: for the pig coronary vein, 990 ~ 2550 mN/mm^2; and for human subcutaneous adipose tissue, 10.4 ~ 13.7 mN/mm^2.

Thus, there is a difference of over 100 times in tensile strength. While this is based on research utilizing somewhat imprecise comparison groups, this suggests that based on research findings and clinical experiences, it is easier to pass a cannula through the fat layer during thread lifting than to accidentally cut a blood vessel.

However, some describe the skin layer containing facial muscles as layer 3. However, facial muscles have origins and insertions. They attach to specific areas of bones and pass through intermediate layers before reaching the skin. In other words, they do not exist solely in one layer but traverse through intermediate layers between bones and skin, spanning across multiple layers (Figs. 6.7 and 6.8).

For successful thread lifting outcomes, clinicians need to accurately understand the three-dimensional anatomical structure of the face and have a precise understanding of the facial layers.

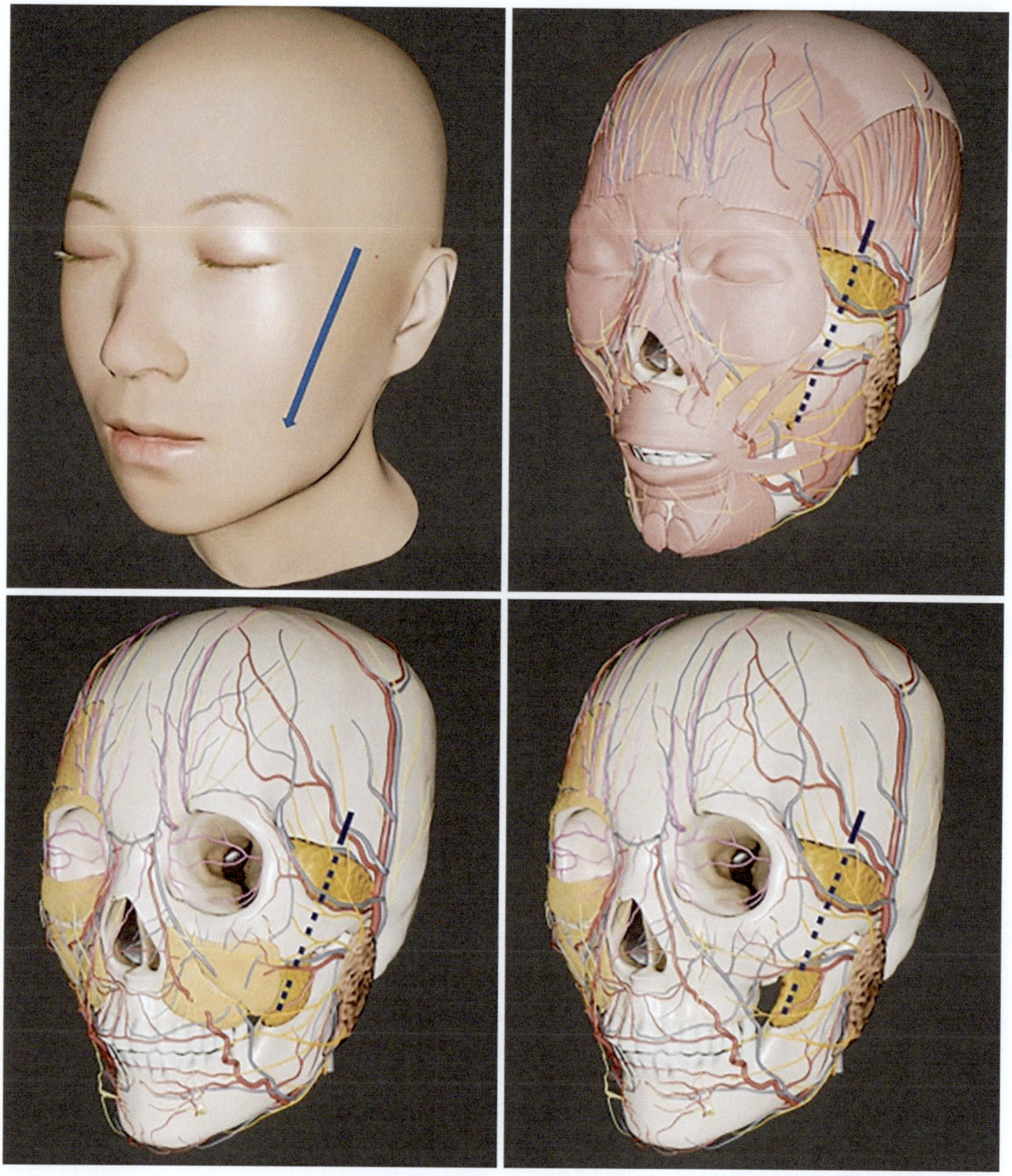

Fig. 6.5 Depth of the facial nerve branches in the lateral cheek area encountered during thread lifting procedures

6.1.2 Main Moving Planes for each Facial Area

Forehead: layer 4—under the frontalis muscle.

Temple: layer 4—under the superficial temporal fascia.

Zygomatic arch: layer 4—under the superficial temporal fascia.

Lateral cheek: layer 2—subcutaneous fat.

Anterior cheek: layer 4—SOOF and preperiosteal fat.

Masseter area: layer 4—under SMAS.

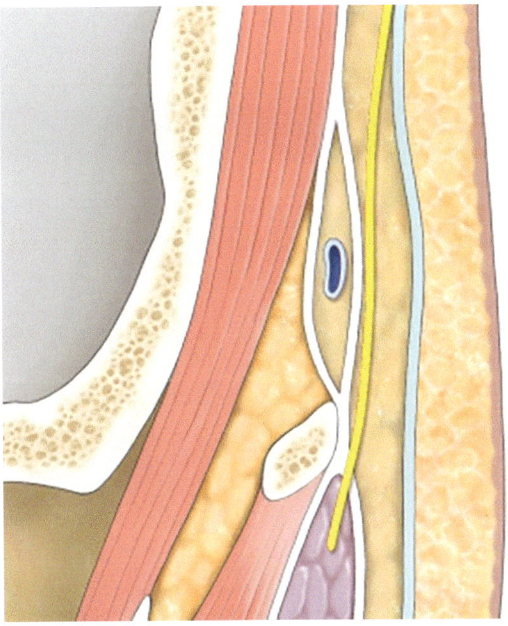

Fig. 6.6 Depth of facial nerve branch at zygomatic arch area

Table 6.2 Calculated mechanical properties of coronary veins

	Transverse sample	Longitudinal sample
Tensile strength mean (MPa)	0.99 +/− 0.19	2.55 +/− 0.38

Table 6.3 Comparison of subcutaneous and omental WAT ECM parameters in healthy obese women compared with those with MetS

	Healthy obese	Metabolic syndrome obese
Tensile strength mean (mN/mm^2)	13.7 +/− 2.5	10.4 +/− 2.3

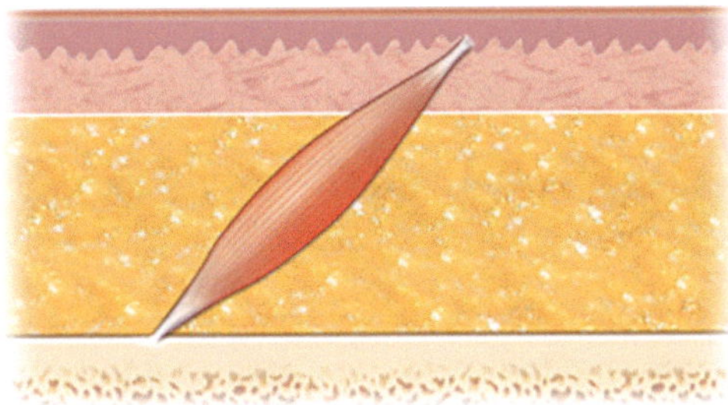

Fig. 6.7 Way muscles connect between bones and skin

6.1.3 Pinch Maneuver and Moving Plane

Efforts to identify the moving area through the pinch maneuver help to enhance the sensitivity of the hands and enable the assessment of the depth of tissues without the aid of imaging devices.

Through cadaver research, the authors found that when performing the pinch maneuver on the cheek area, the soft pinch raises the subcutaneous fat tissue, while the deep pinch raises tissues from deeper layers. Further contemplation arises as to why these areas are lifted during the pinch maneuver. This is likely due to the relatively weak and soft connective tissues in the lifted areas. In other words, the moving plane moves because the tissues are weaker and softer compared to other areas when external force is applied.

Understanding the significance of the moving plane and the moving plane for each area can assist in designing and performing effective thread lifting procedures.

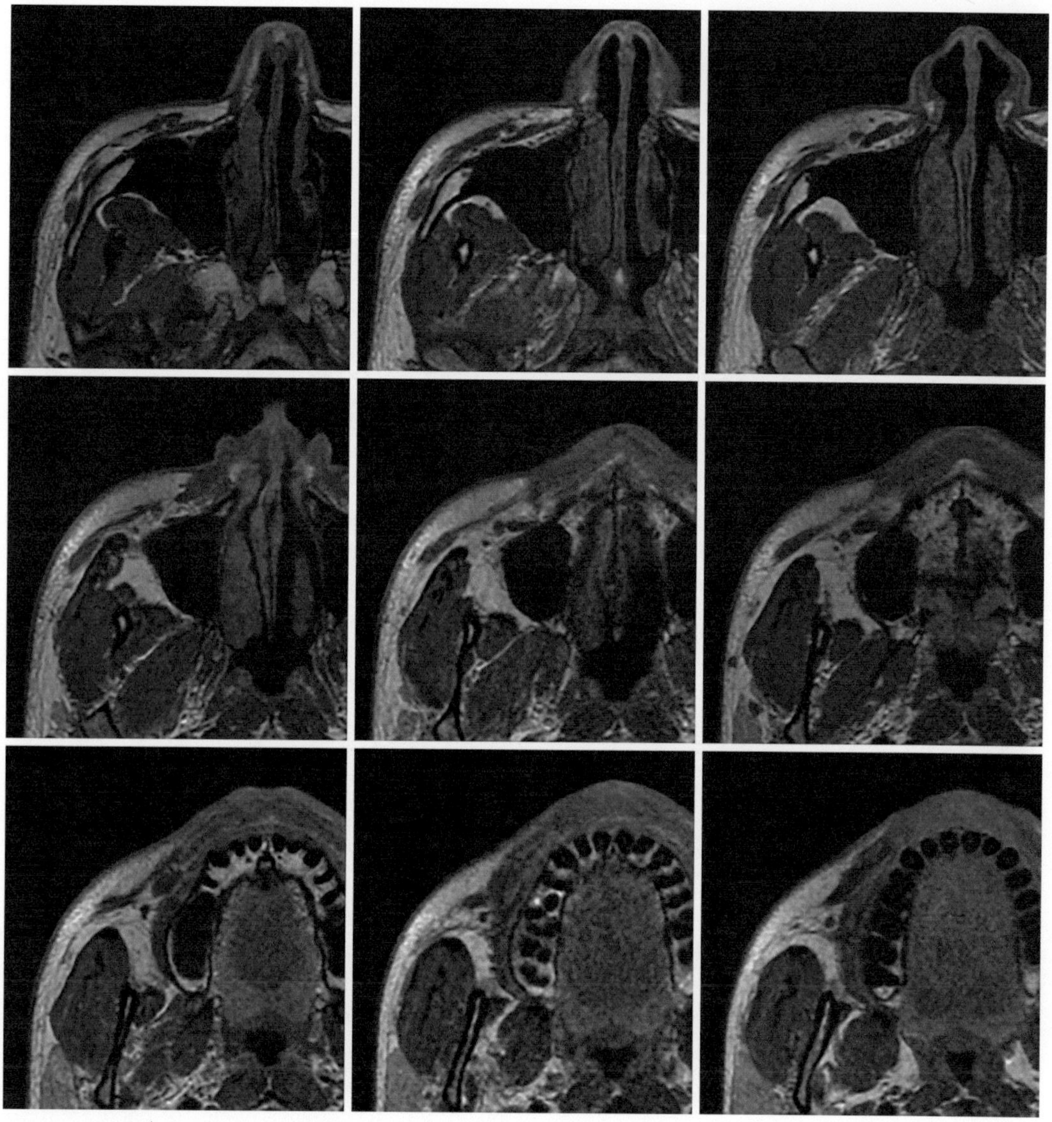

Fig. 6.8 Muscle layer seen in MRI images goes from the bones to the skin

6.2 SMAS Repositioning Technique for Cogged Thread Lifting Based on the Moving Plane Concept

As people enter their sixties, they experience deeper wrinkles and greater sagging in the skin. In the past, many doctors believed that lifting with cogged threads would not generate much effect for such skin conditions that needed face-lift surgery to pull the sagging skin and cut out the extra part of the skin.

Cogged thread-based lifting, however, started to be applied to patients in that age group several years ago. This began with changing the basic concept of cogged thread lifting. The old idea was to simply and unconditionally pull up sagging skin and its subcutaneous tissue. These days, there is a change to the idea of cogged thread lifting. When patients lie down and lift the

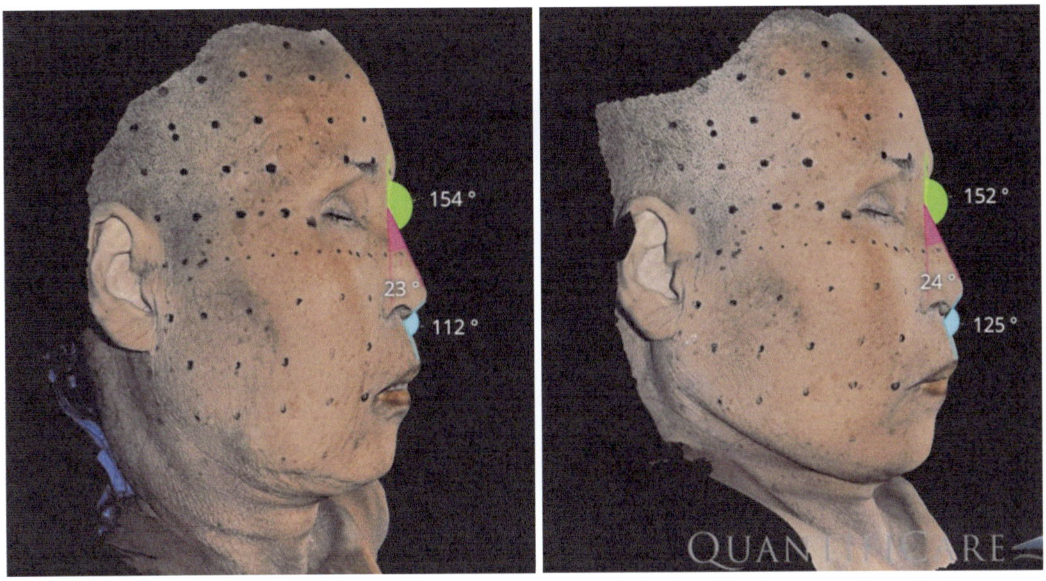

Fig. 6.9 Change of facial skin and soft tissue according to the positional change

tip of the chin a little bit or drop the head further, the tissue of the loose midfacial and lower face areas move to the hard head, ears, and jawlines. The basic purpose of cogged thread lifting is to hold this soft tissue that has become tight to the hard tissue so that it will not move back to its original places. Cadaver studies on the move of facial skin and tissue according to position report that after the head was simply changed from a sitting position to a supine one in a lateral profile view, the entire face became tight with the shapes and angles of the nasion and nose tip altered according to the skin and its soft tissue that was pulled toward the head and ears. Here, changes to the tissue of the lower face area is interesting. When the loose skin and its soft tissue move according to positional changes, the skin and soft tissue of the lower face area, including a double chin, are all pulled toward the head and ears with some of the skin and tissue remaining along the hard tip of the chin, front jawline, and mandibular angle to create their forms and outlines. The outcomes include the tip of the chin and jawlines that have become naturally distinct and also the skin that has become tight. This phenomenon is due to the hard tissue that will not sag over time in the mandibular ligaments along the boundary between the tip of the chin and the jawlines and the angular tract fascia before the SCM muscles inside the mandibular angle and the insertion of mentalis muscles in the tip of the chin. The phenomenon fits the investigator's view that when loose tissue moves toward hard tissue, it can generate natural lifting effects (Fig. 6.9).

Based on this concept, this study examines the outcomes of cogged thread lifting on older patients and found that they had positive outcomes although it did not bring out a complete solution to their heavily sagging skin and deep wrinkles due to aging. The shapes of their faces that looked saggy changed. The texture of their skin and soft tissue improved, and their deep wrinkles became shallow. They looked naturally younger for their age with a soft and gentle impression. If these patients had not received thread lifting, their aging conditions would have grown worse over time. Thread lifting has shown a huge significance in slowing down changes to the face according to aging.

In a natural cogged thread lift based on the moving of tissue according to different positions, importance is placed on the depth of an inserted cogged thread. There are differences in preferred methods of cogged thread lifting among patients.

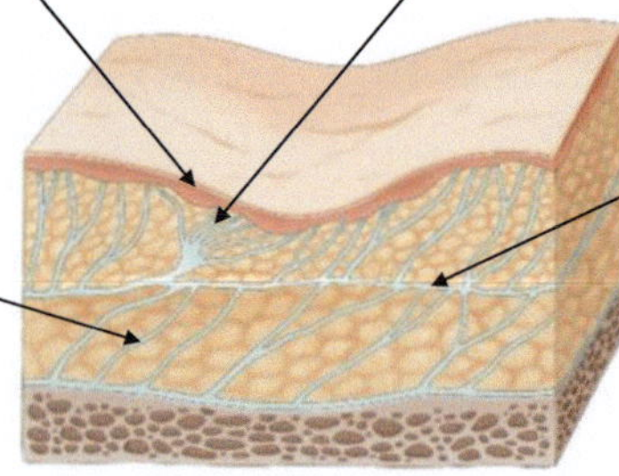

Fig. 6.10 Difference in density of fibrous septa according to facial area

Those who prefer the method of inserting several relatively fine-cogged threads in subcutaneous tissue and pulling them lightly tended to mention the plane to insert a thread softly in the tissue without any resistance. Giving explanations about the dual plane filler procedure, the investigator never fails to mention that the skin and its subcutaneous tissue do not have enough loose space for a filler procedure as they are tightly attached to SMAS below via vertically oriented fibrous septa, except for the medial areas. Then one might wonder how it is possible to create space for a smooth thread lift.

It is possible thanks to empty spaces between fibrous septa connecting the skin and SMAS for threads to get inserted and pass through smoothly in subcutaneous tissue. Under the simple assumption that any other condition is the same, the subcutaneous fat layer can be divided into the top, middle, and bottom parts according to the structural density differences of the fibrous septa. These fibrous septa are comprised lean fibrous tissue, and the ones passing through the SMAS layer gather together densely and look like big branches. As they move up, they tend to spread and taper down gradually. As they get close to dermal tissue, the ones moving toward the skin spread evenly and densely once again to hold the skin firmly. They show a pattern of numerous twigs that are thickly divided. According to this logic, the fibrous septa passing through the SMAS layer have fibrous tissue that is densely holding it together and feeling hard like big branches. The fibrous septa in the middle part of the subcutaneous fat layer include thin twigs; thus, they lack firmness. The retinacular cutis under the dermis has many twigs that are very thin but dense, thus feeling tough. Different areas of the face vary in the density of fibrous septa in subcutaneous tissue and thus hardness. The areas strongly dominated by ligaments or ligament tissue have dense fibrous septa and are thus hard. When threads pass through these areas, they feel tight. In the areas where the fibers of ligament tissue gather together loosely, threads pass through more smoothly. When the zygomatic ligaments, which are the most powerful ligaments in the face, pass under the zygomatic arch holding the skin, they feel huge resistance due to the density of fibrous septa (Fig. 6.10).

After cogged threads pass through the middle part of the subcutaneous tissue to pull and hold together the skin and subcutaneous tissue, the skin may seem to have moved a lot at first. The skin is, however, still attached to the SMAS layer via fibrous septa. When the skin and subcutaneous tissue are pulled with the SMAS layer unmoved, the client will feel pulled in the face at first. The skin will, however, return to its original place, being connected to the SMAS layer that has not moved at all. The client will thus feel that the initial pull has weakened soon. It is better to generate lifting effects of the SMAS layer getting properly attached toward the head and ears than an excessive pull of the skin in the first place. This approach will ensure that the effects from the procedure last longer.

Plastic surgeons perform face-lift surgery by exfoliating, pulling, and fixing the SMAS layer to make the effects last longer. One cannot enjoy long-lasting lifting effects by exfoliating and pulling only the skin and subcutaneous tissue.

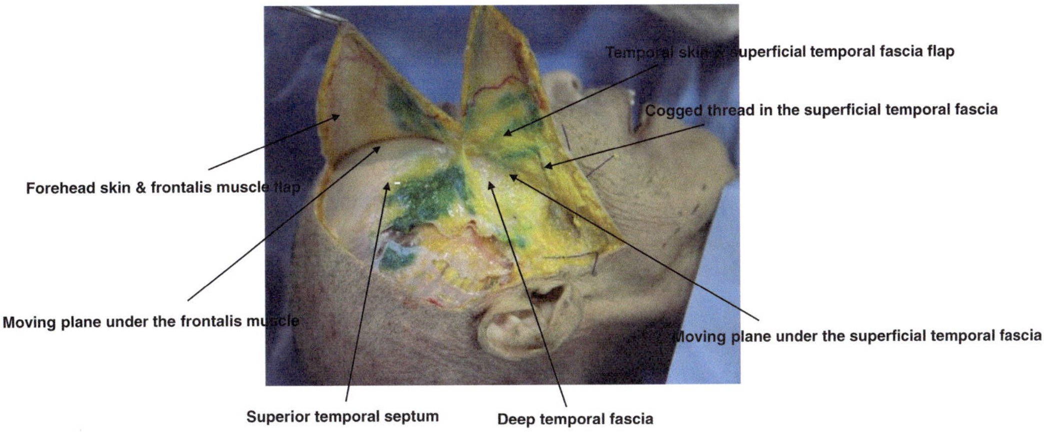

Fig. 6.11 Moving plane under the SMAS layer for cogged thread lifting

This means that the skin will sag again even after it is exfoliated and pulled in surgery. When the skin is pulled only with threads, it will soon return to its original place attached to the SMAS layer, however, strongly it is pulled at first. When the skin is forced and pulled strongly, it will actually cause more issues.

Even recent explanations about the cogged thread lifting method, however, state that the main intended direction of a cannula after its insertion is subcutaneous tissue under the skin. This direction will guarantee that the cannula will go in smoothly without causing any problems. If the cannula moves in deeper than that, it will not go in smoothly. In actual practice, cogged threads are inserted deeper and closer to the SMAS layer along the surface above or below it. Even when some of the threads hold the SMAS layer, the cannula will not face serious resistance while moving as long as they are not caught in the head or ear regions to be used as a fixing point for their hardness. When pulling the cogged threads holding the tissue after pulling out the inserted cannula, the doctor will see that the skin and soft tissue, including the SMAS layer, are pulled easily because the deep fat layer under the SMAS layer is comprised of obliquely oriented fibrous septa unlike the superficial fat layer so that the facial expression muscles passing above the periosteum can move smoothly. This part is not connected strongly to the SMAS layer above with its fat layer that is not dense but loose, thus posing no hindrance to the movement of the SMAS layer. Due to the characteristics of its anatomical structure, the SMAS layer has spaces below it. These spaces where the SMAS can move are called moving planes. When inserting or moving a cannula, the doctor can ensure that there is no harm to the important structures inside by adjusting the cannula angle right so that it will not go too deeply in the loose spaces below the SMAS layer (Fig. 6.10).

Therefore, the investigator argues that doctors should target and pull the SMAS layer or its surrounding tissue in a cogged thread lift rather than the skin or subdermal level in order to maximize the lifting and tightening effects based on the natural repositioning of tissue. As explained above, this procedure is possible thanks to the moving planes under the SMAS layer where it can be moved and pulled to some extent. The investigator calls this thread lifting technique the SMAS repositioning technique with cogged threads (Fig. 6.11).

In fresh cadaver studies for cogged thread lifting, doctors smoothly inserted cannula and cogged threads in the same depth as an actual procedure with an actual patient instead of inserting threads close to the skin and exfoliating the skin to check outcomes and found that threads are inside along the surface above or below the SMAS layer or penetrate the layer partially in many cases. When the skin is thin along with subcutaneous tissue, threads are usually inserted

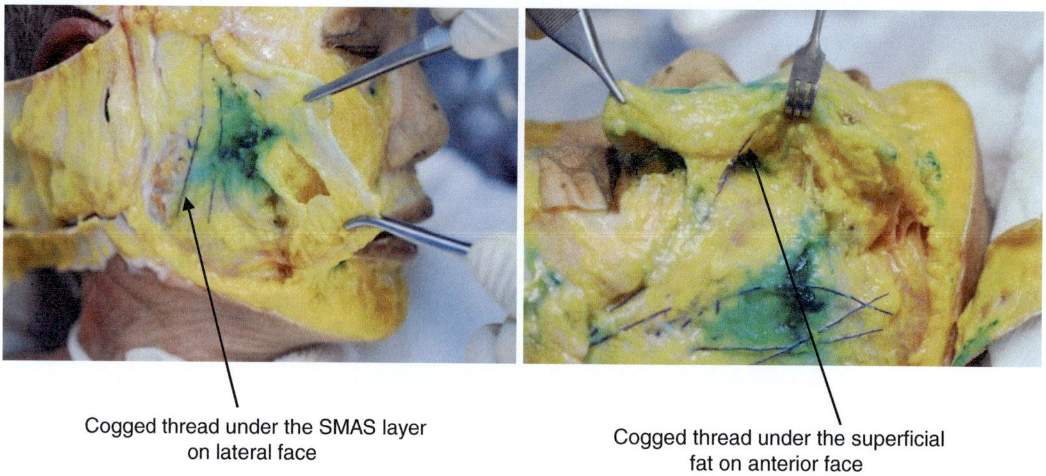

Fig. 6.12 Cogged threads inserted along the periSMAS plane

Fig. 6.13 Structure of the SMAS layer

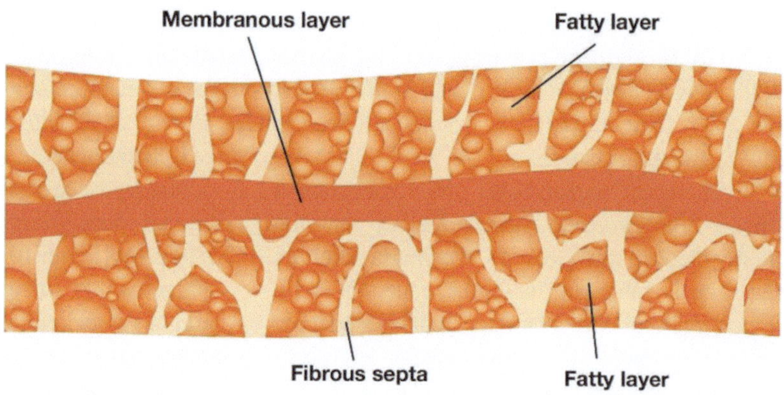

along the surface below the SMAS layer (Fig. 6.12).

Threads can penetrate the SMAS layer itself because the layer is a superficial fascia in three layers, including the fatty layers above and below the thin and tough membranous layer in the middle instead of a thick one layer of fascia (Fig. 6.13).

As mentioned earlier, the skin and the SMAS layer are connected strongly via vertically oriented fibrous septa and retinacular cutis. Cogged threads pass through SMAS or its surrounding parts and pull the SMAS layer around the moving planes below it to reposition it, naturally causing the skin and subcutaneous tissue to move, which generates lifting effects. There has been a shift to the concept that when the SMAS layer moves, the skin and subcutaneous tissue connected to it naturally move along with peri-SMAS tissue. These days, patients in their advanced aging stage receive a cogged thread lift.

In a clinical phenomenon, the skin will have dimples or irregularities when thread cogs are caught in the dermal tissue on the skin surface. When thread cogs are caught and pulled in the deep facial muscle layer, the patient will have awkward facial expressions and feel pain when moving the face. In an actual procedure, when the needle or cannula passes through the fat compartment layer above or below the SMAS layer, the tip of the needle or cannula moves fine without any resistance. When the needle or cannula is inserted in the deep layer of facial muscles, it will not move smoothly and cause the patient to complain about pain.

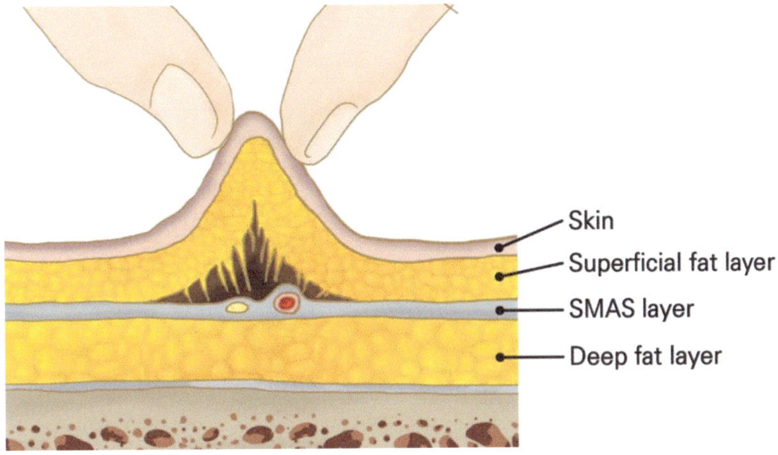

Fig. 6.14 Shallow pinch for subcutaneous tissue traction

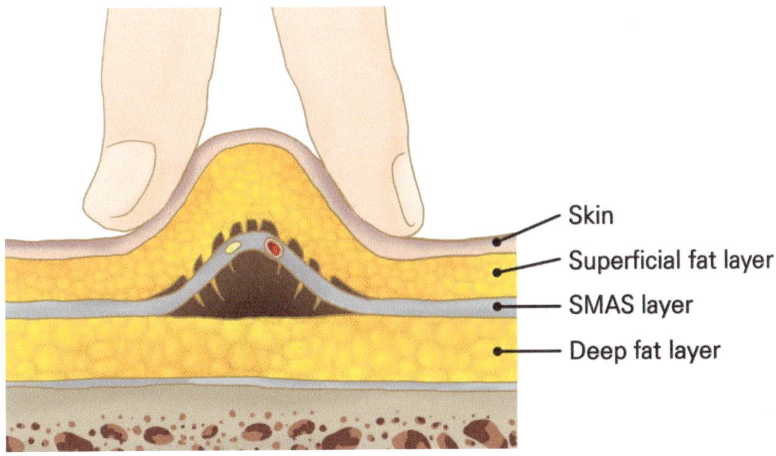

Fig. 6.15 Deep pinch for SMAS layer traction

When the needle or cannula is inserted properly above, below, or in the SMAS layer and is lifted, the skin and soft tissue layer above are lifted in a thickness that corresponds to the length of the needle or cannula. The best way a doctor can figure out the proper depth of a procedure layer is the pinch technique. When he or she is right-handed, the doctor uses the left hand to pull tissue and measure its thickness. According to the pinch anatomy explanations for thread lifting, the doctor can only lift subcutaneous tissue above the SMAS layer by pulling up skin tissue in a small and shallow manner with the thumb and index finger with the SMAS layer below moving up a little bit only at the surface level (Fig. 6.14). When the doctor pulls up the issues in the lateral cheek regions in a wider and thicker manner by using the part with finger lines rather than the thumb and index finger, the skin and soft tissue, including the SMAS layer, will move up in a roughly round manner rather than a V (Fig. 6.15).

Doctors should be careful with this. The SMAS layer is thicker and harder in the lateral part before the ears than in the medial part. You can pinch and pull up the part in a thick manner and will still see that only subcutaneous tissue between the fingers will be lifted downward a little bit with the SMAS layer that is not lifted much upward. As long as a needle or cannula is not inserted too deep under the tissue between the fingers in a thread lift, the likelihood of threads going deep under SMAS is low. The medial part of the face, however, has a shallow SMAS layer and a deep thick fat layer. If a doctor pinches the

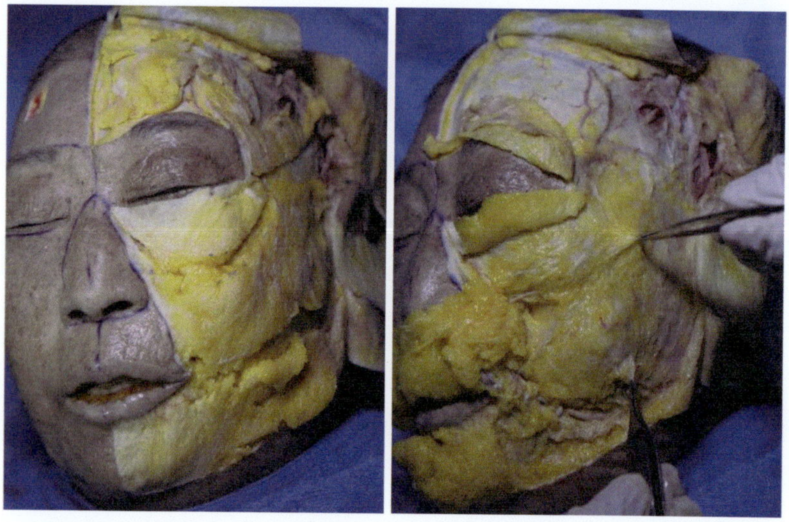

Fig. 6.16 Change of SMAS thickness and tightness depending on facial regio

tissue too thick without thinking, even the deep fat layer will accompany the SMAS layer that is lifted. In this case, the position of the inserted cogged thread will be deeper than expected with the thread penetrating the mucous membrane inside the mouth in bad cases. Most of all, cogged threads hold the tissue too thick, reducing ultimate effects. This definitely calls for a doctor's attention (Fig. 6.16).

This study examined cogged threads as a material for lifting procedures. In their early days, doctors strongly believed that cogged threads should be pulled to the maximum after the cogs were caught in the skin or subcutaneous tissue to ensure that some lifting effects would remain even after the pulling force became weak over time. However, as explained in the previous chapter on considerations in a thread lift, the need to first pull the tissue excessively disappeared with the improved shapes and forms of cogs and the higher quality of cogged threads for a lift. Doctors can now guarantee that lifting effects will not fade soon after by moving the tissue to the extent of natural movement according to positional changes. As mentioned earlier, today's concept of cogged thread lifting is for the natural repositioning of the SMAS layer and its surrounding tissue that are deeper than the surface rather than the forced lifting of the skin and subcutaneous tissue on the surface. After the repositioning of tissue, it is important to stabilize them so that they will not move easily from their repositioned places and keep these places firmly. As a result, the stress of cogged threads has become important rather than traction to hold and pull tissue. The stress of cogged threads helps the tissue keep their changed position, endures the load on the threads in the direction of gravity, and prevents the repositioned tissue from returning to their original place. In the past, long U-type cogged threads were frequently used to meet these requirements. Nowadays, there are many melting PDO threads in various thickness options and with cogs of diverse shapes and forms. The lifting procedure techniques have made great strides along with the manufacturing methods. Doctors can now improve various parts of the face, including sagging eyebrows, sagging skin around the eyes, sagging anterior cheeks, nasolabial folds, marionette lines, and a sagging neck by using the I-type cogged thread that is easy to use in addition to pulling up the sagging lateral jawline upward.

The type of thread used depends on the thickness and weight of the patient's skin and soft tissue, the degree of sagging, the depth of a wrinkle, and the patient's inclination. Different threads can be combined prospered according to different situations. In a cogged thread lift based on SMAS repositioning, the clinical priority is to determine the direction that threads are inserted and go in along the direction of tissue drooping. Once the insertion direction of threads has been decided, the doctor should determine the entry point position of the cogged threads, the thickness, number, and insertion depth of threads, the anatomical tissue to be held by threads, and the major structures that require careful attention. Doctors should always check these considerations in any thread lifting procedures no matter which part of the face is involved.

6.3 Improvement of Sagging and Wrinkles around Nose and Mouth—Reverse Technique Using Cogged Threads and Cross Technique Using Volumizing Non-Cogged Threads

6.3.1 Mechanisms of Nasolabial Folds and Marionette Lines

As explained earlier, different changes happen to the facial skin and soft tissue in different areas over time according to the hardness and thickness of tissue. The tissue around the head and ears has fewer subcutaneous fat tissue and a tough, thick SMAS layer. They do not droop easily with the structures inside the skin holding together tightly. As the basic considerations of thread lifting indicate, they include fixing points to hang sagging tissue on cogged threads, pulling them, and fixing the cogged thread holding the tissue so that they do not move and keep their proper places. However, the skin and soft tissue around the nose, mouth, cheek, and jawline sag easily according to aging since they have a shallow SMAS layer, a lot of a fat tissue, and the medial structures are not holding together tightly. As mentioned in the sections about different factors influencing the outcomes of thread lifting, the ligament tissue that connects and maintains the skin, SMAS layer, and soft tissue in these parts perform their duties to some degree at a young age. Like ligaments in the body, they gradually grow weaker over time. They cannot remain unchanged and solid in the aging process; thus, they fail to endure sagging skin and fat tissue, but rather sag with them. These ligament tissue, however, are comprised of tougher fiber than skin and fat tissue. When the skin and fat tissue are pulled with cogged threads in the sagging target area, they can be hung together. As thread cogs are hung on the tissue more firmly, cogged threads can exercise their maximum pulling and anchoring strength. This makes ligament tissue a good hanging point.

Before offering an explanation about a new thread lifting method to improve sagging tissue and wrinkles around the nose and mouth, the investigator will examine the mechanisms and patterns of nasolabial folds, which are oblique creases from the tip of the nose to the mouth corner, and marionette lines. Doctors should accurately understand the causes of wrinkles to generate optimal effects with proper treatment for them.

Nasolabial folds are creases in a 八 shape that begin from the upper boundary of the tip of the nose between the nose and the cheek and move obliquely toward the cheeks. These creases are commonly called nasolabial folds regardless of their causes, but it is beneficial to categorize them into three types according to mechanism for an accurate procedure fit based on cause (Fig. 6.17).

The cause of the first type is the lack of volume in the paranasal region next to the tip of the nose. In case of patients with the depressed canine fossa of maxillary bones supporting the paranasal region at the bottom, there is fundamentally little superficial fat in the area next to the tip of the nose below the crease compared with plump nasolabial fat above the crease (Fig. 6.18). When this is worsened by the lack of fat in the deep layer, the paranasal region seems depressed in a triangle shape due to a lack of volume. A layer like a step appears along the boundary between the depressed area and the plump fat layer above the nasolabial folds. It is not a real crease, but it similarly resembles a deep line. Creases caused by this can be addressed by filling the depressed paranasal region. In the past, implant insertion and fat transplantation were popular options. These

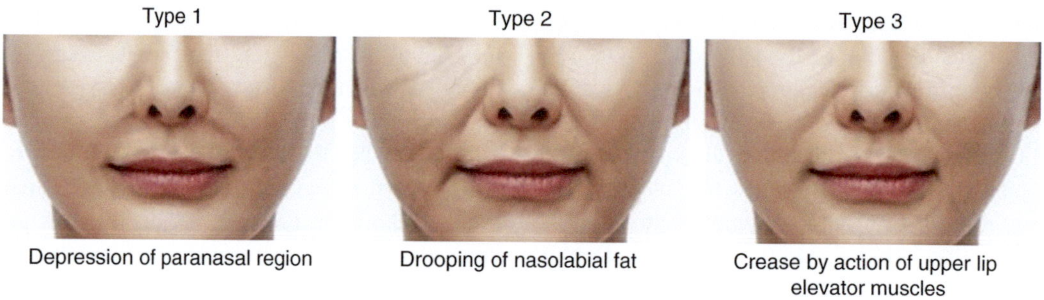

Fig. 6.17 Three types of nasolabial folds

Fig. 6.18 Difference in tissue thickness around nasolabial folds

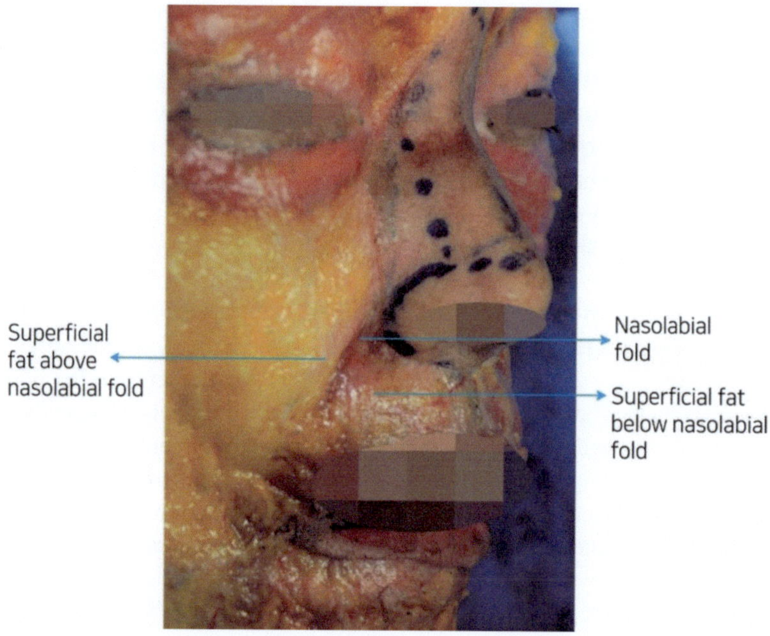

days the most popular option is to correct volume with a filler due to the improved viscoelasticity of filler products.

The mechanism of the second type is as follows: The upper lip area skin above the crease is anchored to the orbicularis oris muscles below in a relatively firm manner, thus causing it to droop less. The skin parts and tissue above the crease are connected in a relatively loose manner and cause subcutaneous fat in the front cheekbone that becomes increasingly plump over time to sag. This causes the second type of nasolabial folds (Fig. 6.19). As people get older, nasolabial fat, which is superficial fat above the crease, grows bigger while the paranasal region below the crease next to the tip of the nose makes a depression. This results in huge thickness differences between the soft tissue above the crease and those below it. Moreover, the skin and soft tissue above the crease that has become plumper lose their elasticity and sag and hang on the paranasal region that is anchored firmly, causing nasolabial folds to look even deeper. The last type is not caused by volume differences among the tissue of different parts or sagging according to aging. It happens when the fibers of some muscles get attached to the skin near nasolabial folds next to the nose before upper lip elevators, including levator labii superioris alaeque nasi, levator labii superioris, and zygomaticus major

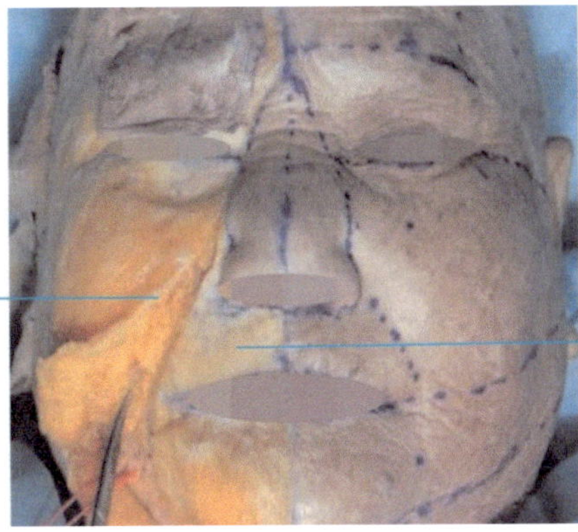

Fig. 6.19 Difference in tissue tightness around nasolabial folds

Fig. 6.20 Musculocutaneous attachment of upper lip elevator muscles under the nasolabial folds

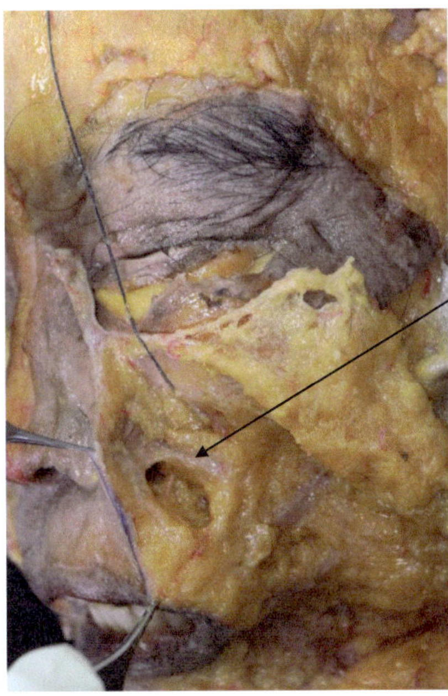

and minor muscle get attached to the upper lip and orbicularis oris muscles. Most of the muscle fibers that get attached to nasolabial folds pull the skin below the lower boundary of nasolabial fat along the crease. When you smile, the musculocutaneous attachment part attached to the skin is pulled according to muscle movements. The part below the crease gets depressed while the fat layer above it gets plump. As a result, the crease becomes deeper. When you are young, it appears deep only when you smile. As you get older, marks are left on the skin by repeated movements and make the crease distinct even when you make no facial expressions (Fig. 6.20). The muscle involved in lip elevation begins in the cheekbone. As they get down, they move in an increasingly superficial way and are combined with SMAS near nasolabial folds, moving to the same layer. Thus, some muscle fibers show a pattern of getting attached to the skin. When the deep tissues, including SMAS, are frequently hung on thread cogs, they can hinder the movement of muscles getting combined with SMAS. It is thus critical to mainly pull the plump superficial fat layer above the SMAS in a cogged thread lift for nasolabial folds (Fig. 6.21).

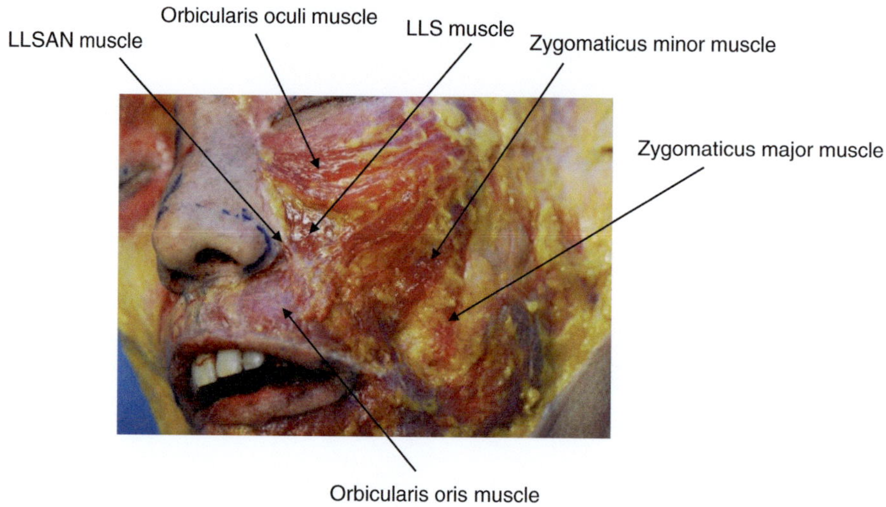

Fig. 6.21 Upper lip elevator muscles on the nasolabial fold

When cogged threads move in a depth that is too shallow and get too close to the skin, they can pull the skin and make a depression like a dimple as the client smiles or makes a facial expression after the procedure. Doctors should make sure that threads get hung on the fat layer in enough thickness.

These three types of nasolabial folds can happen individually, but it is common that two or three of these causes work simultaneously. Doctors pull the drooping skin, soft tissue, and fat above the nasolabial folds as the drooping of nasolabial fat is the cause of the second type, making the plump part above the crease to be pulled flat, generating the effects of faint nasolabial folds. In addition, the paranasal region next to the nose is naturally improved with its relative depression. Patients with the third type of nasolabial folds have a crack and get a deeper crease when making a facial expression due to the fibers of the muscles elevating the upper lip attached to nasolabial folds. This condition can be improved by inserting volumizing non-cogged threads that can generate volume effects along the crease or across it. This procedure makes the skin of the folded crease spread and firm, and the volumizing non-cogged threads push down the loose and plump tissue above the crease and make them flat. Not only does the depressed skin along the crease become revived, but the degree of crease folding is also alleviated when smiling or making a facial expression. After the procedure, the skin becomes firm through collagen regeneration. The creases that are visible even when patients make no facial expression and look like a crack get faint.

The study then examined the causes of wrinkles around the mouth corner. White or black people have the modiolus, which is a small and thick muscular node made of muscles gathering around the mouth corner, and mainly distributed at the corner of the mouth level or above it. Asians, including the Koreans, have the modiolus 11 mm and 9 mm from the mouth corner in the lateral and downward direction, respectively. In many cases, their mouth corners thus appear to be lower than those of Westerners even when they make no facial expressions. Given their lower position, their mouth corners sag easily in the aging process (Fig. 6.22).

The shallow and deep fibrous layers of the most superficial depressor anguli oris muscles and the orbicularis oris muscles in average depth among the muscles of the modiolus create a level due to their depth differences. When level differences are huge, the areas of the mouth corner get a depression and a commissural line that runs vertically obliquely. This line is also frequently found in Asians due to the anatomical position of their modiolus. There are three lateral and central superficial fat compartments below the lips. Of them, the lack of the lateral lower lip fat compartment causes a big difference in thickness between the jowl fat, which is superficial fat in the cheeks, and lower lip tissue. As a consequence, the commissural line caused by level differences between the up and bottom gets deeper, which leads to drooping around the mouth corner (Fig. 6.23).

This line, which is the superficial anatomical boundary between the cheek and lower lip, gets deeper as the thickness difference between the two areas of tissue becomes distinct. It is called the cheek-chin crease or melolabial folds, which create a depressing impression (Fig. 6.24).

As people get older, melolabial folds get deeper due to various causes and extend to the mandible border. The jawline before the extended folds creates a depression, unlike the plump tissue above, creating prejowl sulcus. This type of fold is commonly called the marionette line. It is said that the term was derived from the mouth corners of puppets used in popular puppet plays in Europe, but there is no confirmed information about who started to use the term and when. It is also called static labiomandibular folds as the line is oblique from the area around the mouth corner to the jawline even when one makes no facial expressions (Fig. 6.24).

There are many different causes, including the resorption of the maxillary and mandibular bone, the downward displacement due to the pull of gravity, the loss of the deep fat layer below the muscles under the depressor anguli oris m., the compression of the depressor anguli oris m., the tethering effect of the mandibular ligament, the sagging of the redundant skin and connective tissue, and the sagging of the jowl and buccal fat. Patients may need a combination of different treatments according to relevant causes.

Usual treatments include a filler procedure for the depressed part before a marionette line around the mouth corner and the rugged mandible borderline, including the prejowl sulcus, a toxin procedure to improve the mouth corner depression due to the contraction of the depressor anguli oris m., a procedure or surgery to reduce the volume of the jowl and buccal fat that has become a drooped plump, a cogged thread lift to pull the sagging skin and soft tissue, including fat, to make the area around the mouth corner tight and smooth, and a volumizing non-cogged thread procedure to make the folds less deep for a facial expression by making the oblique line from the mouth corner faint and the skin firm (Fig. 6.25).

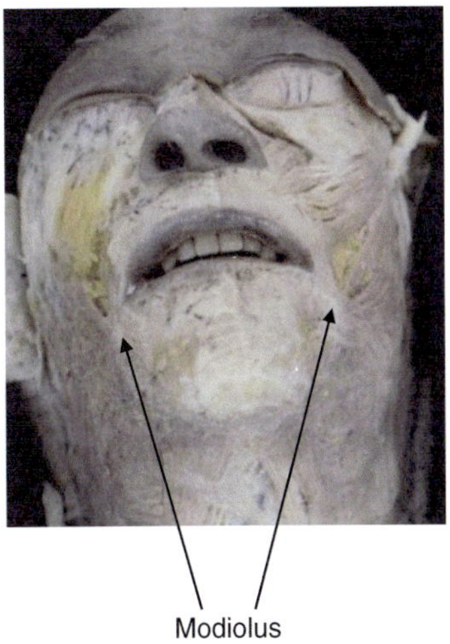

Fig. 6.22 Location of modiolus in Asians

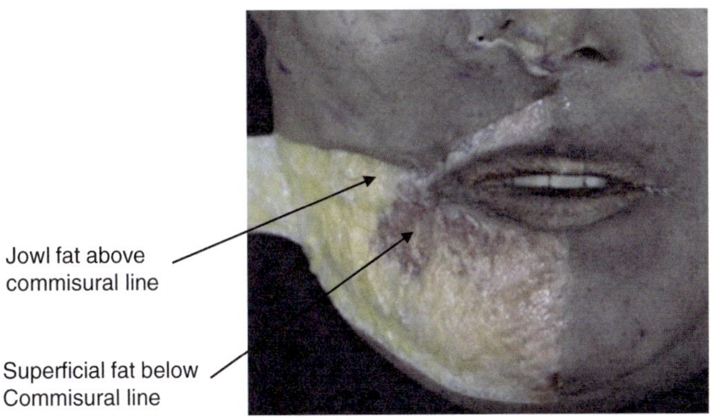

Fig. 6.23 Difference in tissue thickness around mouth corner

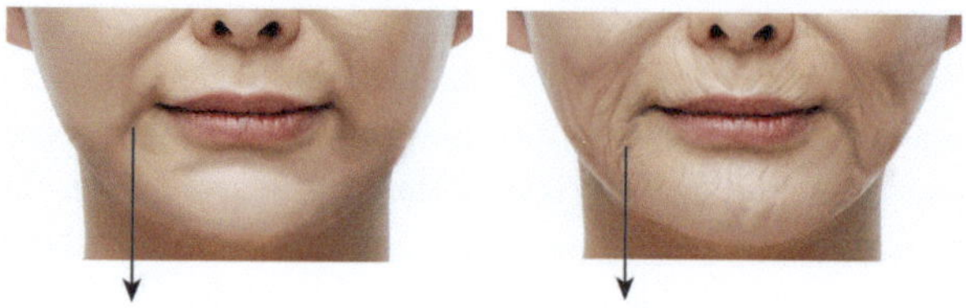

Fig. 6.24 Melolabial fold and Marionette line

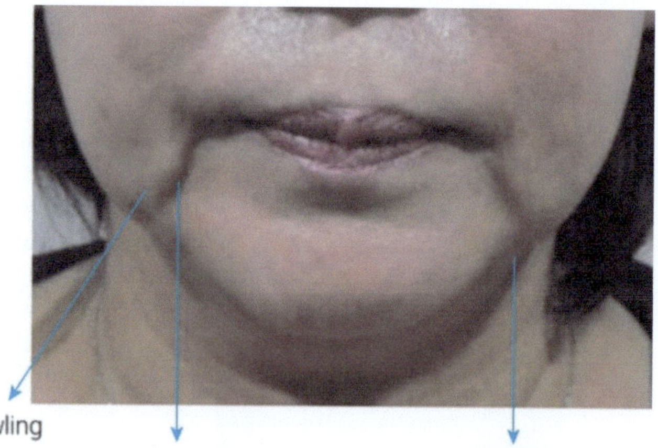

Fig. 6.25 Main symptoms of marionette line

Of these several procedures, the toxin procedure to weaken the depressor anguli oris m. involved in the lowering of the mouth corner reduces the force that pulls on the mouth corner downward and can thus be helpful for a cogged thread lift to pull drooping tissue above the mouth corner line. These days, one of the popular toxin procedures weakens the work of muscles pulling down among the muscles involved in the maintenance of top and bottom balance in the skin and helps the client have a good facial expression that is a relative smile.

6.3.2 Reasons for the Reverse Technique Using Cogged Threads and the Cross Technique Using Volumizing Non-Cogged Threads

Doctors should consider the procedure vectors most efficient to pull drooping tissue, such as how much the skin and nasolabial fat that droop above nasolabial folds should be pulled and in which direct the target tissue should move. As explained above, it is a good approach to make the vectors of a cogged thread lift for nasolabial folds run perpendicularly to the crease. Doctors can maximize the effects of the procedure with the same cogged thread by making it sure that the threads hold and move as many drooping tissue as possible. The old way of inserting a cogged thread according to a lifting vector perpendicular to the crease pushes down a cannula or needle from the lateral to the medial area of the face. Given the anatomical structure of the face, it is difficult to hang the drooping skin and soft tissue next to nasolabial folds fully on the cogged threads. This phenomenon is prominent particularly among Asians.

In an I-type cogged thread lift, a doctor cannot fully pull drooped tissue around the nose and mouth with the old way of inserting threads from the lateral to the medial area. There are a few reasons. The old way inserts a cannula or needle from the lateral to the medial area and makes it

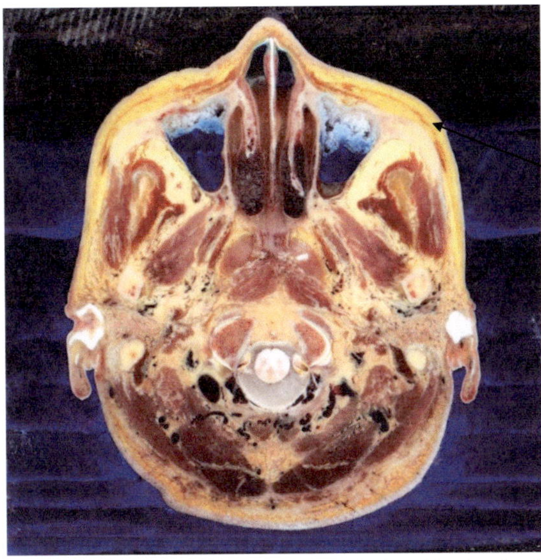

Fig. 6.26 CT scan showing the degree of bending between medial and lateral cheek region

approach nasolabial folds by taking the temporal hairline or the hard tissue of anthelix between the temple and ear as a fixing point. The face has a curve around the boundary between the medial and lateral cheek. The needle or cannula should be bent toward the anterior cheek past the part of the protruding malar eminence, or the cannula should be lifted and bent to have its tip move downward. In its anatomy course, Ajou University provides free anatomy education about how much the medial and lateral cheek of a Korean face is bent. Its CT scan data based on the Browsing Software of the Visible Korean Data Used for Teaching Sectional Anatomy show that there is a curve of almost 70 ~ 80 degrees between the medial and lateral cheek (Fig. 6.26).

It is usually impossible to bend a steel needle or cannula more than a certain degree according to the curve of such a degree. It is also difficult to change the moving direction of the needle or cannula after lifting its tip upward in front of the ear because the lateral face before the ear has hard skin, soft tissue, and a thick SMAS layer. Serving as a moving plane, the deep fat layer below the SMAS layer has little fat and small thickness, unlike other parts of the face with fibrous septa adhering to each other vertically and densely. Overall, the skin and tissue adhere flat. Considering that the skin and tissue where a needle or cannula is inserted are harder and tougher than other parts of the face, it will be a difficult practice to change the direction of the tip of the needle or cannula that has passed them downward by lifting the needle or cannula upward based due to the hardness of tissue to be lifted (Fig. 6.27).

When the insertion plane of the cannula fails to maintain certain depth around the bending section past the protruding malar eminence, the procedure plane can be a problem due to its thinness. On the contrary, the needle or cannula can pass through the bending section too deeply toward nasolabial folds to prevent its moving depth from getting shallow. In this case, it passes the origin area of zygomatic muscles near malar eminence, thus hindering the move of lifting the mouth corner. It can also gather tissue toward malar eminence and make the area more prominent.

In this case, doctors can make an entry point for cogged threads in the loose nasolabial fat lateral to nasolabial folds and lift subcutaneous fat tissue with the free left hand as thick as possible before inserting a cannula to ensure that the cannula passes as fully as possible through the naso-

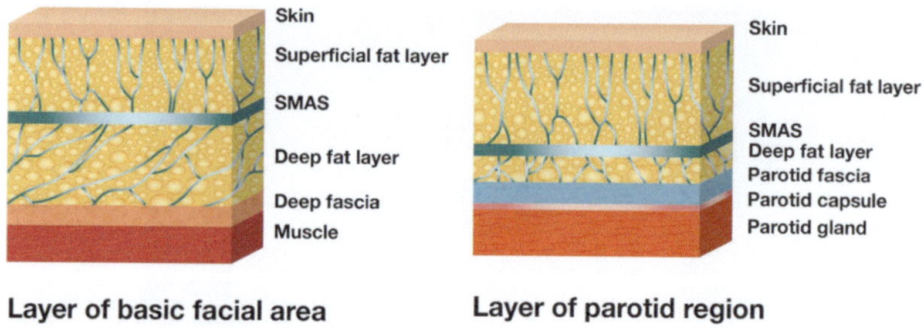

Fig. 6.27 Difference in organization of subcutaneous tissue between basic facial area and parotid region

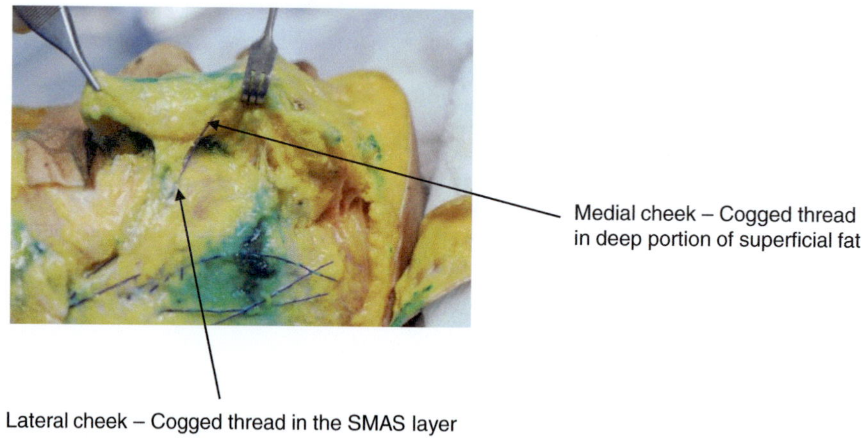

Fig. 6.28 Change of insertion plane of cogged thread between medial and lateral cheek region

labial fat as the target tissue. Then they make sure that the cannula below the superficial fat passes through the bending section of the face above the SMAS layer and keeps moving perpendicular to the crease toward the temporal region and ear. As the medial nasolabial fat is lifted in this way, the cannula passes through the bottom of the fat layer in a lateral direction. The moving depth of the cannula should be adjusted to pass through or around the SMAS layer in the lateral face. The tip of the cannula should be pushed to a fixing point in the hard tissue of the temporal region and ear, and thread cogs should be arranged to hang on hard tissue (Fig. 6.28). This method makes the entry point for a cogged thread in the lower part and inserts a thread from bottom to top, which is called the reverse technique with cogged threads.

The reserve technique with cogged threads has several advantages. It can sufficiently hang the loose tissue of the target area, insert and move a cannula in constant depth even in the bending section of the face, and bury the tip of the thread deep in the hard tissue of the head and ear after hanging enough tissue on the threads below. Thanks to these advantages, the technique can make use of a cogged thread for its maximum length. The traditional way inserts an I-type cogged thread from top to bottom. In this case, it seems natural that the tissue hanging at the end of a thread is pulled to the entry point. One might thus mistake that the upper tissue is pulled downward where a cogged thread is inserted from bottom to top. There are, of course, differences in pulling force according to the number of thread cogs and the direction of each cog, but pulling force is basically from bottom to top with loose tissue moving toward hard tissue when a cogged thread is inserted across loose and hard tissue simultaneously. It does not matter what structure and form the cogs of threads have including the I type.

When pulling force is applied after running the cogged threads through loose and hard tissue for their connection, the direction of force leans

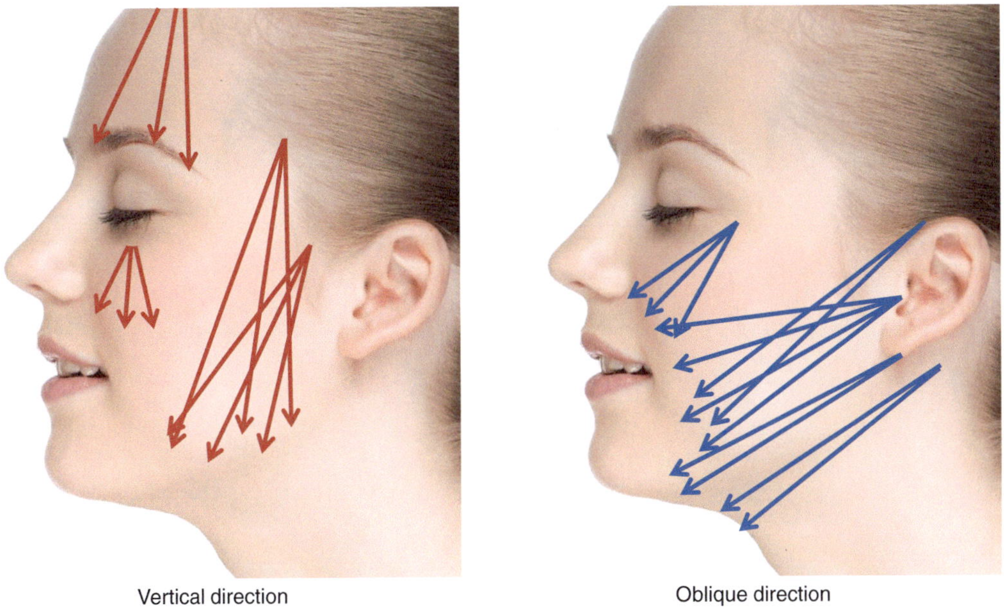

Fig. 6.29 Traditional design and direction of thread lifting using I-type cogged threads (i-THREAD Cog L-Cannula, HEALUX)

on one side with loose tissue moving toward hard tissue. This logic determines the direction of force prioritized over the direction of cog holding tissue, which means that when cog directions are either forward or backward according to the insertion direction of a cannula, the tissue in the forward direction of cogs is not unconditionally moved in the backward direction. For instance, when an I-type bidirectional cogged thread is inserted from bottom to top instead of the old way of from top to bottom, cogs in the forward and backward direction are placed at the head and lower face area, respectively. Even in this arrangement, tissue is pulled toward the head where forward cogs are and the face where backward cogs are instead of the upper tissue being pulled downward.

This principle can easily be understood through daily context. In tug-of-war, two players wind a rope around their waist. The opponent is very powerful and just holds the rope instead of pulling it. Even if one pulls the rope with all one's strength toward oneself, the opponent will not budge. Contrarily, one will move toward the opponent. The same kind of physical force works in this principle. It is thus important to find a fixing point comprised of hard tissue that hardly moves and hangs the thread holding loose tissue on the fixing point so that it will not slip off. This should be done on top of pulling the loose, drooping tissue correctly with a cog for the maximization of thread lifting effects.

Doctors can make beneficial and appropriate use of a fixing point on which to hang cogged threads that are tightly holding drooping tissue by considering the moving direction of the target tissue to be pulled and moved so as to pull the drooping tissue most efficiently. They should also consider the different vectors of thread entry before hanging them accordingly on the fixing point. This figure shows the insertion positions and moving directions of cogged threads in the conventional way of a cogged thread lift in vertical and oblique directions based on lifting vectors for each part of the face (Fig. 6.29). In the case of I-type cogged thread lifting in the reverse technique for the entire face, the insertion position and moving direction of a thread will change as shown in the figure (Fig. 6.30). The overall forms beside the nose and mouth corner will improve after moving the drooping tissue laterally to nasolabial folds and moving the marionette lines

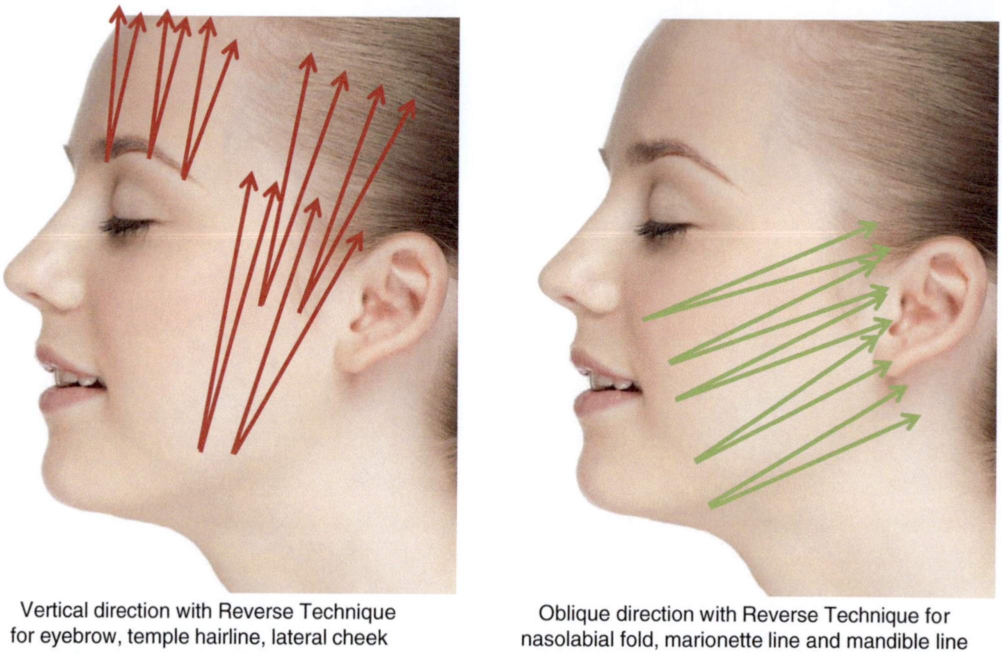

Fig. 6.30 Design and direction of I-type cogged thread lifting for reverse technique (i-THREAD Reverse Cog L-Cannula, HEALUX)

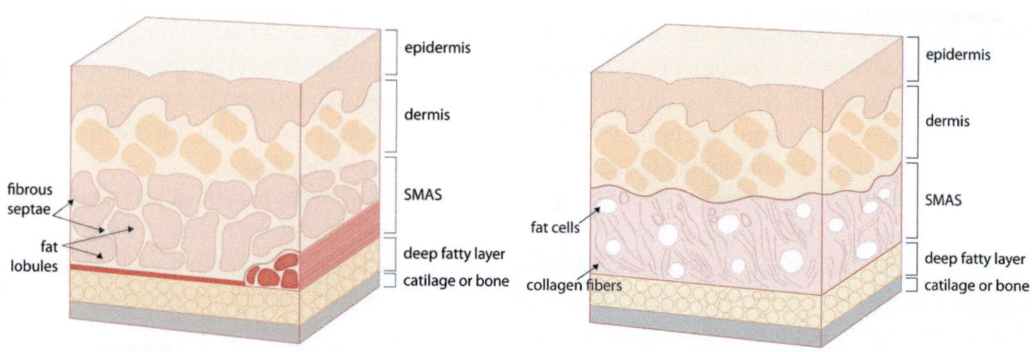

Fig. 6.31 Structural differences of layers between the tissues covering the bones (Lt.) and the tissues not covering them around the nostrils and mouth (Rt.)

obliquely upward in the reverse technique with cogged threads. If doctors try to improve the borders of the remaining creases, they should first consider the differences in thickness and hardness between the upper and lower tissue along the creases around the nose and mouth (Fig. 6.31).

In the past, doctors used various methods of inserting fillers or non-cogged mono-threads along the established crease and filling wrinkles procedures. The investigator inserts non-cogged multi-thread PDO volumizing threads across the crease to make the folded line along the boundary between the hard tissue below the crease and loose tissue above it, such as nasolabial folds and mouth corner lines, and make the boundary smooth. The investigator calls this the cross technique with volumizing non-cogged threads.

In the cross technique with volumizing non-cogged threads, the entry point is a little bit inside the crease next to the nose and mouth corner. Its position down from the crease should be established based on the length of the volumizing non-

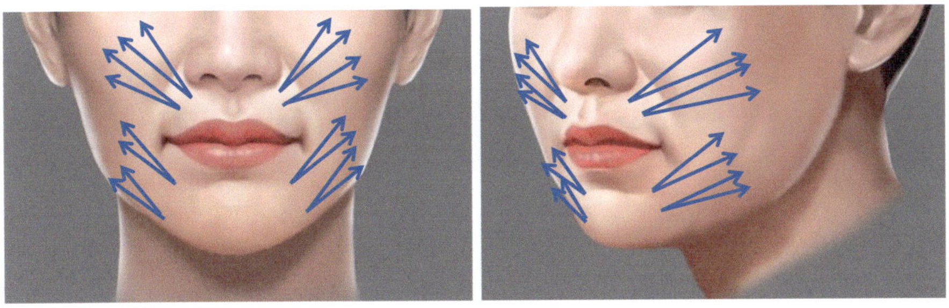

Fig. 6.32 Entry point and direction of cross technique using the volumizing PDO threads for nasolabial folds and marionette lines (i-THREAD Matrix Soft and Hard, HEALUX)

cogged thread to insert. After making a needle puncture, the doctor inserts a thread to firmly pass through thick subcutaneous tissue attached to the skin above the orbicularis oris muscles. The thread will move in from bottom to top perpendicular to the crease across it. After passing the crease, the tip of the cannula should hold the subdermal retinacular cutis below the skin tissue above the loose crease. The area of volumizing non-cogged threads inside the thick tissue below the crease should serve as support, helping the top section of the threads press and push the loose skin tissue above the crease.

As the volumizing non-cogged threads are inserted across the crease, they make the loose tissue above the crease flat by pushing and pressing them, so they can improve the height difference in the skin layers due to the difference in hardness between the upper and lower tissue along the crease. As seen in the figure, several volumizing non-cogged threads are spread perpendicular to the crease. Collagen will grow and move in the thread direction, and the loose skin tissue above the crease will become firm. This will reduce the degree of skin being pressed and folded next to the nose and mouth corner by facial expression muscles as they move (Fig. 6.32).

Volumizing non-cogged threads can also be used along the crease simply to pump up a depressed area in addition to pressing and spreading drooping tissue as support inserted in the hard tissue as described above. Volumizing non-cogged threads in the skin stimulates richer collagen regeneration than simple PDO monothreads, giving remarkable effects of making the skin clear and tight.

6.3.3 The Reverse Technique with Cogged Threads and the Cross Technique with Volumizing Non-Cogged Threads for Nasolabial Folds

6.3.3.1 Anatomical Considerations

During a procedure, doctors should be careful not to hurt a few important blood vessel structures, including the facial arteries moving above the crease in nasolabial folds, the premasseteric branch of a facial artery above the anterior border of masseter m., and the transverse facial artery that branches out from the superficial temporal artery, which is covered with parotid glands in the lateral part and moves up to the subcutaneous tissue below the zygomatic arch in the anterior part of the middle parts of the cheek, and the superficial temporal artery that moves up along the preauricular crease in the lateral faces (Fig. 6.33).

Facial arteries generally move across the facial expression muscles of nasolabial folds above and below the muscles in the same direction as the folds. In a procedure with a cogged thread or volumizing non-cogged thread, the doctor can lower the risk of hurting the arteries by manipulating the cannula as smoothly as possible. The risk grows when using a needle instead

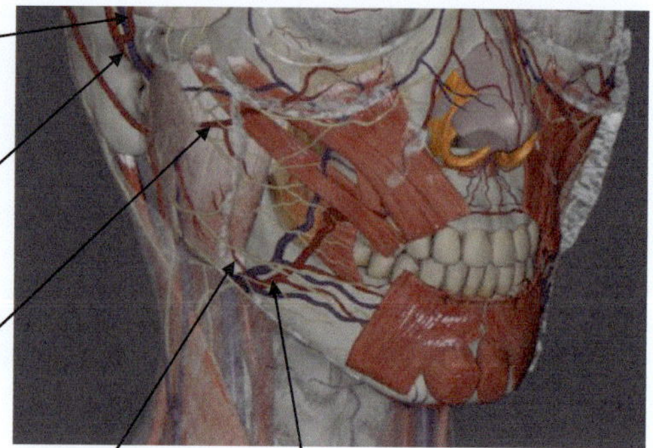

Fig. 6.33 Arteries in the midfacial cheek area

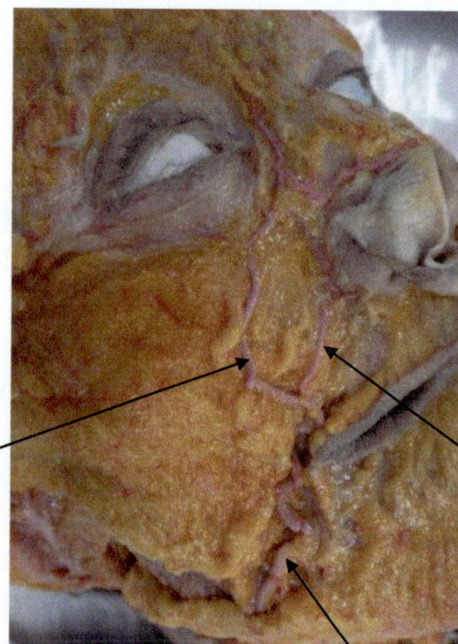

Fig. 6.34 Position of the facial artery around the nasolabial fold

of a cannula in a procedure with mono-threads to make the crease faint.

The reverse technique with cogged threads makes an entry point in the nasolabial fat part lateral to the nasolabial folds. Anatomically speaking, more than 70% of Koreans have the facial arteries passing below nasolabial folds and spread inside them. It is reported that more than 50% have a lateral artery passing within 5 mm from the crease (Fig. 6.34).

The risk of hurting blood vessels can be reduced as much as possible by making an entry point from some millimeters from the crease and inserting the tip of a cannula through it. Since nasolabial fat lies in a long and oblique way only along the nasolabial crease in the lateral part, there is no need to make an entry point for a cogged thread inside the crease to pull drooping fat layers above nasolabial folds (Fig. 6.35).

When using the cross technique with volumizing non-cogged threads, the doctor should make an entry point to insert the thread inside the nasolabial fold line and make the thread pass through thick subcutaneous tissue above the orbicularis oris muscles. In over 50% of Korean people, the facial arteries that move above nasolabial folds, including the section where the superior labial artery branches out from a facial artery, are

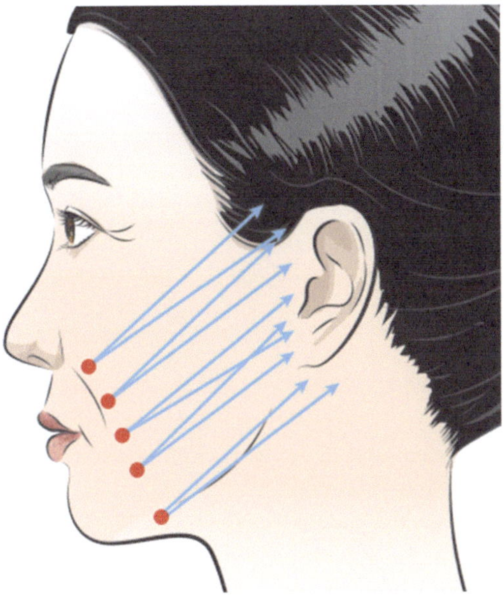

Fig. 6.35 Entry point and direction of reverse technique using I-type cogged threads for nasolabial folds and marionette lines (i-THREAD Reverse Cog L-Cannula, HEALUX)

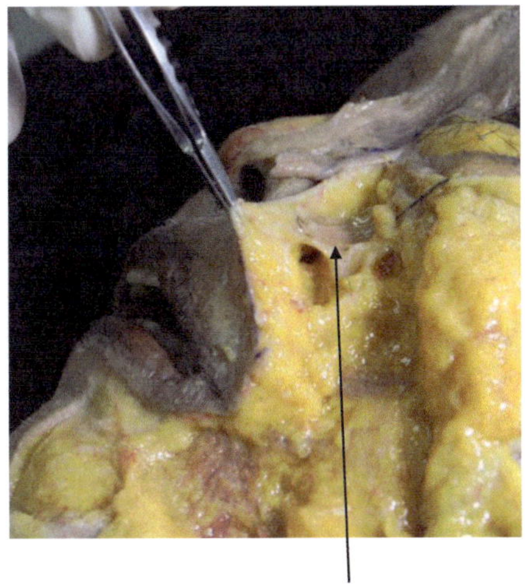

Fig. 6.36 Location of maxillary ligament

exposed shallowly above the orbicularis oris muscles. This means that there is always a risk of hurting a blood vessel during a needle puncture or thread insertion. As explained earlier, facial arteries move near the crease at a high probability. By making an entry point with enough distance from the crease in certain millimeters, doctors can prevent bleeding due to a needle puncture right into a blood vessel (Fig. 6.32).

Doctors should also try to insert a cannula across the crease smoothly in constant depth to reduce the risk of hurting a blood vessel and make the skin smooth rather than uneven after a procedure with a volumizing non-cogged thread.

In the reverse technique with cogged threads, the tip of a cannula is inserted at an entry point and penetrates the part below the nasolabial fat layer. The maxillary ligaments, which are ligament tissue holding the skin and tissue above nasolabial folds, should perform as a hanging point. This tissue should be attached to a fixing point near the ear after being held by cogged threads so that the loose tissue connected to it can move toward the ear easily and maintain its new position for a long time. Lateral maxillary ligaments are also called buccal ligaments. This ligament tissue is lateral to nasolabial folds and connects the fascia tissue inside the skin. The medial maxillary ligaments above nasolabial folds are stronger ligament tissue originating from bones. In a cogged thread lift, they should be pulled correctly to improve the deep nasolabial folds fully due to the plump tissue above the crease next to the tip of the nose (Fig. 6.36).

The procedure layer can be made deeper to penetrate the SMAS layer in the lateral face and move below when the cannula passes the border between the medial and lateral face. This can eliminate the risk of hurting the superficial temporal artery and premasseteric branch when moving threads.

When cogged threads are moved in a perpendicular direction to nasolabial folds as their vector, a fixing point is set in the middle of the ear. Generally, Lore's fascia, which is the very hard fascia tissue right before the ear tragus, is used as a fixing point. As the tip of a cannula approaches the tragus after crossing the lateral face and passing below the SMAS layer, it feels a hard resistance before the tragus, which is due to Lore's fascia. The tough fibers begin at the ear cartilage and pass SMAS of deep and superficial fascia, being connected to ligaments in the skin. Anatomically, there is the upper and lower border of hard rectangular ligament tissue that begins at

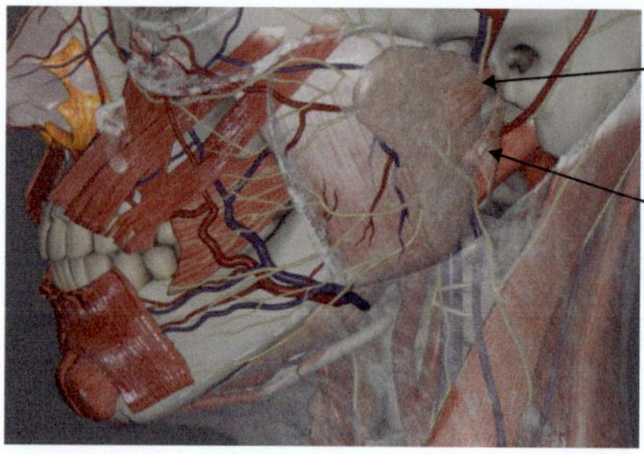

Fig. 6.37 Location of Lore's fascia

the parotid gland and connects to the ear cartilage below the tragus after the parotid fascia is put ahead (Fig. 6.37).

6.3.3.2 Procedure Designs and Techniques

As mentioned earlier, the reverse technique with cogged threads should be performed in a way to hang cogged threads on the loose nasolabial fat part that is lateral to nasolabial folds and push them toward the tragus to almost touch it. Doctors should be careful not to move the treads to the very loose parts without careful consideration since the parts near the nasolabial folds have a less tough feel due to the thin SMAS layer. When threads go in a deep fat layer, they can stimulate the mucous membranes inside the mouth and make the patient feel uncomfortable when opening the mouth as if there are some foreign matters in the deep tissue.

The tip of a cannula can be inserted like running a thread from bottom to top in the fat pad after pinching the skin and soft tissue in the loose drooping nasolabial fat as the thick target area and lifting them up with the left hand.

After the procedure ends, the plump nasolabial fat above the crease moves laterally and becomes even. It looks flat due to its reduced volume. As height differences from the depressed paranasal region next to the nose decrease, the border section resembles a step and becomes smooth with the nasolabial folds growing faint. Tissue moves to the front cheekbone where a midcheek groove appears that seems relatively depressed, and the overall front cheekbone part looks smooth as well.

When the patient lifts the tip of the chin into a bit of a supine position, the drooping tissue above nasolabial folds moves toward the eyes laterally. Under this condition, a cogged thread is inserted at the entry point. Any I-type multidirectional cogged threads with cogs in many directions will generate proper lifting effects. I-type bidirectional cogged threads that are only for the reverse technique can be used to emphasize tensile force. As seen in the figure, these threads have more cogs on the handle. As they are inserted from bottom to top, more cogs hang on loose tissue below and pull them as much as possible. Doctors should be careful with the tip of a cogged thread since it has relatively fewer cogs. They need to find the hard tissue that will serve as a fixing point and hang the upper cogs on them so that loose tissue is pulled and maintain that state so as not to droop again (Fig. 6.38).

The thickness and number of bidirectional cogged threads for the reverse technique depend on the thickness and elasticity of the skin and the drooping and volume of the skin and tissue.

After inserting a cogged thread for the reverse technique in the medial face and moving it to the lateral face, doctors should change the cannula insertion layer at the border of the medial and lateral face as explained above. In general, they can change the thread insertion plane from a deep subcutaneous fat layer to the one below the SMAS layer while moving it lateral to a vertical line from the lateral orbital rim (Fig. 6.39).

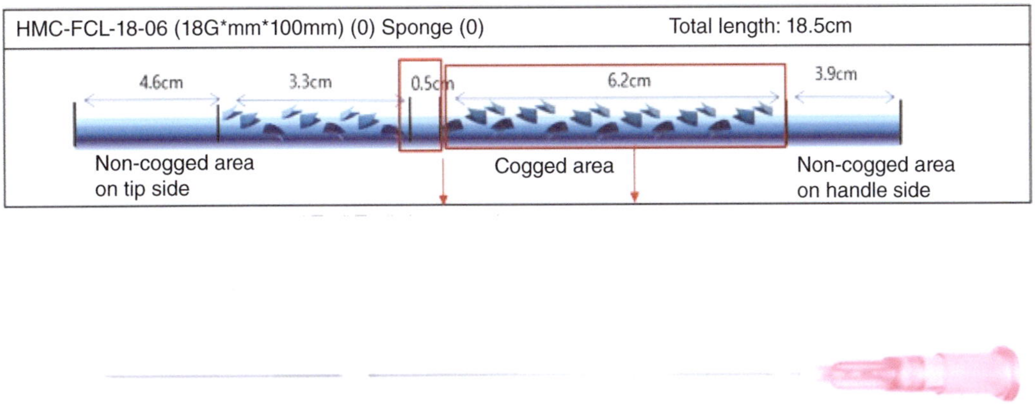

Fig. 6.38 Advanced I-type bidirectional cogged thread for reverse technique (i-THREAD Reverse Cog L-Cannula, HEALUX)

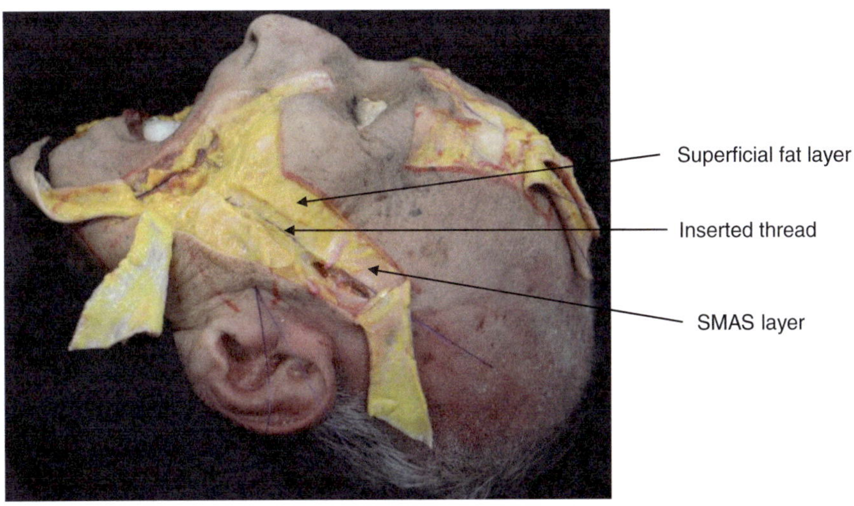

Fig. 6.39 Difference in insertion plane of cogged threads between the medial and lateral cheek regions

Doctors occasionally have patients that have a plump band at the beginning of the nasolabial folds where the tip of the nose meets the cheek. In these cases, doctors cannot pull the drooping skin and soft tissue at this beginning section easily just by pulling the middle part of the nasolabial folds. They should pull the part right next to the tip of the nose. Since many Koreans have the protruding malar eminence, the cogged thread cannula should move right above the malar eminence to pull this part before the ear. Just like an entry point along the temple hairline, the cannula should bend to pass the cheekbone area, which makes it difficult to maintain the procedure plane accurately. In this case, it is a good approach to use the lateral orbital thickening of the orbital rim around the eye as a fixing point and pull the fat layer medial to the front cheek. After making an entry point in the drooping fat layer band near the tip of the nose, doctors can insert a short bidirectional cogged thread for the reverse technique, move it toward the eye without touching the area near the malar eminence, and tightly hang it on the lateral orbital thickening so as not to droop again (Fig. 6.40).

After the procedure, the drooping tissue becomes tight with an improved form due to volume differences between the parts. There are

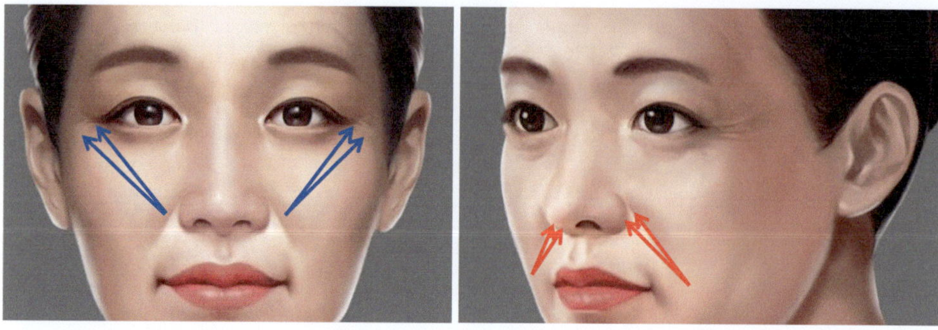

1. Insertion sites and directions of cogged threads for prominent medial nasolabial fat

2. Insertion sites and directions of volumizing threads for nasolabial crease

Fig. 6.40 1 Design of cogged thread insertion for prominent medial nasolabial fat 2. Design of volumizing thread insertion for nasolabial crease

marks of folded tissue left at the border between the cheek and paranasal region after a cogged thread procedure. The cross technique with volumizing non-cogged threads explained above can be applied to these marks to improve lines such as folded marks and make the skin firm.

When the goal is to improve only the crease with no big depression in the paranasal region next to the nose, doctors can target the part a little medial to the crease and insert volumizing non-cogged threads along the crease. Considering the length of thread to insert, doctors should make an entry to insert a thread at the lower tip of the crease. Following a needle puncture, the doctor will insert a thread in subcutaneous tissue above the orbicularis oris muscles and move the thread along the crease from bottom to top (Fig. 6.40).

6.3.4 The Reverse Technique with Cogged Threads and the Cross Technique with Volumizing Non-Cogged Threads for Marionette Lines

6.3.4.1 Anatomical Considerations

In a thread life for a marionette line and jowl, a needle or cannula can meet certain blood vessels and nerves around the mouth corner in its course including the facial arteries that pass the jawline, move up toward nasolabial folds, and make branches that move up and down the mouth corner and premasseteric branches that move along the anterior border of the masseter muscles after branching out from the facial artery near the jawline. Doctors should always be careful to manipulate a cannula or needle softly where these blood vessels pass so as not to cause damage to them.

When performing the cross technique with volumizing non-cogged threads to make creases on the skin surface faint, doctors should make an entry point inside the marionette line and insert a volumizing non-cogged thread. Here, they should be careful not to hurt the mental arteries and nerves coming from the mental foramen below the mouth corner. In many cases, the mental foramen is approximately in the middle of a vertical line from the mouth corner to the borderline of the mandible (Fig. 6.41).

6.3.4.2 Procedure Designs and Techniques

In the reverse technique with cogged threads to pull and smooth out marionette lines oblique from the mouth corner to the jawline and jowl fat drooping plump above them, a procedure vector aims to pull toward the ear perpendicular to the crease.

An entry point to insert a cogged thread can be made near the inferior margin of jowl fat upward perpendicular to a marionette line. A fixing point can be made in the temporal fascia near the ear anthelix or near Lore's fascia before the tragus in the middle of the ear (Fig. 6.42).

After pinching and lifting the jowl fat with the left hand following a needle puncture at the entry

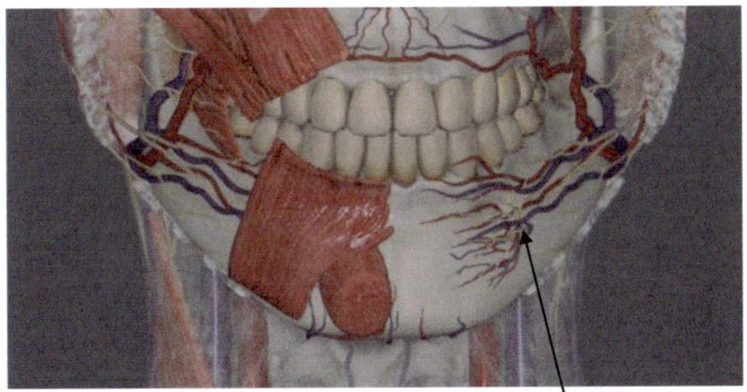

Fig. 6.41 Location of mental foramen

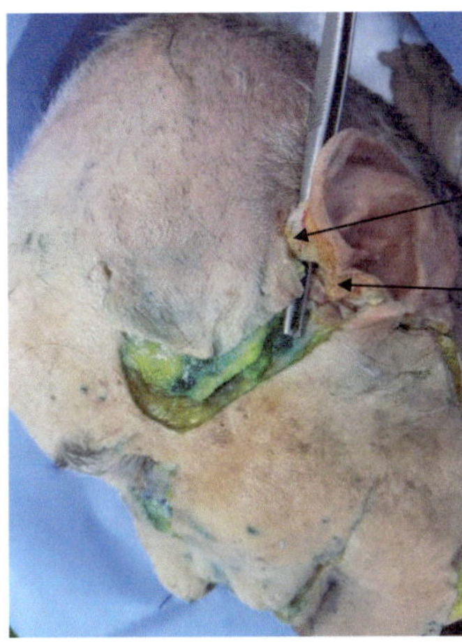

Fig. 6.42 Fixing points for reverse technique using I-type bidirectional cogged threads

point and inserting and passing the cannula through the bottom of the jowl fat in a thick pinch, doctors should move the cannula along the thread vector that has been designed in advance such as the reverse technique for nasolabial folds, which can move along the thick and tough SMAS layer in the lateral face. SMAS becomes thick and tough as it moves over the vertical line of the lateral orbital rim from the anterior face to the lateral face; thus, the cannula of the cogged thread can feel that it is passing through a stiffer part.

After being inserted at the entry point, the cannula should hold jowl fat tissue, which is the target tissue, as thick as possible. For this, doctors might push the cannula too deep toward the buccal fat pad and the mucous membranes inside the mouth. It is thus important to be careful not to make the tip of a cannula move too far downward. It is a better approach to move the tip of a cannula to thread the jowl fat with the drooping jowl fat above a marionette line lifted a little bit by a hand. Unlike the nasolabial fat of nasolabial folds, jowl fat should be pinched with fingers along with the skin before a marionette line for an enough lift. The part below the mouth corner causes no big hindrance to such moves as opening the mouth or lifting the mouth corner. As long as the moving direction and depth of a cogged thread are observed correctly, doctors can make an entry point a little medial to a marionette line instead of lateral without facing huge issues after the procedure.

When a patient lifts the tip of the chin a little in a supine position, the drooping tissue above a marionette line moves toward the ear. As seen in the figure, a cogged thread for the reverse technique is inserted at an entry point. The thickness

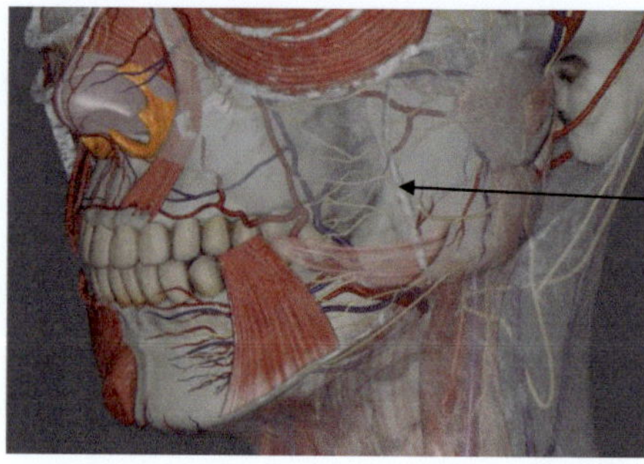

Fig. 6.43 Hanging points for reverse technique using I-type bidirectional cogged threads

of a cogged thread is determined based on the degree of wrinkles, the skin thickness of the patient, and the degree of movement around the mouth (Fig. 6.35).

There are masseteric-cutaneous ligaments, which are ligament tissue, perpendicular to the procedure area where a cogged thread passes. If cogged threads hold these ligament tissue along with the SMAS layer in the lateral face and move them along with the drooping tissue around the mouth corner before or above the ear by using them as a hanging point, their effects of tissue movement and the period of their duration can be maximized (Fig. 6.43).

Volumizing non-cogged threads can be used to create the folded line along the border between faint hard and loose tissue after the overall form around the mouth corner improves thanks to the upward movement of drooping tissue lateral to a marionette line.

For the cross technique with volumizing non-cogged threads, doctors can make an entry point a little bit inside the crease and insert a thread from bottom to top across the crease in a perpendicular direction. The volumizing non-cogged thread part inside the thick tissue below the crease will serve as support and make the upper section press and push the loose tissue of skin above the crease.

After several volumizing non-cogged threads are spread perpendicular to the crease as seen in the figure, collagen will be produced and come in along the thread direction. As the loose skin tissue above the crease becomes firm, the degree to which the skin around the mouth corner that is being pressed and folded by facial expression muscles will be reduced when there is movement around the mouth (Fig. 6.32).

6.4 Procedures Possible to Be Used in Combination

Liposuction, transplantation, and filler procedures are often performed along with thread lifting. This is because as important as lifting the soft tissue up by gravity is to create a three-dimensional face with the right volume. Therefore, before thread lifting, it is recommended to fill up the volume of the face, such as filler or fat transplantation, and to reduce the volume, such as liposuction or laser lipolysis, for those with too much facial volume.

Until now, questions have been raised that liposuction will reduce the effect of cogged thread lifting, and some physicians who think liposuction will reduce the anchoring and holding strength of the cogged threads have waited for a period of stabilization after liposuction. However, if the procedure is divided into two times, there has been an inconvenience of having to go through two elapsed periods such as swelling.

The results of the experiments conducted to see how liposuction actually affects the effect of cogged thread lifting are as follows. First, it was found that the traction force of the cogged thread lifting was significantly reduced when the cogged thread was placed parallel to the direction of the cannula used during suction in the same layer as the liposuction layer. The reason is that a tunnel was created in the direction in which the cannula moved during the liposuction, creating a loose space. More importantly, liposuction has damaged the septa between fats, reducing the hard tissue that the cogs of the cogged threads have to hang.

Second, when the cogged thread was placed in the layer where the fat was suctioned at an angle of 90 degrees to the direction of the cannula subjected to liposuction, the traction force of the cogged thread was similarly reduced.

In order not to be affected by the tunnel made by the movement of the cannula during liposuction, even if the cogged thread enters at a 90-degree angle to the direction of the tunnel, the traction force of the thread seems to have also decreased because there are fewer rigid tissues to be held due to the already loose space and reduced the septa between fat tissues.

From the above results, it can be seen that cogged thread lifting at the same time on the liposuction layer is not good, and when liposuction and cogged thread lifting are performed at the same time, the tissue layer that is not affected by liposuction should be targeted. In the study experimented with fresh cadaver, cogged thread lifting was performed to allow the cogged thread to pass through the SMAS layer, not the same subcutaneous fat layer, without liposuction on the other half of the face.

Therefore, when pulling the drooping tissue using the cogged thread at the same time as liposuction, the cogged thread should be inserted along the SMAS layer, which is deeper than the subcutaneous fat layer, which has been loosely changed due to liposuction, to show sufficient traction force. One of the good reasons for cogged thread lifting after liposuction is that while the surface layer including the skin separated from deep layer around the SMAS to some extent due to liposuction is adhered again through adhesion, the cogged threads pulled the SMAS layer upward, so the surface layer adheres to the deep tissue layer moved upward and can positively affect the effect of cogged thread lifting. One thing to note is that if liposuction is performed before the thread absorbs after cogged thread lifting, the thread may break. Therefore, in situations where liposuction is required after cogged thread lifting, the procedure should be planned for a sufficient period of time.

If the volume of the face is insufficient, filling up the insufficient volume of the face by filler treatment or fat transplant along with the cogged thread lifting can maximize the effect of lifting, especially the part that needs to be supplemented is a lateral cheek hollow. If there is a severe lateral cheek depression in front of the ear, it is recommended to create a smooth line through additional filler injection and fat transplantation because no matter how much tissue is pulled up by cogged thread lifting. These days, many good-quality fillers with high viscoelastic values are released, so the author personally uses fillers to fill the insufficient volume when necessary while cogged thread lifting. In addition, invasive laser lipolysis equipment that melts and removes fat, such as Accusculpt and Venus, can also be done with cogged thread lifting, and these procedures are recommended before cogged thread lifting to prevent the threads from breaking. Recently, as energy-based lifting devices have been widely distributed, various equipment such as Ulthera, Shurink, HIFU, and Doublo are being used. These lifting devices are equipment that tightens skin and soft tissues rather than lifting them in a strict sense, and the target layer is mainly about the subcutaneous fat layer or the SMAS layer. It is not yet clear how the cogged threads are deformed when treated with this energy-based equipment while the cogged threads are inserted, but theoretically, it will not significantly weaken the tensile strength of the threads or the anchoring and holding strength of the cogged threads. In the case of absorbable threads, heat energy may be applied to cause some deformation of the threads, and some say that such a change may increase the effect of thread lifting in reverse, but it is not certain yet. However, I think the overall treatment satisfaction can be increased when combined with cogged thread lifting due to the incidental tightening effect that these procedures using energy-based devices have on the skin.

6.5 Evolution of Absorbable Thread Type

6.5.1 Generational Differences in Absorbable Thread Lifting

The evolution of threads used in absorbable thread lifting has undergone several changes (Table 6.4).

Table 6.4 Threads used in absorbable thread lifting

Types of threads used in absorbable thread lifting				
Shape	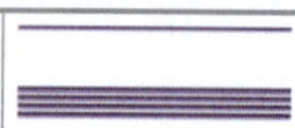	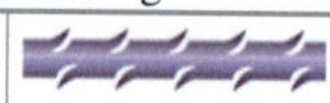		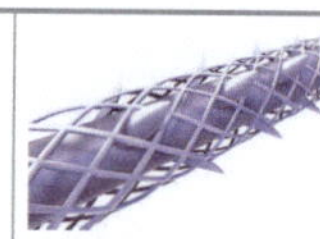
Characteristics	Non-cogged threads and bundles of them	Cutting-type cogged thread	Molding-type cogged thread	Threads mixed with mesh or multifilament in cogged sutures
Effect	Wrinkle Skin elasticity	Lifting effect Wrinkle Rejuvenation Skin elasticity	Lifting effect Wrinkle Rejuvenation Skin elasticity	Lifting effect Neo-collagenesis

In the first generation, fine threads without barbs were used, and there were cases where these threads were twisted or combined into one. Threads were also processed to create a mesh-like structure.

In the second generation, barbed threads with cutting on the surface were used. Threads with cutting were widely used due to the ease of manufacturing and use.

With the introduction of third-generation threads, molded threads without cutting emerged, raising expectations for durability and longevity. In fact, third-generation molded threads are still the most widely used today. Although there may be slight differences in molding method or shape of the barbs, these products can be considered as one group.

The fourth-generation threads, which have recently emerged, have been modified in shape or designed to perform complex functions compared to conventional threads.

For example, they may incorporate barbed threads into mesh-type threads, have different shapes on each side of the thread, or process the threads into a sturdy spring-like coiled shape. These advancements aim not only to provide lifting effects by simply pulling but also to effectively induce tissue reactions through the threads, thus enhancing the lifting effect.

The types and classifications of absorbable threads vary depending on factors such as manufacturing method, shape of the cogs, and presence of barbs. The criteria for distinguishing them are broadly as follows (Table 6.5).

Table 6.5 Classification of absorbable threads

Classification criteria		
1. Presence of cog	Mono-thread	Cog thread
2. Cog direction	Unidirectional	Bidirectional
3. Variety of cog orientations	Zigzag type	Bidirectional
4. Depending on the twist of the thread	Simple type	Coiling type
5. Depending on the manufacturing method of the cog	Cutting manufacturing	Molding manufacturing
6. Depending on the length	Long thread	Short thread
7. Depending on the shape of tip	Cannula type	Needle type
8. According to the material and duration	PDO	PLLA, PCL

Based on these classification criteria, we can explore the characteristics and expected effects of various actual products.

6.5.2 Various Types of Absorbable Threads

The above illustration shows the difference between mono-thread and cog thread. It varies depending on the presence or absence of cogs, with threads without cogs demonstrating their effects through chemical changes in the tissue after injection. In contrast, cog threads additionally exhibit traction and fixation effects due to the cogs themselves (Fig. 6.44).

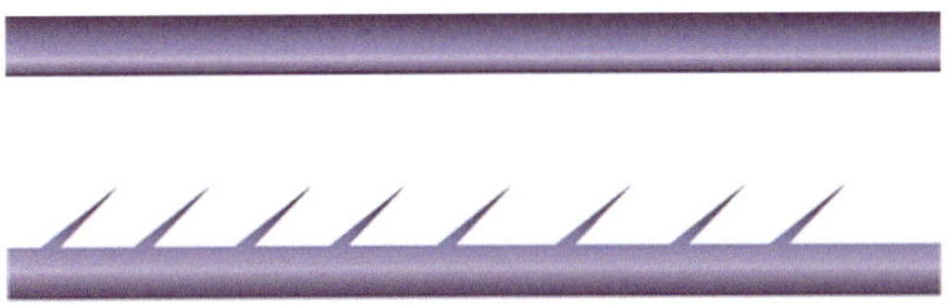

Fig. 6.44 Mono-thread vs cog thread

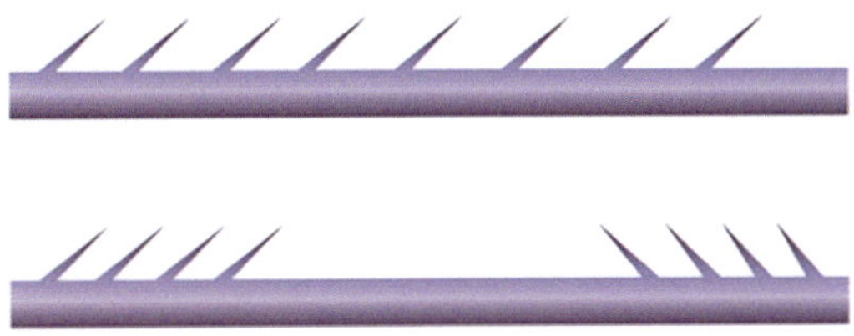

Fig. 6.45 Unidirectional vs bidirectional cog thread

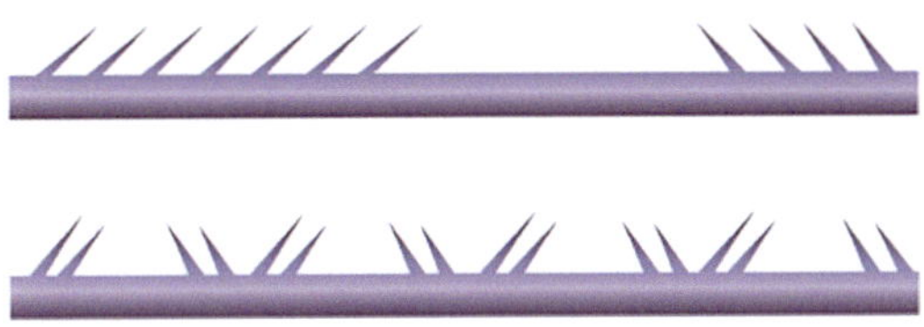

Fig. 6.46 Bidirectional vs zigzag-type cog thread

The above illustration shows unidirectional cog threads and bidirectional cog threads. Unidirectional cog threads are rarely used nowadays because they lack the function of forming fixing points, although they can pull tissues depending on the shape and function of the cogs. Below, bidirectional cog threads are the most commonly used threads as they have the function of collecting tissues in the center of the cog (Fig. 6.45).

The above figure illustrates the difference between bidirectional cog threads and zigzag-type threads (Fig. 6.46). Bidirectional cog threads gather tissues toward the center without cogs. This can be seen in Fig. 6.47 below.

Classification based on the length of the thread and surgical skill is also possible, as shown in Fig. 6.48. It depicts bidirectional threads, commonly known as long threads. They effectively lift tissues by fixing the middle part without cogs to firm tissues such as fascia.

The method involves placing the midsection over dense fascia or firm fascial areas. With needles attached at both ends of the thread, the procedure can be performed simply without additional equipment. Particularly, the technique of securing the midsection to the deep layer of the fascia produces superior effectiveness and longevity compared to other methods. In contrast to the longer threads depicted in the upper part of the diagram, shorter threads are referred to as "short threads" and are mostly seen in bidirectional cog threads. When properly utilized, the function of gathering tissues demonstrated in Fig. 6.47 enables effective lifting. Additionally, classification based on thread shape is feasible (Fig. 6.49).

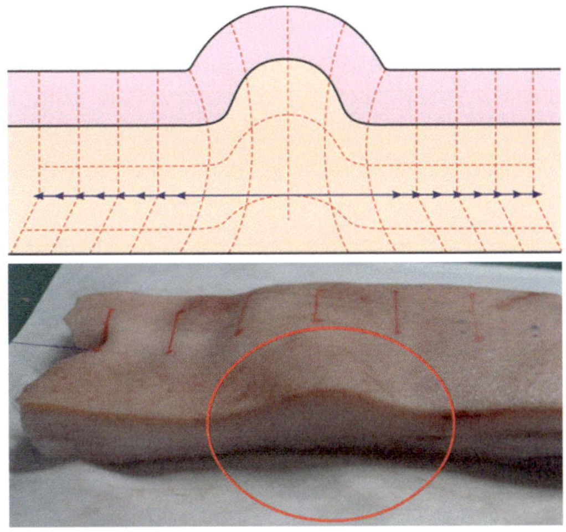

Fig. 6.47 Function of bidirectional cog threads

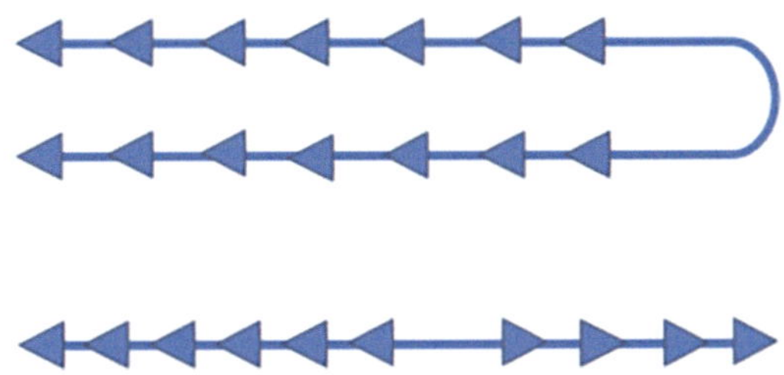

Fig. 6.48 Long vs short thread

The top portion of Fig. 6.49 depicts the mono-thread, while the bottom shows the coiling-type thread. Furthermore, various modifications are possible, such as creating multifilament threads or mesh-type threads. In actual production, when manufacturing coiling-type threads, special manipulations are often applied to make the threads somewhat firmer than the original yarn. Firm coiling-shaped threads exert a compressive and fixation effect on the tissue rather than a lifting effect. It is similar to inserting a firm rod-like filler.

The effects of threads made by combining multifilament or multiple strands of mono-thread into a multifilament form can be explained by volumization and fibrosis. The amount of fibrosis due to foreign substances is proportional to the contact area, assuming the injection of biocompatible materials. Therefore, multifilament or mesh-type threads, which have a larger contact area with the tissue, activate collagen formation, allowing us to predict the resulting outcomes accordingly.

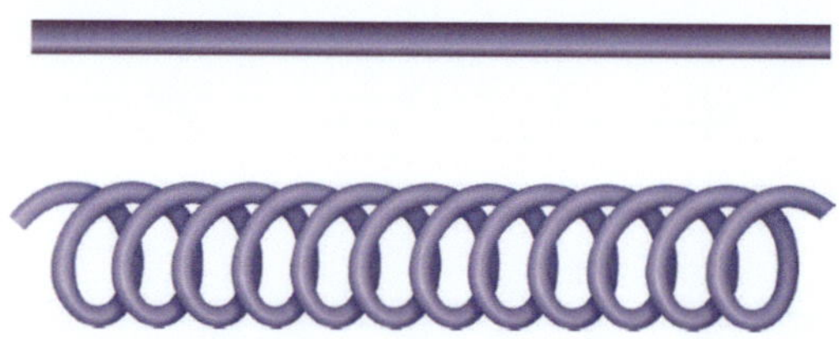

Fig. 6.49 Mono vs coiled-type thread

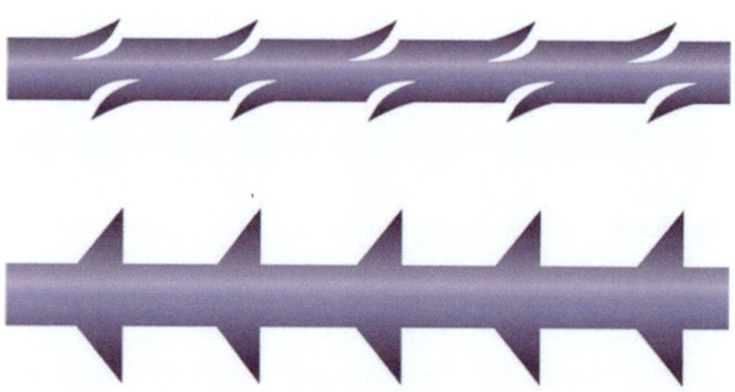

Fig. 6.50 Cutting vs molding thread

Above figure illustrates the difference between cutting threads and molding threads (Fig. 6.50). In the early days, threads were manufactured by making cogs on the thread surface using sharp blades to produce cutting-type cogs. Subsequently, molding threads, which are produced by pressing the thread itself with a press machine, became widely used. It was naturally assumed that molding threads would have much higher tensile strength than cutting threads. However, recent research suggests that the tensile strength of threads may be more related to manufacturing techniques rather than whether they are cutting or molding threads. Matthias M. Aitzetmeueller et al. conducted tests on the tensile strength and pulling force of commercially available cogged threads and demonstrated that some cutting threads exhibit stronger tensile strength than molding threads. Therefore, selecting high-quality products with well-controlled quality control in the production process has become more important than whether they are cutting or molding threads.

Spring-type threads are made by special processing of PDO threads. During the processing, the threads become firmer and can maintain their original shape without bending after insertion (Fig. 6.51).

Fig. 6.51 Spring-type vs mesh-type thread

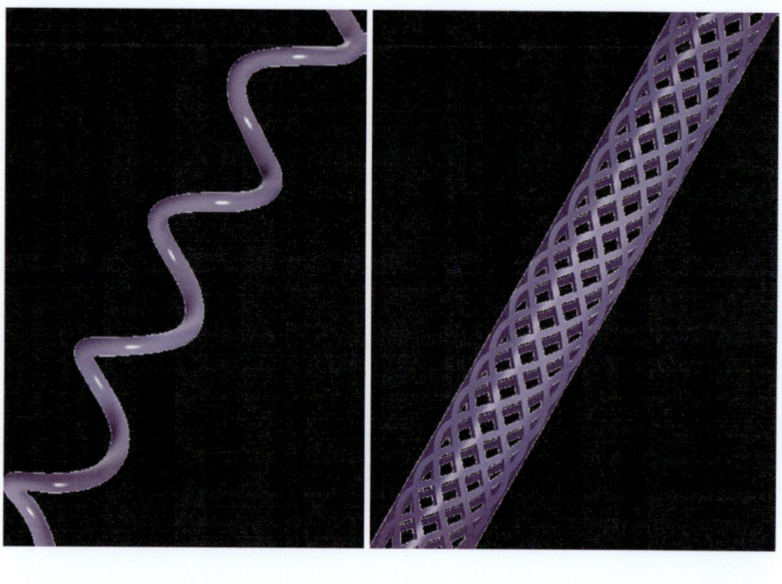

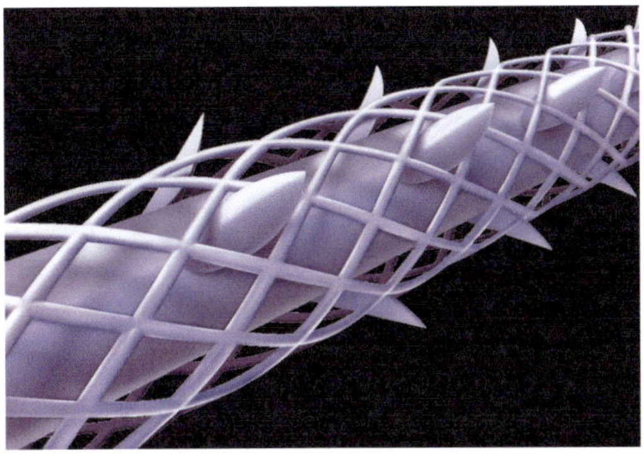

Fig. 6.52 Combined cog and mesh-type thread

Mesh-type threads are made by combining multiple threads to increase the contact area between the thread and the tissue while also helping to maintain the original shape of the thread for a longer period (Fig. 6.51). As the collagen tissues are formed around the mesh and inside the cylinder, a strong supporting structure can be created. Considering research suggesting that the amount of collagen formed around the thread after injection is proportional to the contact area between the thread and the tissue, mesh-type threads are suitable for procedures aimed at producing a large amount of collagen.

Recently, research on tissue responses to PDO has led to the development and use of new types of threads that combine cog and mesh threads to target increased tensile strength and collagen synthesis (Fig. 6.52).

At this point, human comparative clinical studies are needed to determine which types are more effective in actual clinical practice. However, in reality, conducting such studies is not easy.

6.6 Introducing the Structure of the Latest Absorbable Thread Products

6.6.1 I-THREAD

There are cutting thread and molding thread types, and in the case of cutting threads, their tensile strength is similar to or stronger than molding-type threads of the same diameter (Tables 6.6 and 6.7). A characteristic feature of two-way cog threads is the reverse-type cog thread, designed to allow insertions from below the face to upward by placing the cogs in the opposite direction to conventional threads (Figs. 6.53 and 6.54). There are also types that attach needles to both ends of the threads for easier use (Fig. 6.55).

With the introduction of molding threads, there was a general belief that molding threads would have higher tensile strength compared to cutting threads. This belief stemmed partly from the fact that molding threads appeared sturdier due to the consistent thickness of their body, unlike cutting threads where the thickness of the thread body decreases. However, Matthias M and others conducted experimental studies comparing the tensile strength and anchoring capacity of PDO threads. Through this research, they demonstrated that cutting threads are not inferior to molding threads. This proved that the quality of the thread is crucial, rather than whether it is a molding or cutting type. In other words, even cutting threads, if precisely manufactured to maintain the thickness of the thread body above a certain level, can demonstrate superior tensile strength and lifting capacity compared to molding threads.

6.6.2 Reversed Trapezoidal PDO Cogged Thread

Regardless of the method or principle of production, the shape of preexisting cogs was usually triangular such as leaves, thorns of flowers, or arrowheads with sharp ends and forms of barbs from the threads. However, the recently developed product was manufactured to have reversed trapezoid-shaped cogs made by inner punch method, cutting a groove inwards of the threads. The cogs were known as reversed trapezoid-shaped multidirectional cogs because the way the cogs cut inward of the thread held the tissues seemed like reversed trapezoid (Fig. 6.56).

Because there were no sharp structures on the outside of threads, it was initially concerned if the cogs with shape of furrow were enough to

Table 6.6 Various i-THREAD types

i-THREAD types			
Shape	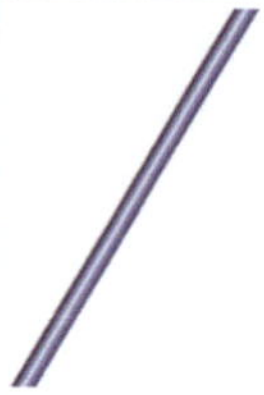	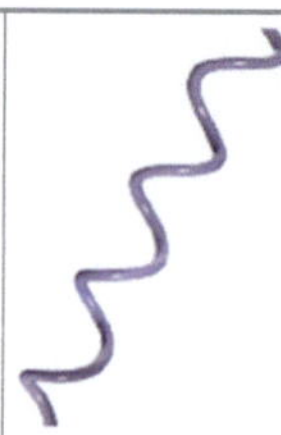	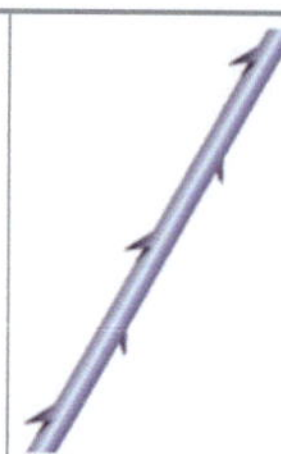
Naming	Mono-thread	Screw or coiled thread	Cogged thread
Characteristics	Linear	Spiral	Cog

Table 6.7 Various i-THREAD types

i-THREAD types				
Shape	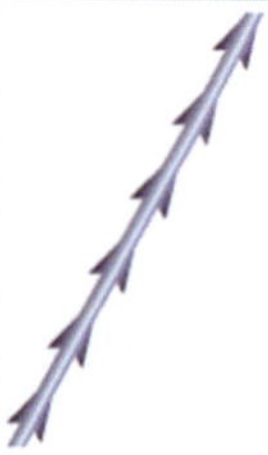	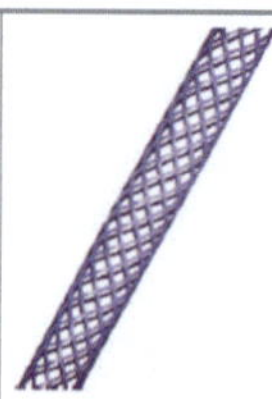	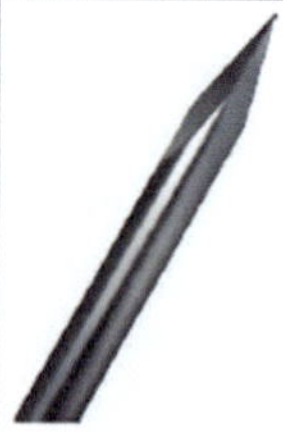	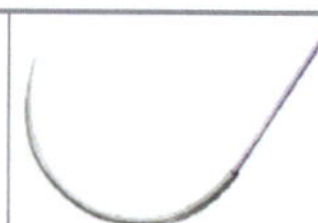
Characteristics	Molding-type thread	Mesh type	Needle attached to both ends of the thread (long needle type)	Needle attached to both ends of the thread (suture type)

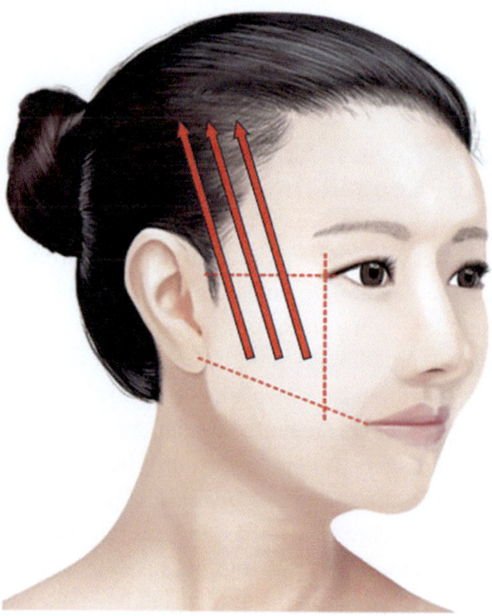

Fig. 6.53 Reverse cog-type thread technique

hold the tissues. However, it was identified later that these types of cogs had much stronger anchoring and holding strength that may firmly hold and retain the tissues because once soft tissues under the skin are held and interlocked into the groove, the holding effects of cogs on the both sides of a groove are superimposed. In order to achieve such superimposition effect, however, it is important to select products that have appropriately positioned grooves with appropriate depth and width (Fig. 6.57).

One of the advantages of reversed trapezoid-shaped cogged threads is that the outer surface of the thread feels smooth when touched by hands since the groove, which serves as a cog of the thread, is cut inward of the thread. Therefore, it may reduce lancinating pain or irritation when pulling the inserted threads while pressing the skin tissues even it may feel like the tissues digging into the grooves (Fig. 6.58).

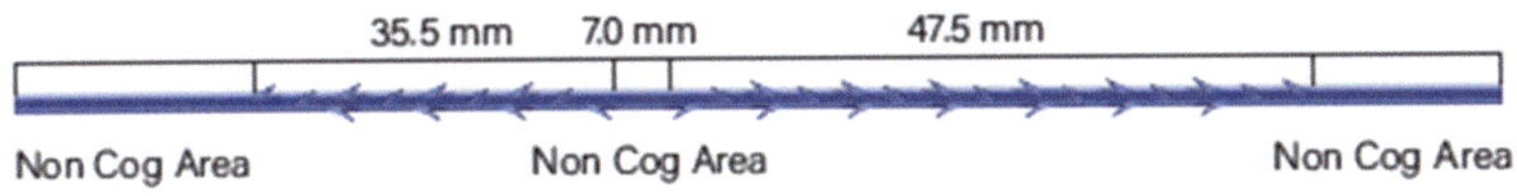

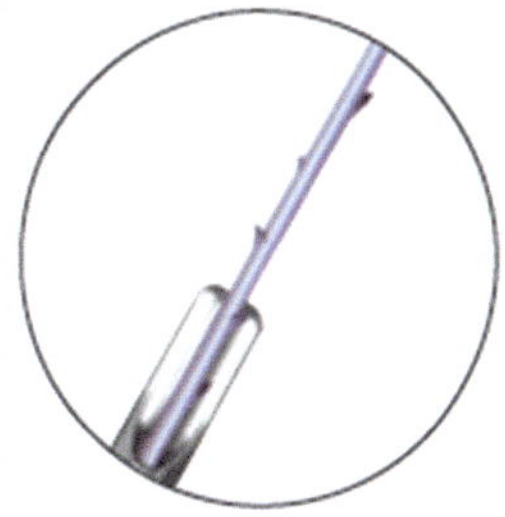

Needle gauge	Needle length (mm)	Thread length (mm)	Thread thickness (USP)
18G	70 mm	162 mm	2
	100 mm	185 mm	2
19G	70 mm	162 mm	0–0
	100 mm	185 mm	0–0

Fig. 6.54 Reverse cog L-cannula type

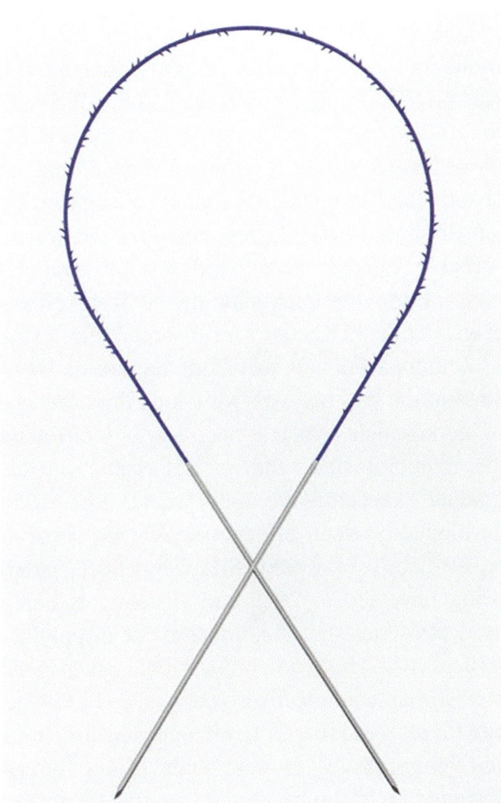

Fig. 6.55 Double-arm needle cogged thread: i-THREAD Magic Plus

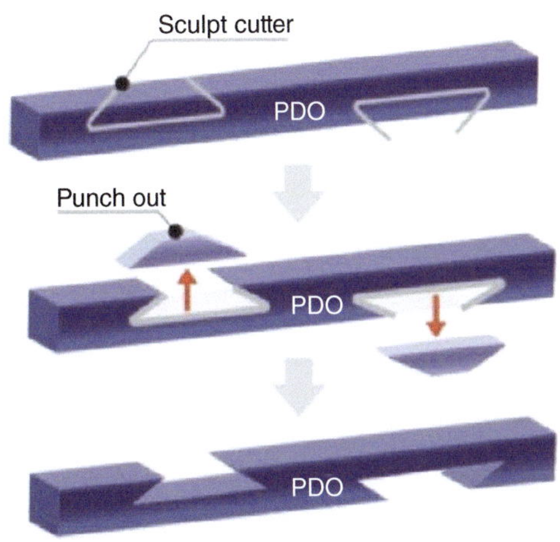

Fig. 6.56 Inner punching-type cogged thread

Also, it has advantage of not deforming the original shape of the thread, except for the grooved parts when producing the cogs. When cutting out the original threads in the shape of thorn or barb, it is inevitable to make the threads thinner as much as the thickness of thorn or barb, causing shortening of effect duration according to the thickness of the threads. However, in case of reversed trapezoid-shaped cogged thread, since the thickness of the thread is maintained except for the grooved portion, it causes little damage to tensile strength or the duration of effectiveness of thread lifting (Fig. 6.59).

Threads with thorn-like cogs require cannula that is thicker than threads to have sufficient space in the cannula to place the threads without damaging the cogs that are positioned to be outward. However, with reversed trapezoid-shaped cogged thread, which has cogs inwardly formed, cannula with same thickness of thread can be

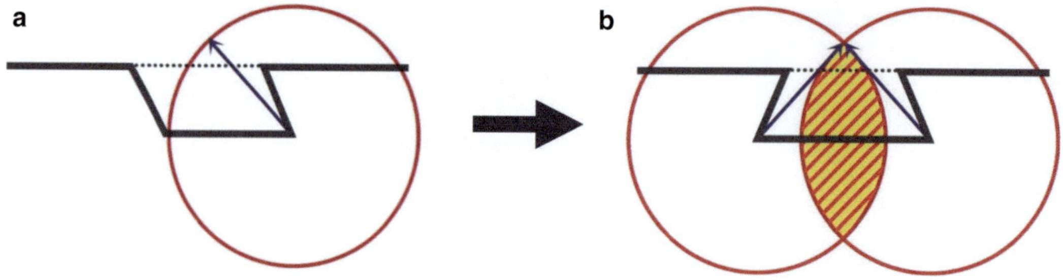

Fig. 6.57 In comparison to (**a**), the overlapped traction and holding power are significantly higher in (**b**)

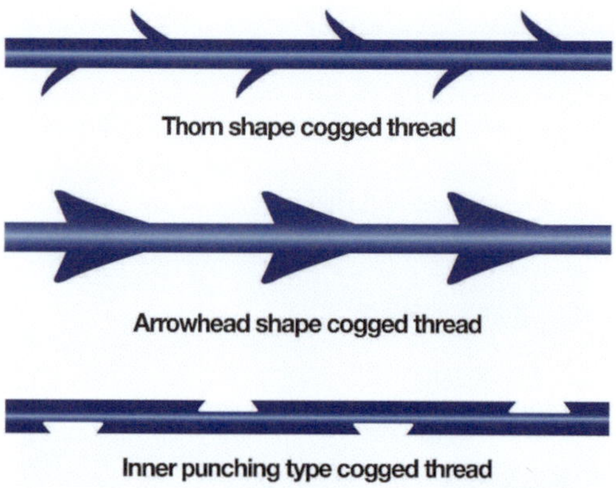

Fig. 6.58 Comparison of outer surface of each cogged type

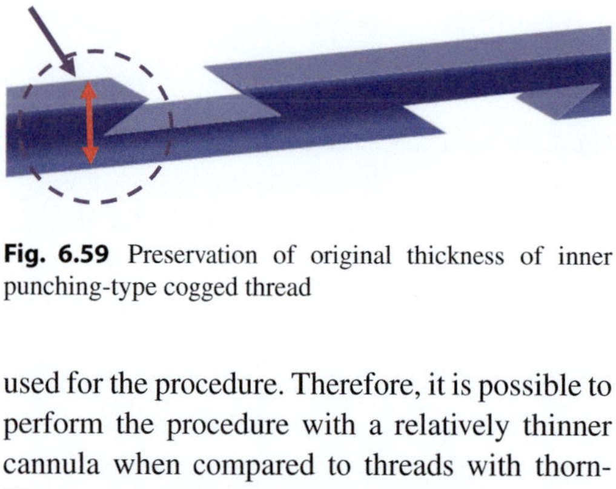

Fig. 6.59 Preservation of original thickness of inner punching-type cogged thread

used for the procedure. Therefore, it is possible to perform the procedure with a relatively thinner cannula when compared to threads with thorn-like cogs same in thickness (Fig. 6.60).

As described above, multiple or spiral directional cogs, which may distribute the tension applied to the cogs, are needed to naturally reposition the sagging tissue and efficiently retain it on the spot. Reversed trapezoid-shaped cogged thread is an optimized type of product for cogged thread lifting using the string and repositioning method in that it has greater capacity to distribute the tension applied to the cogs than any other type of cogged threads (Fig. 6.61).

6.6.3 Cone Mixed-Type PLLA Thread

In the mid-2000s, a thread called a Silhouette Lift was firstly introduced to lift skin and soft tissues in different way. Unlike other cogged threads, the tissues were pulled by a funnel-shaped cone on absorbable PDO, which is capable of transferring tensile force in 360-degree, and then, the nonabsorbable threads were fixed on the temporal region using mesh, maintaining the lifting effects even after the PDO cones are absorbed (Fig. 6.62).

Although the new technique received a lot of attention, it was not used for a long time because of inconvenience such as necessity of incision on the temporal side, and as absorbable threads gradually became the main trend, the newly developed product, Silhouette Soft, has come to be available. In Korea, Silhouette Soft started being imported in 2015 and currently is being used. It is consisted of a thread made of polylactic acid (PLA) material, bidirectional cones made of absorbable polylactic glycolic acid (PLGA) to pull the skin and soft tissues in opposite directions and long needles at both ends of the thread designed to lift the tissues by inserting the thread without the aid of other equipment. Silhouette Soft is available in three different types of products depending on the number of cones—8, 12, and 16 (Fig. 6.63).

Since it is not possible to insert the thread into the cannula guide due to the size of the cone, even applied with the basic application of principle of long-length cannula-guided bidirectional

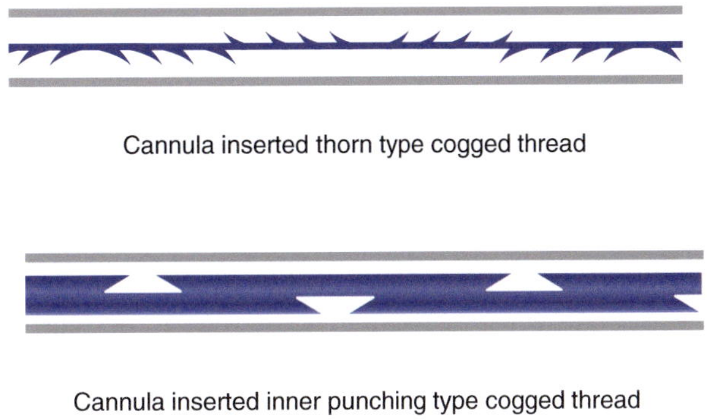

Fig. 6.60 Comparison of cannula size and thread diameter

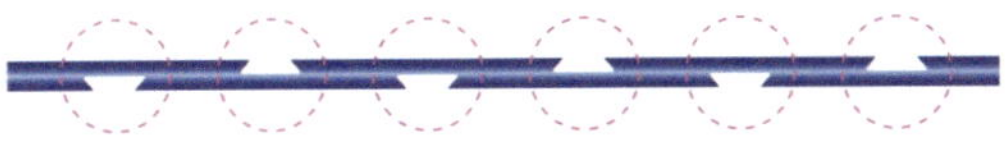

Fig. 6.61 Multiple dispersion of tension and tissue holding force

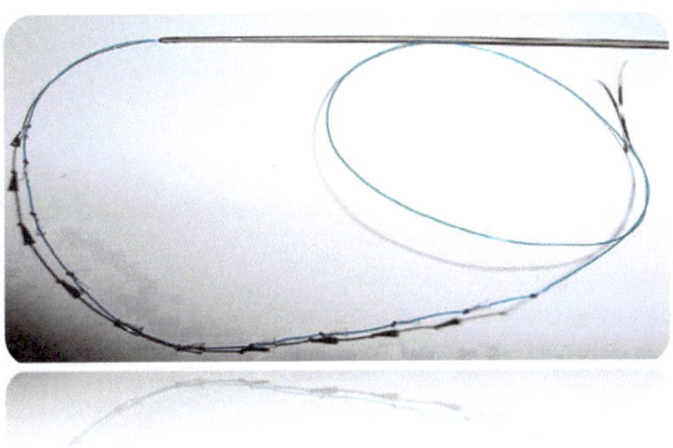

Fig. 6.62 Silhouette Lift

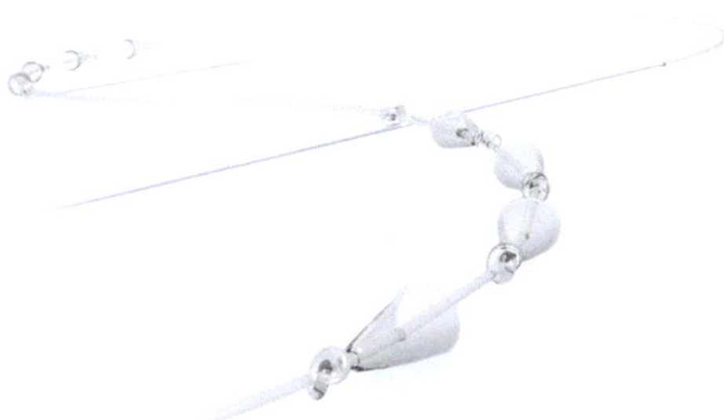

Fig. 6.63 Silhouette Soft

cogged threads. So, the product was made to be used easily without help of cannula guide by attaching long needle on both sides of the thread like long-length double-needle cogged threads. However, in the course of needle passing through, there was a higher risk of bleeding as compared with the cannula, and when passing through the curved region, as the long needle gets bent, it was difficult to handle the needle to maintain the plane accurately.

Since the basic purpose of the procedure was not to lift and fix the tissue of the lower facial part firmly to the temporal region, the product had advantages of being applied to various sites with various designs of I, U, V, L shapes according to its purpose and the procedural area.

Some people may say that the lifting force of cones of this thread is stronger than other cogged threads, but since the number of cones is actually limited, and cone is somewhat mobile between the knots of the thread, it is hard to say that the thread would exert strong force that is sufficient enough to lift the lower facial tissue like long-length cannula-guided bidirectional cogged threads. Therefore, a patient whose main purpose is to lift the drooped lower facial tissues as much as possible is not an appropriate subject for cone-type thread lifting procedure. In my personal view, cone-type thread lifting is a suitable for patients whose overall skin loses elasticity, by lifting the whole tissue naturally, repositioning the skin and soft tissues and resultantly improving the condition and resilience of skins through tissue reactions.

The most important advantage of the Silhouette Soft, when compared to PDO threads, is that it has longer retention period, taking about 18 ~ 24 months until absorption. In addition, the size of the cones is larger than that of cogs of conventional PDO threads, which may lead to a more accurate lifting effect in the area where the tissue is held by the cones of thread. However, since the threads have small number of cones and thus, the loads applied on each cone may increase, the possibility of dimple formation may increase, and cones can be touched and stand out through the thin skin. As such, the Silhouette Soft with certain properties that are different from ordinary PDO cogged threads can be used in combination with the general PDO threads, inducing synergy effect and long-term effect.

7 Basic Treatment Process for Thread Lifting

Contents

7.1 Patient Selection and Design

One of the most important points in patient selection is that the stronger the skin and subcutaneous tissues, the better the effect. As previously discussed in the concept of the moving plane, the skin layer is connected to layer 3, the fascial layer, through fibrous connective tissue present in the subcutaneous fat layer.

Since the visible effects of lifting depend on how much the skin has moved, ultimately, it is important to consider how to design and perform the procedure based on the moving plane of each area.

Design is the most fundamental step in thread lifting procedures and is a crucial factor in determining the results of the procedure. Since the direction and extent of sagging vary

S. M. Oh et al., *The Art and Science of Thread Lifting Based on Pinch Anatomy and Moving Plane*,
https://doi.org/10.1007/978-981-97-5516-5_7

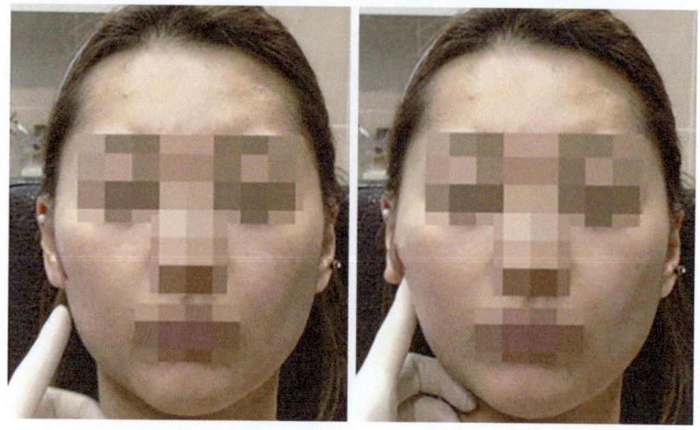

Fig. 7.1 Finding vector

from person to person, it is desirable to design accordingly. However, in clinical practice, there are cases where patients first decide on the type and number of threads they want before undergoing the procedure. Although it may be challenging to achieve good results in such cases, it is essential to create the best outcome under the given conditions through meticulous design.

To do this, the practitioner should use their hands to pull the patient's face in various directions and select the optimal vector (key vector) among them (Fig. 7.1). It is necessary to show the patient a mirror and confirm whether the desired vector by the practitioner matches the desired vector by the patient.

Sometimes, the direction of lifting envisioned by the practitioner may differ from what the patient desires. When it comes to cheek lifting, the vectors commonly used by the author are broadly the following three.

The vector from the marionette line to the ear lobule.

→ Referred to as the oblique vector in this chapter.

The vector from the lower cheekbone through the zygomatic arch to the temple.

→ Designated as the vertical vector in this chapter.

The vector from the nasolabial fold through the zygoma to the hairline.

→ Named the nasolabial vector in this chapter.

7.1.1 Finding Vector

Pushing in the direction intended for lifting using one or both hands to confirm if lifting occurs is a practice referred to as "simulation."

During consultation, lifting the skin using two or three fingers or the palm of the hand tends to result in better lifting compared to using just one finger. Explaining the difference between the results obtained using one finger versus using the palm of the hand in terms of the expected outcomes based on the type and number of threads helps patients understand more easily. Showing the patient their reflection in the mirror to confirm.

During the procedure, once the type and number of threads are determined, identifying the key vector, which is the direction where lifting occurs most effectively, through simulation; then, drawing a reference line, whether horizontal, vertical, or diagonal; and marking the starting and ending points on the key vector according to the length of the thread are done.

7.1.2 Making Reference Points (Fig. 7.2)

Draw a horizontal line from the lateral canthus (the outer corner of the eye)—(a).

Draw a vertical line from the lateral canthus—(b).

Draw a line connecting the oral commissure (corner of the mouth) to the lobule (earlobe)—(c).

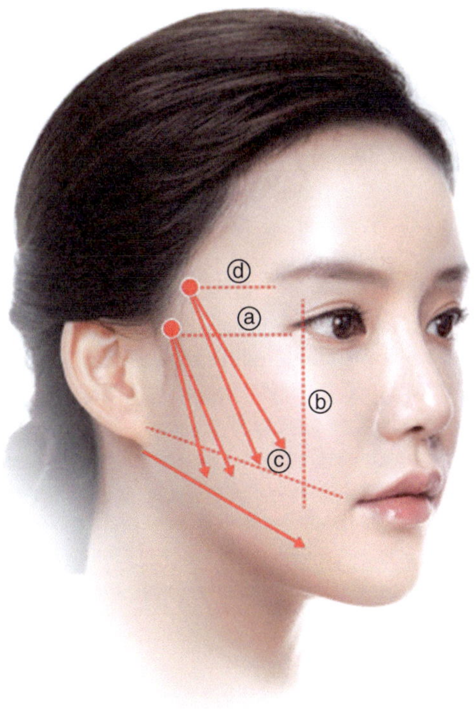

Fig. 7.2 Design baselines and fundamental vectors

Draw a horizontal line from the end of the eyebrow—(d).

Meaning of (a): Near the point where this line meets the hairline, an entry point for the nasolabial vector (often referred to as the "smile lines vector") can be determined.

Meaning of (b): When performing smile lines lifting or marionette lines lifting, there is no need to extend the end point (the point of suspension) of the thread all the way to the desired area. The effect can still be sufficiently achieved without placing the end point more medially (toward the middle) than the (b) line.

There may be differing opinions among clinicians about threading inside the (b) line. My reason for avoiding threading inside the (b) line is due to the elasticity of the thread; if the thread traverses a curved surface, there is a high likelihood of it protruding.

Since all facial tissues are connected, lifting the entire face is entirely possible by positioning and pulling the thread outside the (b) line alone. However, an important consideration in this case is that the tissues inside the (b) line must be firm enough so that pulling the thread outside the (b) line also draws the tissues inside the (b) line along.

In patients with good facial tissue elasticity, pulling just outside the (b) line is sufficient. However, this is not the case for patients with weak facial tissue elasticity. In such cases, additional treatments to improve the elasticity of the facial area inside the (b) line are required. This should be carefully considered when selecting patients and designing treatments, as failure to do so can lead to lower patient satisfaction.

Tip

Reasons not to place the endpoint more medially than the (b) line:

If the thread traverses a curve, there is an increased likelihood of complications such as dimpling or protrusion.

The subcutaneous fat layer is very dense, with more fibrous tissue than fat, making depth control challenging.

However, in patients with reduced elasticity where a lifting effect is anticipated to be less effective, a design considering the lifting of tissues inside the (b) line may be necessary. Sometimes, additional procedures inside the (b) line are also considered.

Meaning of (c): When lifting sagging cheeks using the vertical vector, there is no need to extend the hanging point of the thread all the way to the desired area (as previously explained, the desired lifting area and the thread's hanging point do not necessarily have to match). The effect can still be sufficiently achieved without placing the hanging point lower than the (c) line. This does not mean that one should never go below this baseline; going down about 1 finger breadth (FB) below the line is generally not problematic.

However, if the thread is placed too low, it could make opening the mouth or eating difficult. This also subjects the thread to continuous external forces, making it difficult to maintain the lifted tissue and potentially shortening the duration of the procedure's effects.

Meaning of (d): When determining the entry point at the intersection of this baseline and the hairline (d'), care must be taken with the superficial temporal artery (STA). The STA typically runs more laterally (outside) between points a' and d' along the hairline and then turns medially (inside) past point d'. However, variations in the STA can also run more medially between points a' and d'. Therefore, it is crucial to palpate the STA's pulse around the hairline when setting the entry point and to avoid that area accordingly.

7.1.3 Marking Hazardous Areas

Marking the path of the superficial temporal artery (STA).

7.1.3.1 The Importance of Thread and Patient Selection

Before designing, the type and number of threads are determined through consultation with the patient. Sometimes, if the consultation reveals that the patient's expectations are too high or only a minimal effect is anticipated, it may be necessary to recommend referral to another hospital for surgical options instead of thread lifting. Therefore, it is crucial to develop the ability to select patients who are expected to achieve a satisfactory outcome from thread lifting.

7.1.3.2 The Importance of Design and Vectors

If I were to choose the most crucial aspect of the thread lifting procedure, I would say it is the design. I often teach this to beginners through thread lifting hands-on courses. Once the patient is selected and the type of thread is determined, the post-procedure outcome becomes somewhat predictable. Typically, the number of threads is decided during the design phase. Usually, as the trainer, I design both sides, or I design one side and the trainee follows by designing the opposite side. Then, I insert the threads, and the trainee performs the procedure on the other side. What would be the result of the procedure? To give the conclusion first, there is hardly any difference between the results on the right and left sides. Differences in bleeding during the procedure or post-procedure dimple occurrence may arise. However, if the optimal vector is identified for the design and the procedure is performed accordingly, the results on both sides are generally satisfactory. However, if the trainee designs and performs the procedure without the trainer's design (using a vector other than the optimal one), the outcomes mostly fall short of expectations. Therefore, finding the optimal vector during the design phase is the most crucial part of the procedure.

7.2 Anesthesia

7.2.1 Anesthesia with Dental Lidocaine

When using dental lidocaine, it is injected focally into multiple areas (Figs. 7.3 and 7.4).

7.2.2 Anesthesia with Cannula

After creating the entry point, the cannula is inserted into the area where the thread is planned

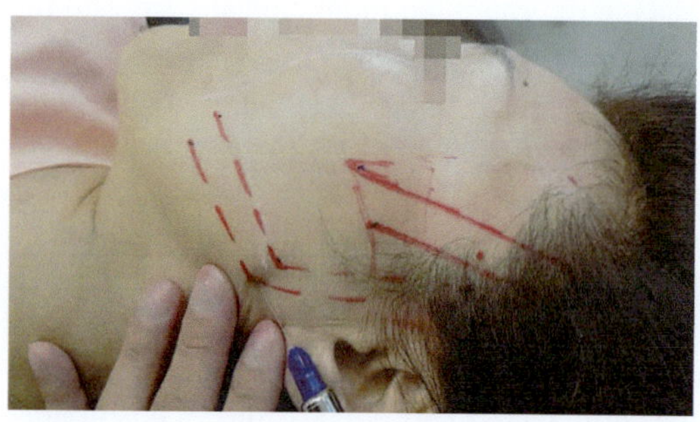

Fig. 7.3 Anesthesia with dental lidocaine

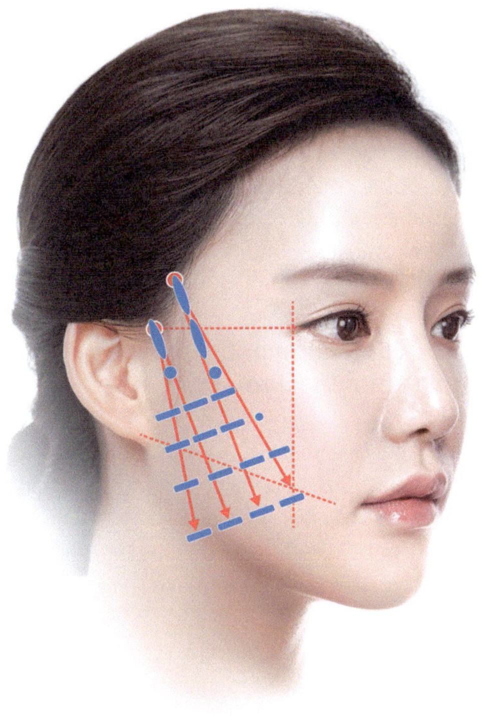

Fig. 7.4 Anesthesia pathway using dental lidocaine

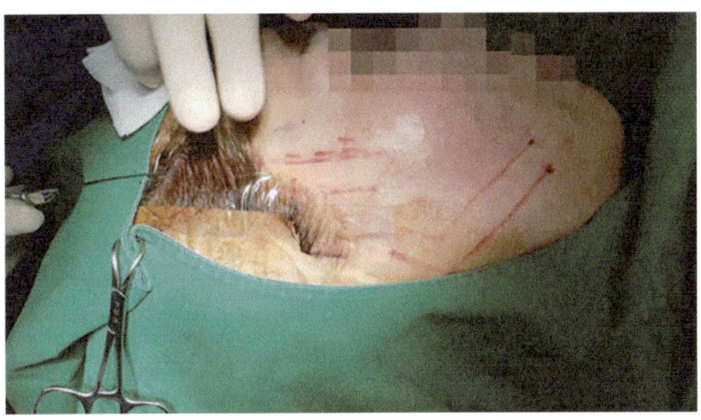

Fig. 7.5 Anesthesia with cannula

to be placed, and then, the anesthetic solution is injected (Figs. 7.5 and 7.6).

When using a needle for anesthesia, there are instances where unexpected bruising at the anesthesia point can cause discomfort.

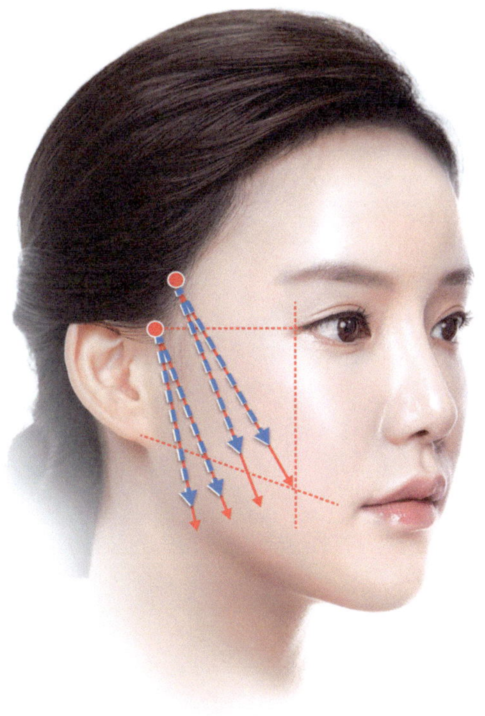

Fig. 7.6 Anesthesia pathway with cannula

However, by injecting the anesthetic through the entry point using a cannula, bruising can almost be 100% prevented, and there is less pain.

However, using a cannula for anesthesia takes more time than using a needle.

7.3 Entry Points

7.3.1 The Position of Entry Point

Lifting essentially involves pulling the skin outward, so it is common to create entry points on the outside of the face (Fig. 7.7). However, recently, instead of pulling the tissue after inserting the thread, a technique that drags the tissue along as the thread is inserted is also widely used (Fig. 7.8). In this case, while the direction of the pull remains the same as in traditional thread lifting, the entry points are created on the opposite side of the classic entry points.

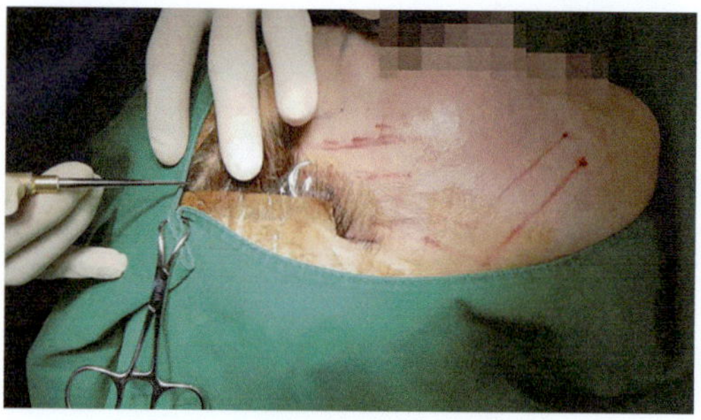

Fig. 7.7 Creating an entry point using an awl

7.3.2 The Number of Entry Point

Once the vector and number of threads to be inserted are determined, the entry point is established, broadly categorized into two types:

Inserting one thread through one hole or inserting multiple threads through one hole (which is most common).

7.3.3 Selection of Entry Point Making Tools

There are two main tools used for creating an entry point: One is a disposable needle, and the other is an awl (Fig. 7.9).

By using an awl to create a hole of the appropriate size, it is possible to make an entry point of the right size while preventing bleeding. The depth should only reach the SQ (subcutaneous) layer; there is no need to make the hole too deep to reach the fascia and muscles.

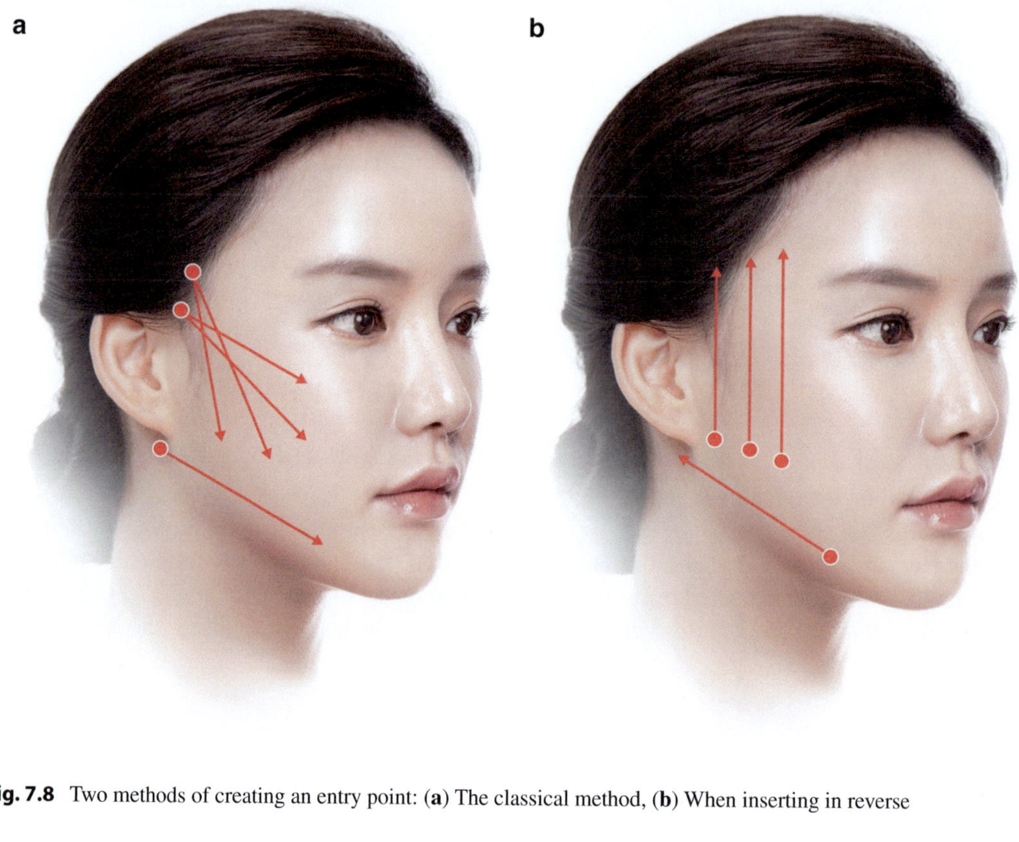

Fig. 7.8 Two methods of creating an entry point: (**a**) The classical method, (**b**) When inserting in reverse

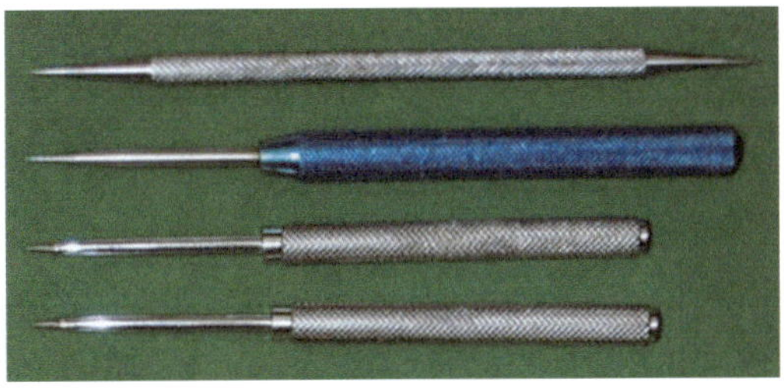

Fig. 7.9 Tools used for creating an entry point

7.3.4 Precautions During Entry Point Puncture—Bleeding (Superficial Temporal Artery and Vein) (Figs. 7.10, 7.11 and 7.12)

Summary

Solutions for bleeding at the entry point

1. Bleeding when creating the entry point—if it stops easily (within seconds to 1 min):
   (a) Small-sized vessel injury.
   (b) It is safe to proceed with thread insertion.
2. Bleeding when creating the entry point—if it does not stop quickly (2–3 min or more):
   (a) Medium-sized vessel injury or damage to the superficial temporal artery (STA)/superficial temporal vein (STV) should be considered. In this case, it is better to create a new entry point.
   (b) Generally, there is a higher chance of no blood vessels area medially to the hairline. Move about 5 mm medially to create a new entry point.
3. Bleeding after thread insertion:
   (a) This is bleeding along the insertion path. It can occur if the blunt cannula is handled too roughly or if a sharp needle is used.
   (b) First, stop the bleeding by pressing and leave the thread as is.
4. Bulging due to bleeding during cannula insertion:
   (a) Occasionally, bulging due to bleeding can occur at the site where the cannula (blunt/sharp) is advancing. In such cases, remove the cannula and do not insert the thread. Extensive hemostasis may be required.

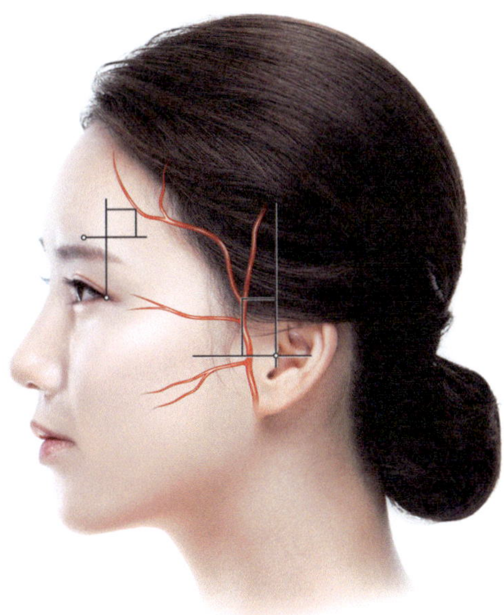

Fig. 7.10 Pathway of superficial temporal artery

Fig. 7.11 Pathway of superficial temporal artery and sentinel vein

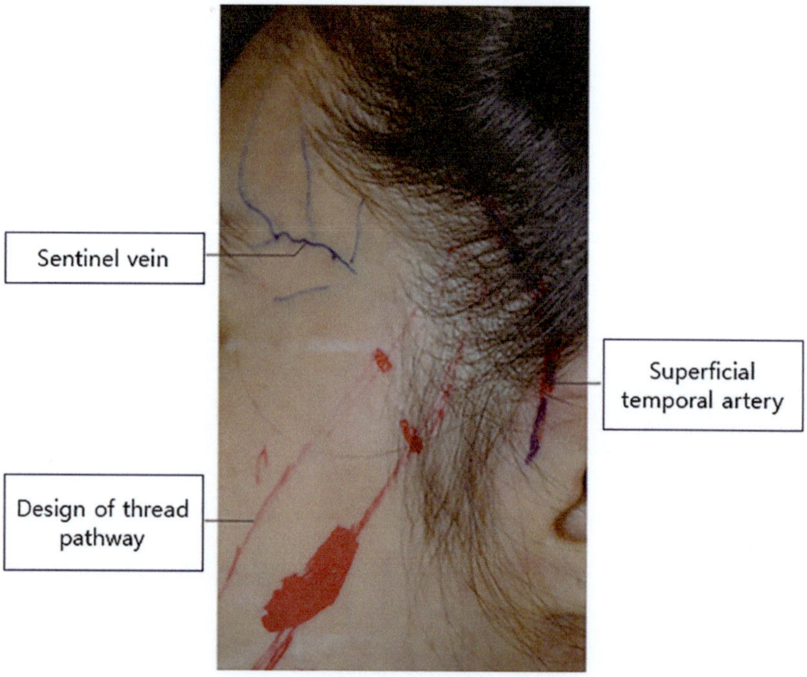

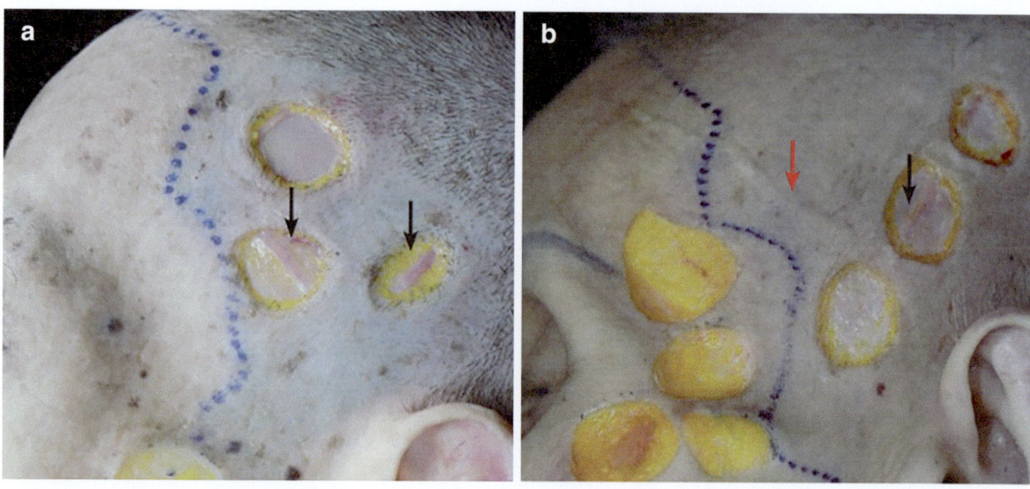

Fig. 7.12 (**a**) Course of the superficial temporal artery near the hairline, (**b**) Depth of the superficial temporal artery near the hairline

7.4 Insertion of Threads

7.4.1 Various Techniques and Insertion Tools

The following classification refers to the level of difficulty in approach and procedure based on the extent of experience, not the quality of the procedure itself. In other words, a skillful advanced user can achieve excellent results with the relatively simple technique of using a disposable cannula, even surpassing those of more advanced techniques.

For beginners.

Insertion using a disposable cannula (Fig. 7.13).

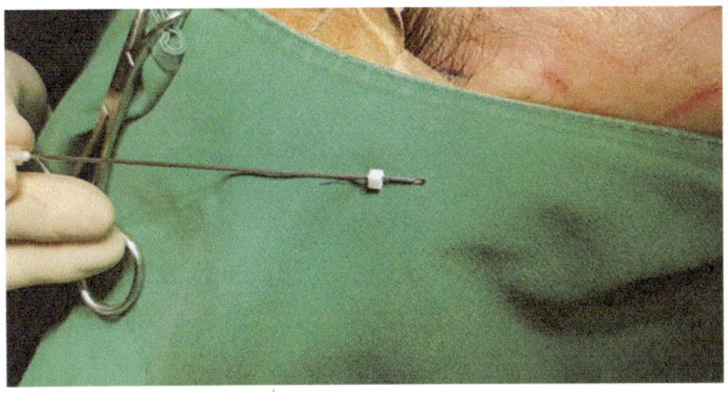

Fig. 7.13 Disposable cannula

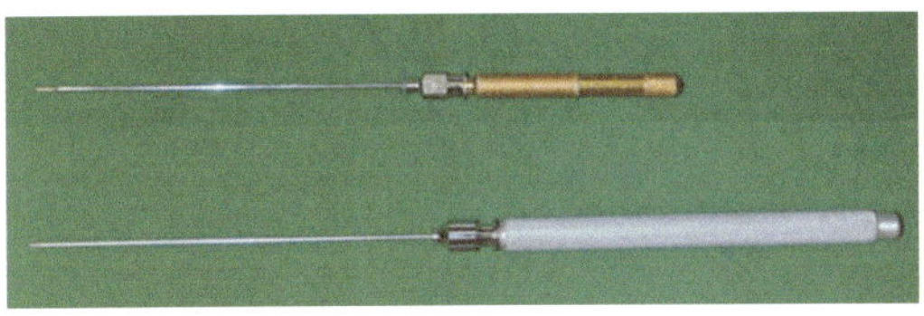

Fig. 7.14 Surgical cannula

For intermediate users.

Inserting the cannula first, followed by the thread.

Insertion using double-arm needle bidirectional cogged threads.

For advanced users.

Temporal fixation (using long threads—longer than 41 cm).

7.4.1.1 Disposable Cannula (Blunt/Sharp Cannula)

The differences between a blunt cannula and a sharp cannula are as follows:

Blunt Cannula

- Lower risk of bleeding.
- More difficult to pass through tissues compared to a sharp cannula.

Sharp Cannula

- Risk of bleeding and nerve damage.
- Can pass through easily (with less force) if depth is well controlled (however, in cases of severe acne scarring, even a sharp cannula may not pass through easily).

The differences between disposable and surgical cannulas are as follows:

Disposable Cannula

- Can potentially reduce procedure time.
- Cannot repeatedly advance and retract the cannula during insertion. Once advanced, it cannot be retracted or removed from the hole. Attempting to retract after advancing can result in the cog threads becoming anchored in the tissue, with only the cannula being pulled out (this becomes problematic if depth control is incorrect mid-procedure). However, slight retraction is possible by pressing on the proximal head of the cannula (the entrance of the cannula and the thread) with the thumb. If even one cog of the thread is already bonded with the tissue, further retraction becomes difficult. Incorrect anchoring of the cogs can occur, necessitating the removal of both the thread and the cannula.
- However, recently, products have been developed that allow for repeated advancement and retraction by equipping a fixed cap on the proximal part where the thread enters the cannula.

Surgical Cannula

- Since separate insertions for the cannula and the thread are required, the procedure time may be longer (Fig. 7.14).
- The cannula can be advanced and retracted repeatedly. If it advances to an unintended depth, it can be pulled back and advanced again.

7.4.2 Insertion of the Thread After Cannula Insertion

The method of inserting a surgical cannula involves first inserting the entire cannula (guide needle + sheath), then removing the guide needle first, and placing the thread into the sheath (in the figure, the long thread is already inserted in a U shape) (Fig. 7.15).

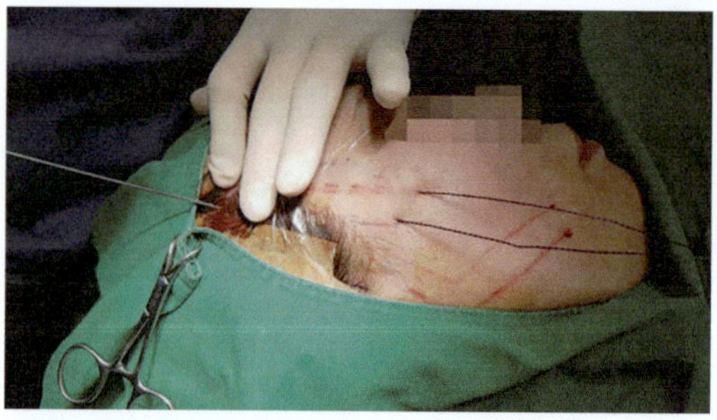

Fig. 7.15 Insertion of surgical cannula

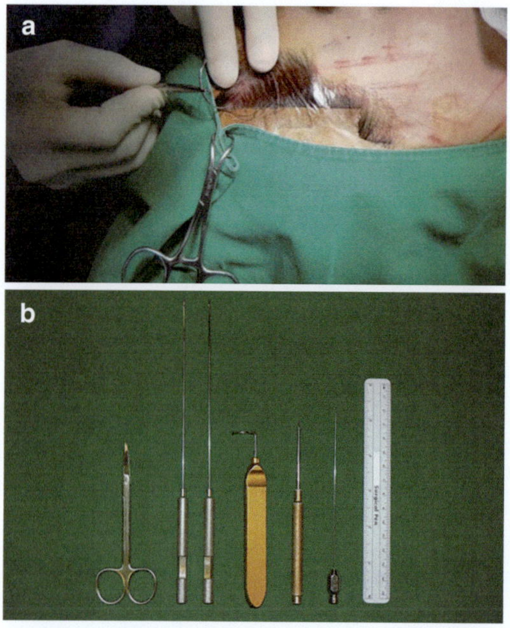

Fig. 7.16 (**a**, **b**) Fixation method in the temple area using a long cannula. (**a**) Scene of anchoring in the temple area using a long needle to insert a long thread. (**b**) Tools required for the procedure. From the left: sterilizing scissors, long cannula set (17 G), temporal ring, awl, cannula for anesthetic injection, and a ruler for design

7.4.3 Temporal Fixation (Long Thread—41 Cm)—U Pattern (Fig. 7.16)

7.4.4 Insertion Using a Thread with Needles Attached at both Ends

Although it is a long thread, it does not require separate tools for insertion, making the procedure simple. It is a bidirectional cog thread, with a section in the middle of the thread that does not have cogs. The thread ends are equipped with needles, making the procedure convenient (Fig. 7.17).

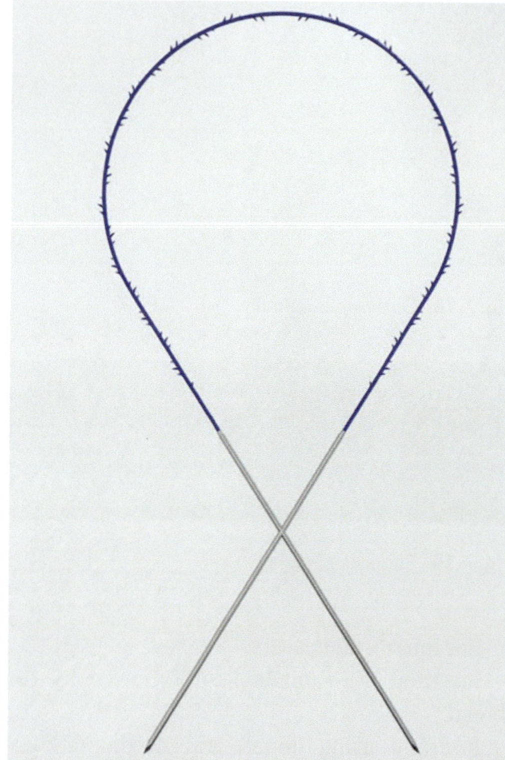

Fig. 7.17 A cogged thread with needles attached in both directions

7.5 Cutting and Finishing

7.5.1 Removal of Cannula

After the thread is secured, use the opposite hand to push the skin upward while removing the cannula. (In the area intended for lifting, push the skin upward using the opposite hand, at a point more superficial than the depth where the thread and cannula are inserted.)

7.5.2 Cutting

7.5.2.1 Cutting while Pulling

Points to Watch

Inconsistent tension on the threads can lead to complications. For example, if one thread is pulled too tightly, the middle of the bidirectional thread may rise, while the other thread remains unchanged, leading to localized bulging or depression. This can cause patient dissatisfaction.

Prevention of Complication

When pulling the thread, the procedure assistant should press down about 2–3 cm below the entry point and cut while pushing the skin with sterilizing scissors.

If the midpoint of the thread is positioned at the zygomatic bone level, dissatisfaction can increase due to the prominence of the zygomatic area. Therefore, design and perform the procedure so that the midpoint of the bidirectional cog thread does not coincide with the zygomatic bone level.

7.5.2.2 Cutting with Sterilizing Scissors while Slightly Pushing the Skin

Cut the thread without pulling it, using sterilizing scissors while pushing the skin, and then, cover the thread well with skin to ensure the end of the thread is not exposed (embedding). The end of the thread should not be close to the exit point. To prevent dimpling, ensure that the end of the thread maintains a distance of at least 5 mm from the exit point through proper embedding.

Various Techniques for Thread Lifting

8

Contents

S. M. Oh et al., *The Art and Science of Thread Lifting Based on Pinch Anatomy and Moving Plane*,
https://doi.org/10.1007/978-981-97-5516-5_8

8.1 Basic Techniques Using the Mono-Thread

8.1.1 Mono-Thread Insertion

In traditional thread lifting theory, it is explained that directionality occurs toward the side where more threads are inserted (Figs. 8.1 and 8.2).

It is challenging to regard the mono-thread injection method as effective procedure for lifting. The concept of a fixing point is fundamentally unclear, and the theoretical basis for directionality is presumed to arise from the contraction of subcutaneous fat tissue, suggesting that the lifting force may not be substantial. The authors will provide a more detailed discussion on this matter later.

Consequently, efficacy, consistency, and durability of procedure may vary depending on the practitioner (Fig. 8.3). However, from an empirical standpoint, when an adequate amount of threads is inserted in the right location and manner, the cosmetic outcomes have generally been favorable. This technique has been used for an extended period and is still widely used today.

The theoretical explanation for this procedure is illustrated in Figs. 8.1 and 8.2. It shows when threads are placed in two areas, the tissue is drawn toward the side where more threads have been inserted.

Based on tissue experiment results presented in the book "Dissolvable Threads: Regenerative Medicine Using Physical Stimuli" by Yoon Jeong-hyun et al., and papers written by the authors, we aim to deduce the theoretical foundation for mono-thread injection. The histological changes resulting from PDO thread insertion can be summarized as follows (Table 8.1).

The effect of mono-thread insertion for thread lifting can be considered more as a restoration of elasticity by inducing neocollagenesis in sagging tissues, rather than true lifting in its strictest sense. Considering the changes due to aging in adipose tissue, fibrous tissue, and skin, and taking into account the tissue changes after thread insertion, the following transformations can be inferred:

1. The insertion of mono-threads can lead to a reduction in the protrusion of the fat layer due to the fat cell denaturation with the proliferation and contraction of fibrous tissue. The decrease in the size of the fat layer results in a reduction of the protruding parts of the face, leading to a tightening effect as the face appears more contoured inward.
2. New fibrous tissues are formed and simultaneously connect with the existing surrounding

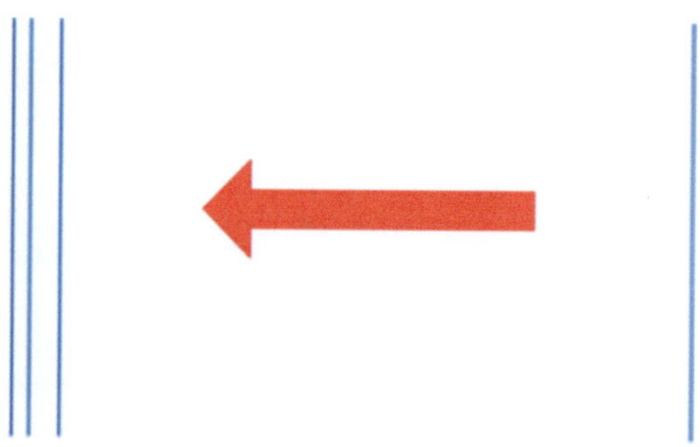

Fig. 8.2 Direction of tissue movement after mono-thread insertion according to the difference of thread numbers on the same plane

Fig. 8.1 Direction of tissue movement after mono-thread insertion according to the difference of thread numbers depending on the depth

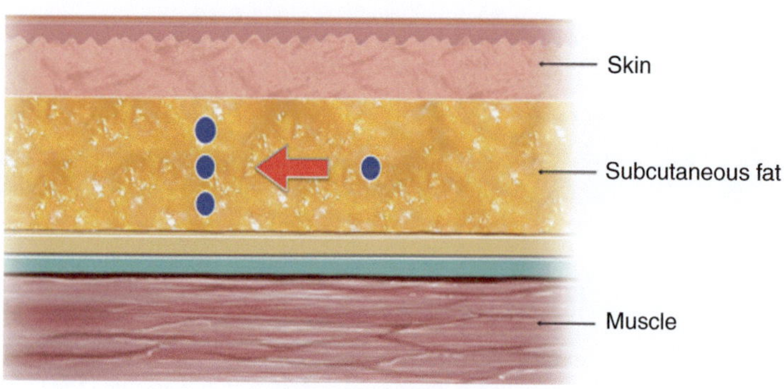

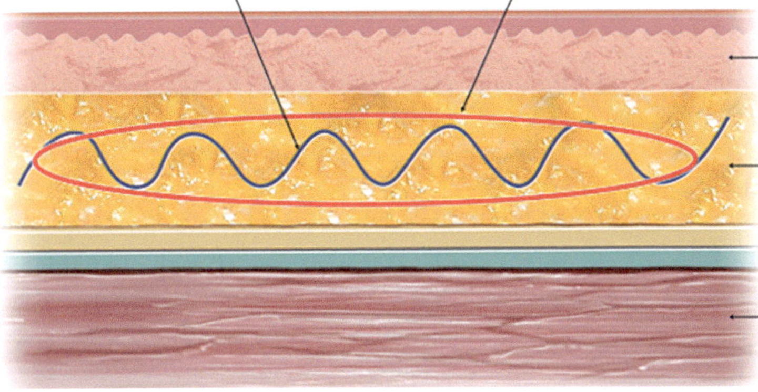

Fig. 8.3 When inserting into the subcutaneous fat layer, the thread is placed in a wavy pattern to maximize contact with the fat layer

Table 8.1 Tissue changes after PDO thread insertion

Newly developed fibrous connective tissue
Merging effect with existing fibrous connective tissue
Tissue contraction by myofibroblast
Increased capillary vessel size
Fat cell denaturation

fibrous tissues. As a result, the structure of the subcutaneous fibrous tissue becomes denser and stronger.

3. Tissue contraction effects occur due to myofibroblasts formed around the inserted threads, pulling the sagging facial skin inward.
4. An increase in neovascularization improves the environment of the skin layer and surrounding tissues.

8.1.2 Expected Outcomes Based on the Mono-Thread Procedure

Based on the tissue changes after mono-thread injection mentioned above, when the thread is injected into the fat layer, it is expected to cause adipocyte degeneration, fibrosis, and tissue contraction changes. The various changes observed by clinicians in the actual clinical setting after mono-thread insertion can be explained through this mechanism.

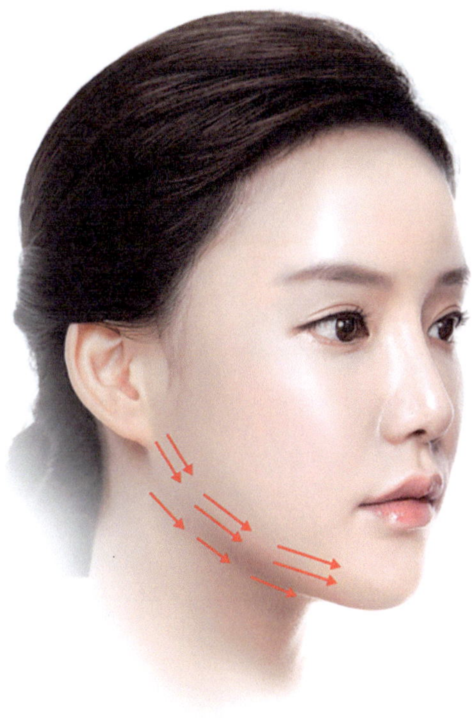

Fig. 8.4 Mono-threads are inserted above and below along the neckline

8.1.3 Procedure Method

8.1.3.1 Treatment of Neck Line

To enhance the jawline, PDO mono-threads are inserted above and below the jawline (Fig. 8.4).

By inducing adipose tissue degeneration and fibrous tissue adhesion, a more defined jawline is created.

When PDO is inserted in a wavy pattern traversing the subcutaneous fat layer and the SMAS layer, as the thread dissolves, it undergoes a fibrosis process, which can lead to the formation of fibrous tissue over a broader area and an increase in tissue elasticity (Fig. 8.3).

In practice, there has been a trend of injecting in a wavy pattern, moving through the upper and lower parts of the fat layer, rather than injecting at a uniform depth.

8.1.3.2 Mono-Thread Technique for Inner Cheek

The anatomical explanations about the reason for bulging of the inner cheek area are as follows—due to an empty space between the risorius m. and zygomaticus major, the SMAS is not continuous and an empty space is created. Deep fat tissues which are stretched from aging push and come out mainly through this area (Fig. 8.5).

The mechanism of procedures on the inner cheek using the PDO mono-threads is using the effect of fat denaturation, fibrosis effect, and tissue contraction effect of the PDO (Fig. 8.6).

On one hand, in case of using a hard PDO twister-type thread in a spring form, an effect of pressing fat which sticks out like by causing the muscles to cover fat in this area may be expected. In reality, the twister-type PDO in a spring form is expected to have an effect of pressing tissues and volumizing effects and is used in various areas.

8.1.3.3 Mono-Thread Technique—Frontal Cheek and Nasolabial Area

Drooping frontal cheek areas are elements which aggravate the nasolabial folds. Through inserting mono-threads in the area where the frontal cheek

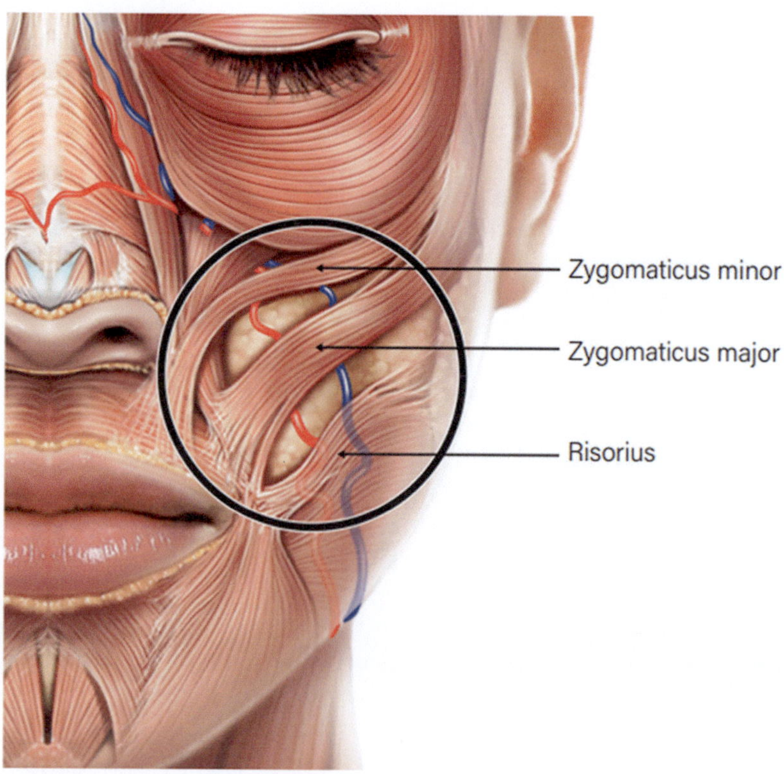

Fig. 8.5 Anatomical finding about the fat bulging of inner cheek

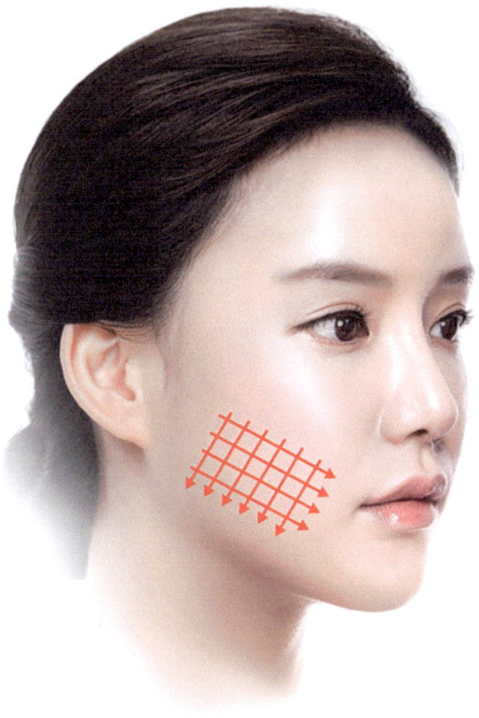

Fig. 8.6 Mono-thread technique—method of performing procedures to make entering of jowl

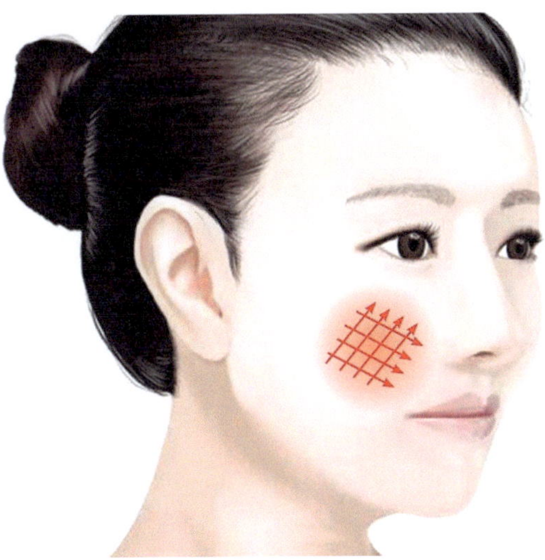

Fig. 8.7 Mono-thread technique—frontal cheek and nasolabial area

droops above the nasolabial fold, conglutination of fibrotic tissues and contraction of fat cells may be expected. As a result, there is effect of pushing the bulging frontal cheek in slightly.

If a slightly thicker and harder spring-type mono-filament is inserted from the cheek to over the nasolabial fold area, an effect of reducing the frontal cheek is by pressing with the force of the hard PDO thread (Fig. 8.7).

8.2 Basic Techniques Using the Cogged Threads

8.2.1 Unidirectional Cog Thread

After inserting the cogs to be hung on tissues, pull them in one direction. The lifting effect is maintained only if the fixing point of thread is made in anyway.However, based on the structure and mechanism of the thread, it is difficult to maintain lifting effect. Nowadays, this type of thread is used for limited cases (Fig. 8.8).

8.2.2 Spike-Type Cog Thread

Threads in a spike form are used for fixing after performing lifting using bidirectional cog threads, etc. First, among various techniques of thread lifting, after dissecting of the layer to which the thread is to be inserted, if the thread in a spike form is inserted into such layer after adjusting the up and down direction well, it plays the function of fixing the dissected and dislocated plane. When lifting through plane dissection is performed, spike form thread is useful rather than cog thread (Fig. 8.9).

The following matters need to be considered in performing a spike thread procedure.

- It is advisable to insert for fixing in the area where tissues are dislocated through dissection.

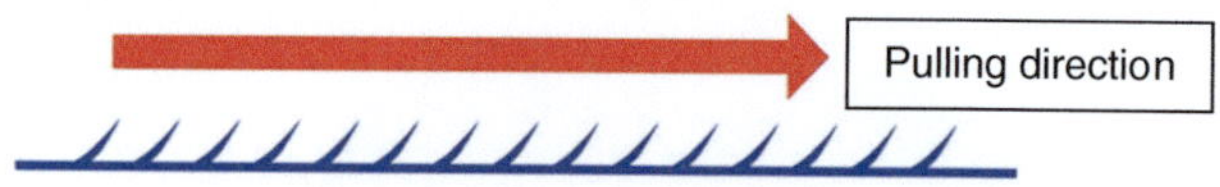

Fig. 8.8 Unidirectional cog. It can be fixed after pulling tissue in one direction

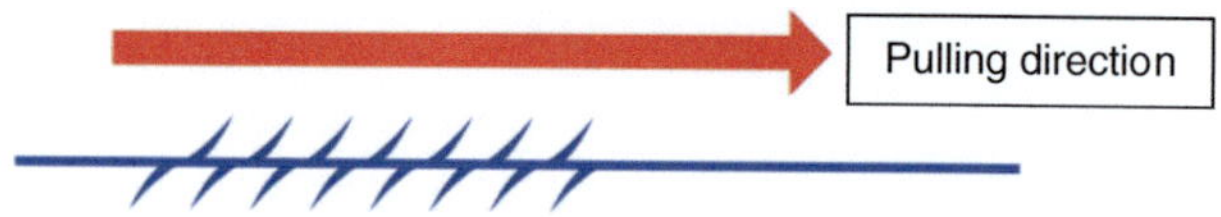

Fig. 8.9 Spike-type cog thread. Rather than the function of pulling tissue, it stabilizes already pulled tissue, and the up and down direction is important

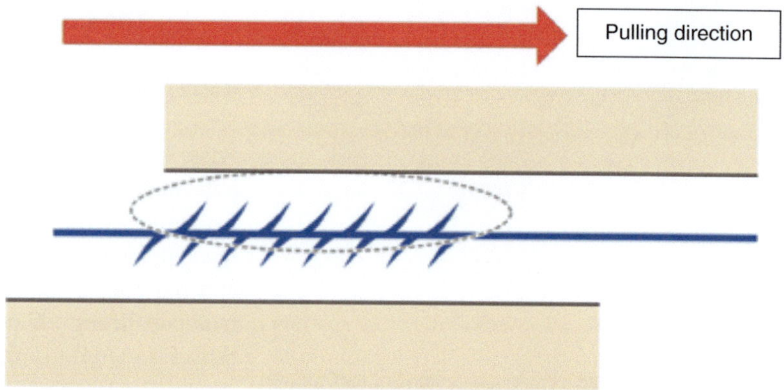

Fig. 8.10 Right insertion direction: pulled tissues can be stabilized

- It is advisable to insert accurately on the surface where the upper board and the lower board are separated through dissection and the direction of cogs is very important. After accurately finding out the direction of lifting, the spike thread must be inserted. The pulled direction and the lying direction of cogs in the upper side of the thread must coincide (Fig. 8.10).
- If it is inserted into an opposite direction, fixing does not occur and it slips, not stabilizing the pulled tissues (Fig. 8.11). Surely, this will not be able to maintain the lifting effect.

Through Fig. 8.10, it can be seen well which side the top and bottom of spike cogs must be. Lifting can be maintained only if the spike cog is inserted in the direction which prevents driving which returns in the direction that is opposite from the pulled direction.

On the other hand, based on Fig. 8.11, if the direction of cogs cannot prevent the movement of the tissue to return to the original position, pulled tissue would be slipped. Therefore, when spike threads are used, direction is very important.

8.2.3 Zigzag Method

The mechanism of the bidirectional zigzag cog method is as follows:

- The cog thread of the zigzag method is largely used for fixing pulled tissues after performing lifting rather than for lifting itself.
- After lifting procedure using bidirectional cog threads, to prevent side effects like sinking, zigzag threads are sometimes inserted supplementary (Fig. 8.12).

8.2.4 Engraved Thread

This thread does not rely on the physical anchoring of tissue by the cog's force; instead, it allows new collagen to grow into the engraved areas within the thread, securing the lifted tissue in place. The amount of collagen produced around such threads is proportional to the surface area of the thread. Therefore, threads with an engraved design, having relatively larger contact surfaces

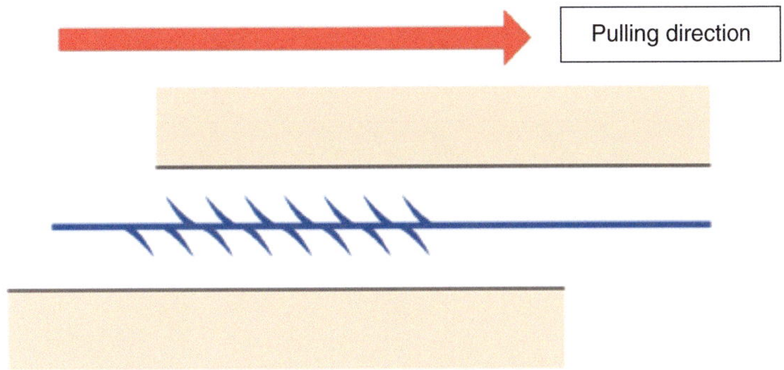

Fig. 8.11 Wrong insertion direction. This cannot stabilize the pulled tissues

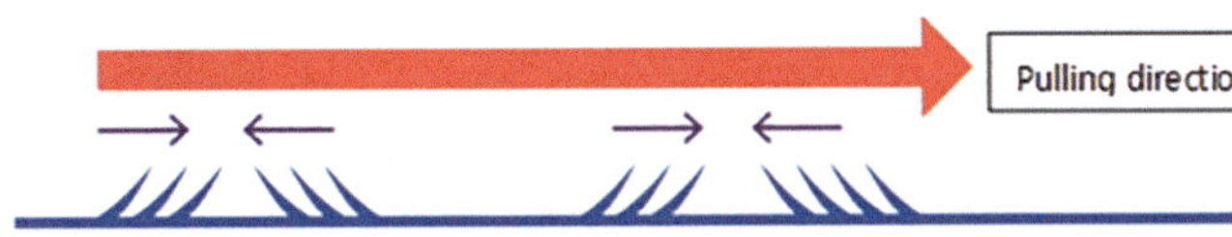

Fig. 8.12 Zigzag method (multi-bidirectional cog). It holds the pulled tissue in place throughout the midsection

Fig. 8.13 Engraved cog thread

with surrounding tissues, facilitate the formation of a significant amount of collagen through neo-collagenesis. As a result, this leads to a robust tissue fixation effect (Fig. 8.13).

8.2.5 Bidirectional Cog

8.2.5.1 Understanding Bidirectional Cog

Bidirectional cogs consist of forward cogs which plays the role of pulling and reverse cogs which play the role of fixing the pulled tissues not to go down (Fig. 8.14).

In the end, it has effects of lifting the tissues in both sides to the middle part without any cog. It has better effect than unidirectional cogs (Figs. 8.15, 8.16 and 8.17).

By causing the tissues in the middle part to be gathered, the bidirectional cogs show lifting effects. In actual practice, it is also important to understand the function of the area where the cog thread enters subcutaneous. The entry point area of the thread inevitably passes beneath of the dermis, the cog thread tends to be hung hard at that point. Lifting effects can be maximized by using the effect of gathering tissues to the middle area and the effect of cogs in the opposite direction of the cog thread hanging in the bottom of the dermis well.

As seen in the figure, the accurate function of bidirectional cog threads is not to pulling one direction, but to gather to the middle part. Namely, it can be understood as a method of pulling both sides to the middle area. If design and procedures are performed with well understanding of this mechanism, good result can be expected.

By using such characteristics of the bidirectional cogs, the sunken facial area can be adjusted. If there are adequate design and technical support for the facial shape, lifting in any form is possible.

Experiment on actual bidirectional cogs (Fig. 8.18)

1. After preparing a wide area in the subcutaneous fat layer of pork, areas below the muscle layer were removed.
2. After inserting a 19 G bidirectional cog thread to the skin perpendicularly, progress was made in a consistent depth through the subcutaneous layer by changing the direction horizontally.
3. After removing the cannula, the cog thread was pulled.
4. Changes were observed thereafter.

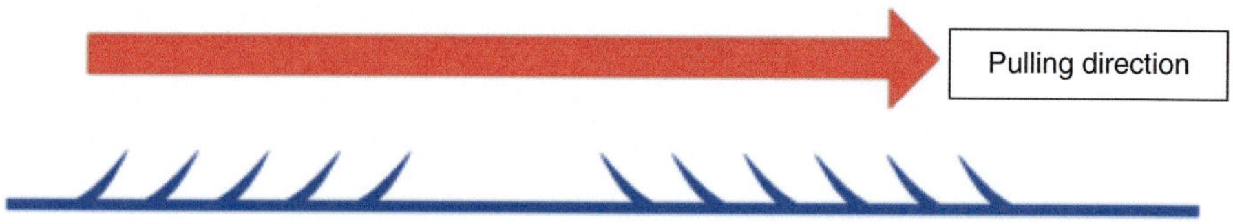

Fig. 8.14 Bidirectional cog

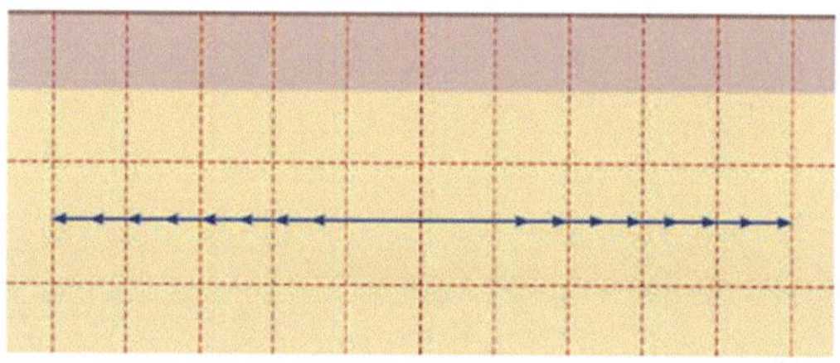

Fig. 8.15 After simple insertion

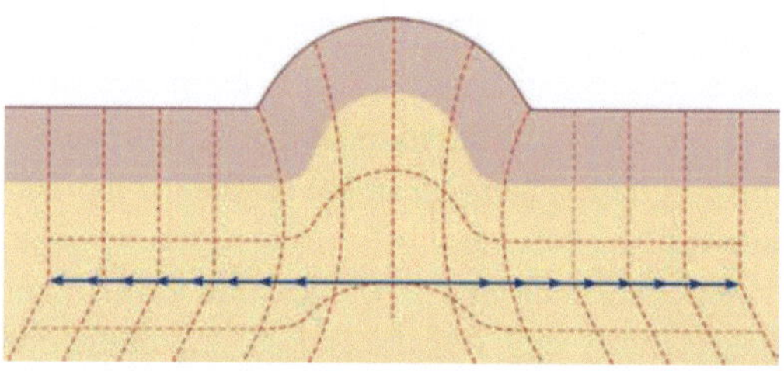

Fig. 8.16 Pulled after insertion. If this is used wrongly, it can be a cause of side effect

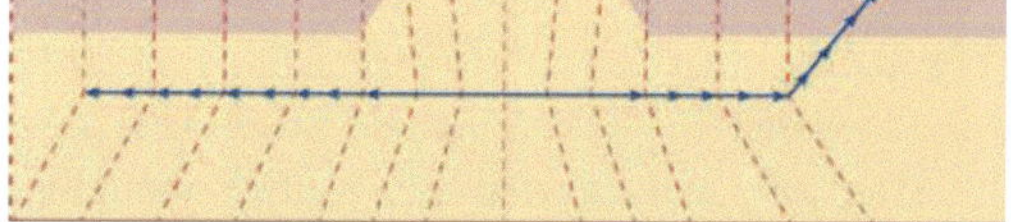

Fig. 8.17 Actual practice with bidirectional cogs

The appearance after inserting the bidirectional cog thread into the subcutaneous layer and pulling in one direction can be seen. Although it is slightly distant from the thread entry site, when it is seen through a cutting surface, it can be seen that the subcutaneous fat layer that coincides with the middle area of the cogs is gathered and inflated. If the procedures are performed after

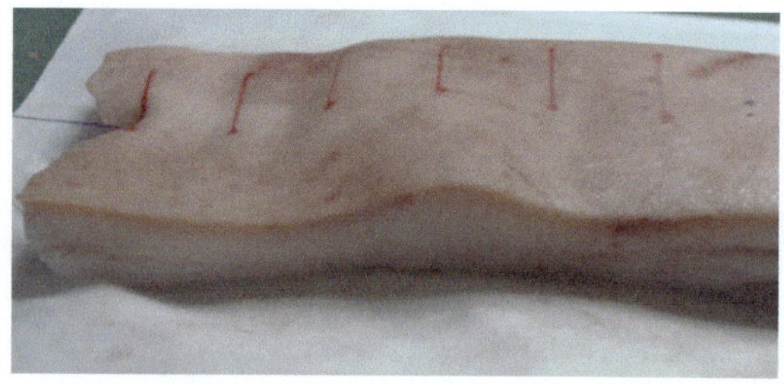

Fig. 8.18 Traction test of bidirectional cogs

understanding the mechanism well, it has the effect of gathering tissues as well as the effect of lifting, namely, the effect of volumizing through re-disposition.

8.2.5.2 Angle Technique Using Bidirectional Cogs

The angle technique can be understood as an expansion of bidirectional cogs. As mentioned previously, bidirectional cogs create lifting effects by repositioning tissues to the middle where there is no cog. In case of the angle technique, by causing the angle to be slightly bent, rather than in straight line, it is a method of causing the tissues inside the bent angle to gather (Fig. 8.19).

It has effects of adjusting sinking, together with lifting effects and various designs are possible. Insert the cannula with threads and proceed, then deflect the direction at angle point and insert to the end (Fig. 8.20). Remove the cannula from the skin and pull the thread to make the tissue inflated.

8.2.5.3 V Technique (Bending and Fixing) (Fig. 8.21)

8.2.5.4 Tying Method

Tying method means that tying of the cog thread at the fixing point. Thickened tie enters inside the

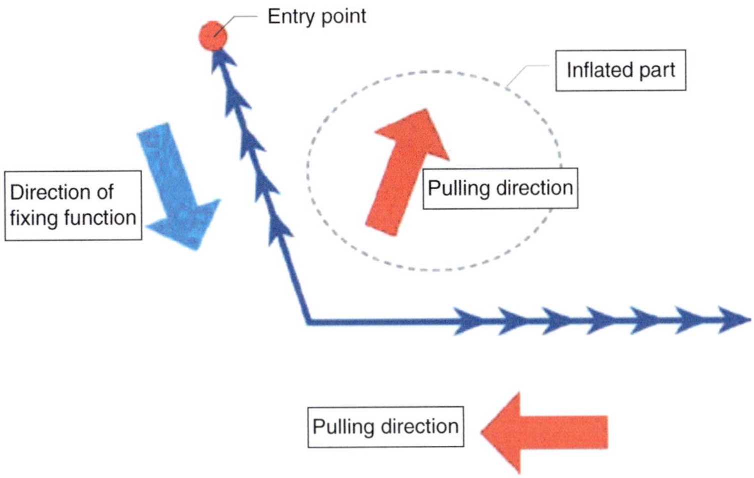

Fig. 8.19 Bidirectional cog thread technique—concept of angle technique

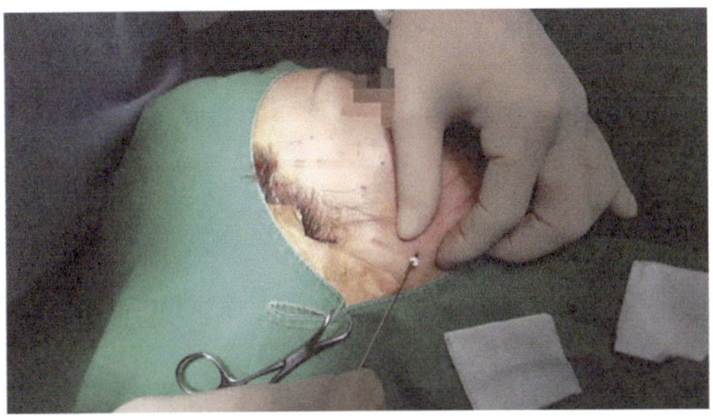

Fig. 8.20 Technique of bidirectional cog thread—insertion of angle technique

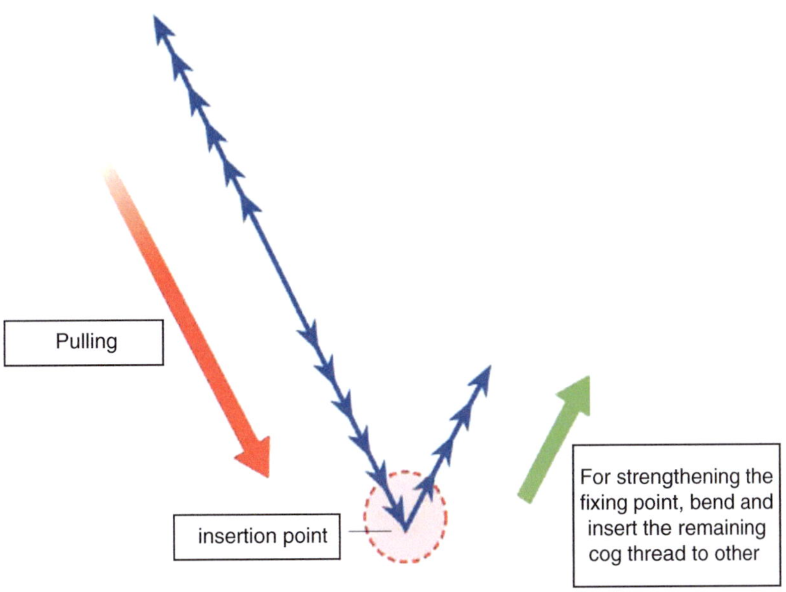

Fig. 8.21 The remaining cog is not discarded but used for its fixing function

skin thereafter and acts as a stronger fixing point than simple cog thread insertion using uni- or bidirectional cogs (Fig. 8.22).

8.2.5.5 X-Cross Technique

To strengthen and maintain the lifting effect, it is important to utilize reverse directional cogs. In general, remaining cogs are removed after desired length of insertion. In some case, a significant amount of reverse directional cogs is cut out.

To optimize the lifting effect, it is important to vitalize the function of reverse cogs. In such case, without removing the remaining cogs, the method of pushing them toward the opposite direction can be used. In addition, by tying the middle part of the cog thread, it can be combined with the method of making one more area which can act as a fixing point. By using the two skills together, it is a method of strengthening the function of the fixing points (Fig. 8.23).

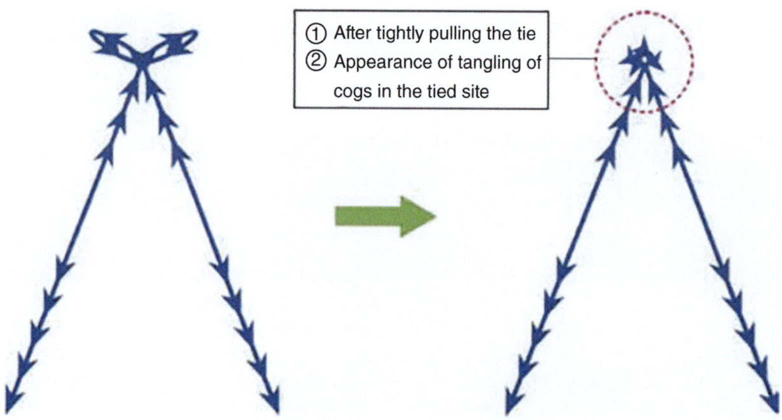

Fig. 8.22 Method of tying cog thread

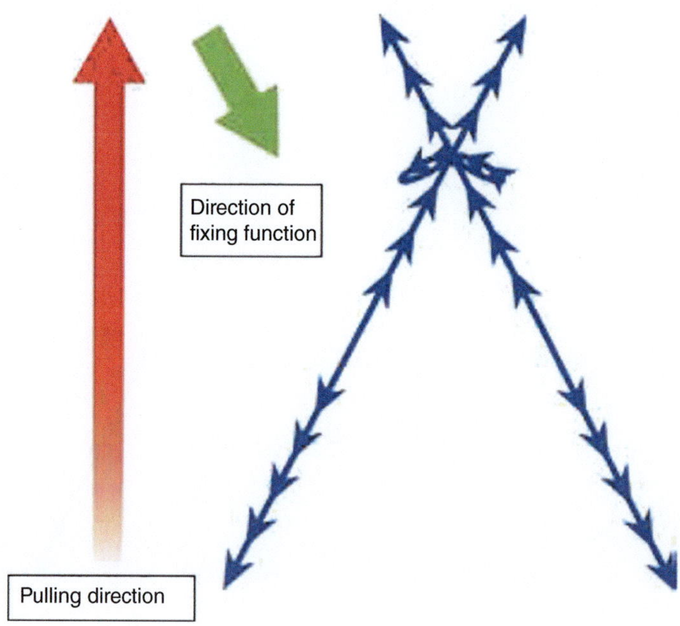

Fig. 8.23 Bidirectional cog thread technique—the X-cross technique concept has the advantage of using the remaining opposite-directional cogs without having to throw them out

8.3 Techniques of Tagging the Long Cogged Threads to the Temples

8.3.1 Mechanism

The difference between the lifting of the anchoring method and others using mono-thread or cog thread is that it can make strong fixing point (Fig. 8.24).

It is ideal to anchor a thread in the fascia of the anchoring site. If the thread is anchored in the subcutaneous fat layer, the fixing force is weak. Understanding the changes in the tissues that occur when pinch manipulation is performed at the temple area, the thread can be reliably anchored to the fascia layer. Thread should be appropriately anchored to temple area fascia by pinch manipulation where there are no large vessels. After the anchoring is done properly, the remaining thread is inserted to the subcutaneous layer and exit out to perform the lifting procedure (Fig. 8.25). The pulled skin is placed in a folded state at the anchored area. And it is maintained by cogs of thread. The instant result is stronger than the mono-thread method and the simple cog thread lifting procedures. The longevity is determined by the strength of the cogs, efficiency of the cogs, sustainability of threads, and expertise of the physician.

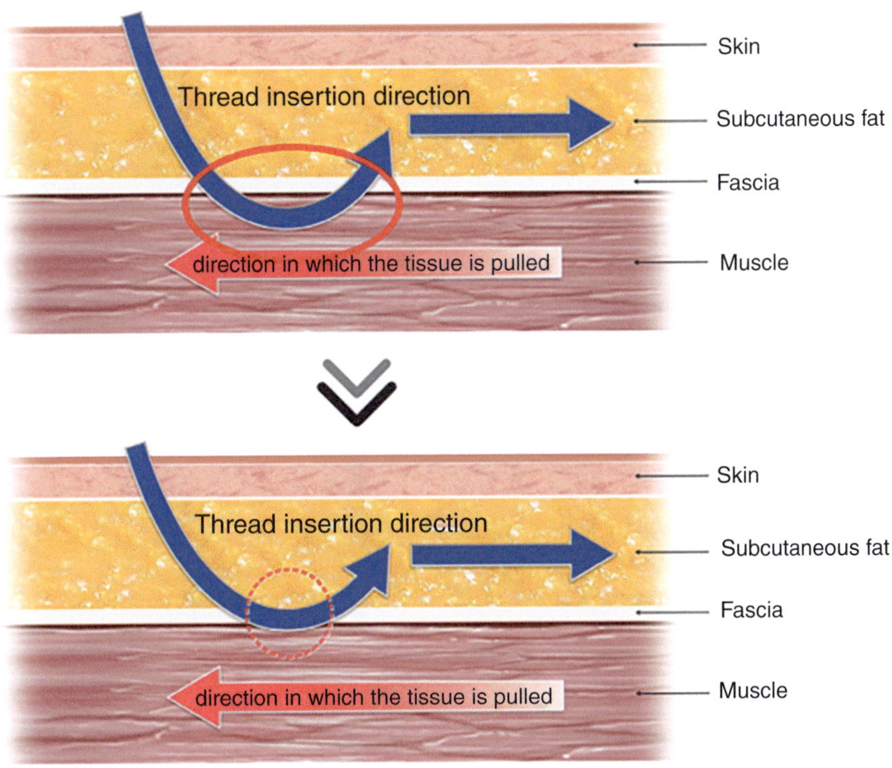

Fig. 8.24 Fascia anchoring method: This shows the mechanism of hanging the thread in the fascia and making a fixing point

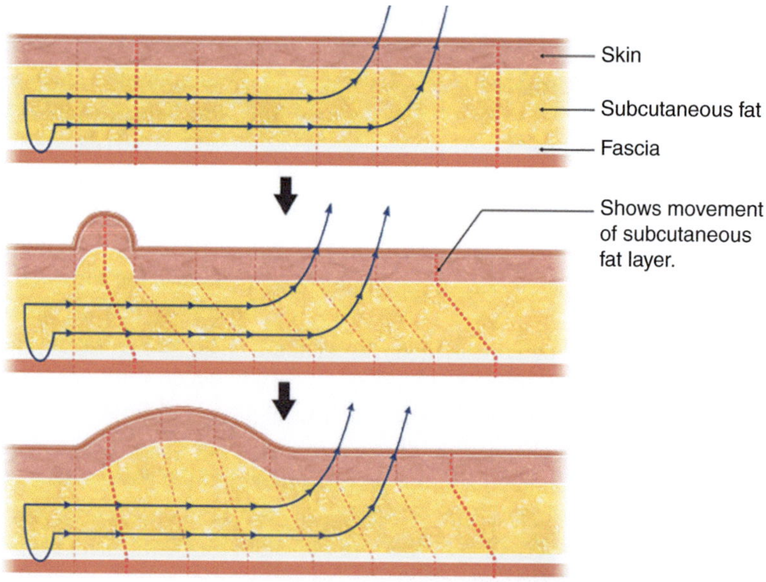

Fig. 8.25 Understanding of lifting mechanisms about fascia anchoring method: Pulled tissues gather in at some point between the fixing point and the exit

8.3.2 Insertion Method

8.3.2.1 Design

Summary Design Method (Fig. 8.26)

Facial landmarks and reference line

(a) Horizontal line at the lateral canthus

(b) Perpendicular line at the lateral canthus(c) Line connecting from the oral commissure to the lobule

(d) Horizontal line from the end of the eyebrow

Mark a reference line inside the hairline

Perpendicular line (h) at the center of the tragus (e),

(f) Temporal crest it appears simultaneously with masseter muscle contraction.

Entry point

Assuming that the quad circle located from approximately 2 finger breadth from the crossing point of (e) and (f), is (h), it is convenient to set an entry point therein. If you make an entry point higher than this, it is difficult to handle the cannula because of the curved surface of the skull. If lower than this, you may cause damage to the anterior branch of the STA(superficial temporal artery) resulting in massive bleeding.

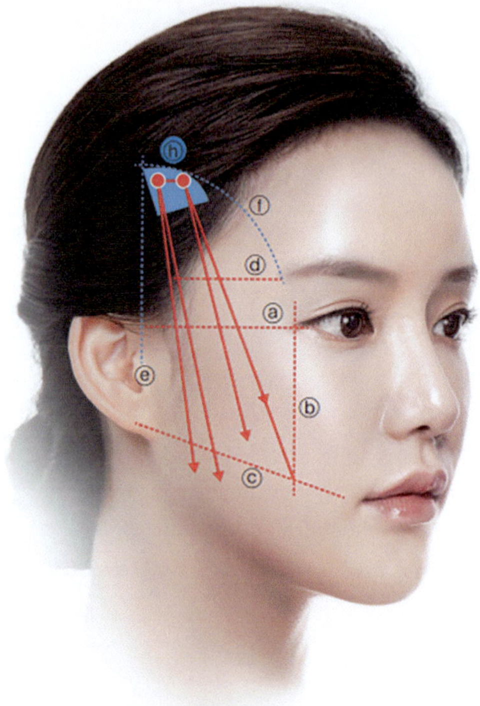

Fig. 8.26 Design of the fascia anchoring method

Summary Key Considerations when Designing

Prevention of slanted eyes and sentinel vein rupture

If the innermost thread is near to the lateral canthus, the lateral canthus may be lifted after the procedure. In some cases with young patients, they desire lifting of the lateral canthus, but patients in their mid to elder ages generally consider lifting of the lateral canthus to be unnatural. Therefore, it is necessary to explain about the lateral canthus rising and if that is not desired, the design of thread pathway should not be done so closed to the lateral canthus. It is advisable to distance at least two finger breadths away from the lateral canthus (Fig. 8.27). When designing as above, it will not overlap the running of sentinel vein.Prevention of aggravation of fine wrinkles under the eyes

With the rising of the lateral canthus, when the infra-orbital skin is pulled, the fine wrinkles below the eyes may appear deeper. This can be prevented to a certain extent by designing the thread to pass through two finger breadths away from the lateral canthus. During designing, by actually pulling the skin with the finger, check whether the under-eye wrinkles become deeper together with whether the lateral canthus lifts or not.

Passing the sunken cheek must be prevented

Cautions to be taken at the area of frequent dimples

When the exit of the thread is located medially, it is advisable to stay within the crossing points of the blue dotted line (limit line) and Fig. 8.28 (3) and (4). If the exit is medial passing the crossing point, the lifting effect of the mouth sagging may become better but due to occurrence of dimples, patient's satisfaction level is more likely to decrease.

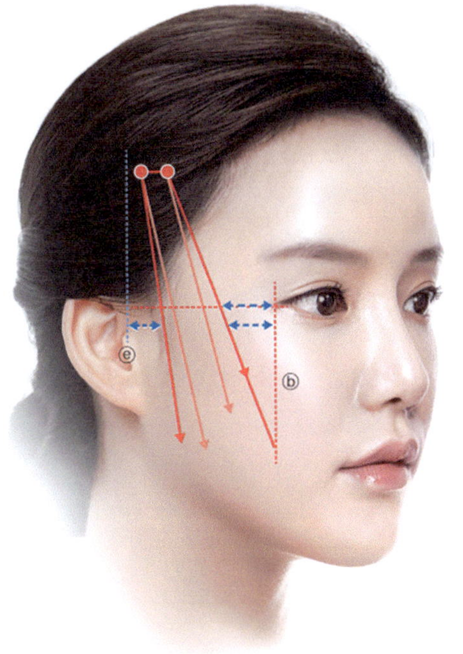

Fig. 8.27 Cautions to be taken in designing the fascia anchoring method—slanted eyes

Be cautious of STA (superficial temporal artery)—1

When designing the pathway of the outermost thread, do not design in the space between the tragus and inner 1 finger breadth where the pulse of STA is strongest. It is advisable to design at least 1.5-2 finger breadth away from center of the tragus (Fig. 8.27). If the distance is closer than this, the likelihood of STA damage becomes high and also, there may be claim of "wrinkling of the skin in front of the ear" after the procedure in patients with skin laxity (Fig. 8.29).

Be cautious of STA—2

The entry point should be within range (h). In some cases, an anterior or parietal branch of STA may run within that range. Before you make entry points, you must check whether you feel pulse (Fig. 8.26).

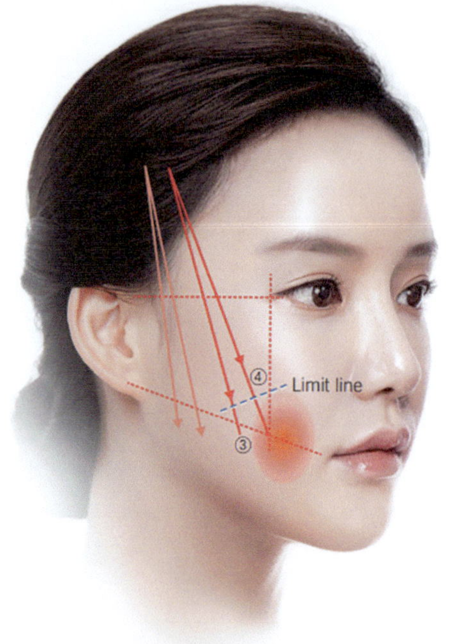

Fig. 8.28 Cautions to be taken in designing the fascia anchoring method—area of frequent dimples

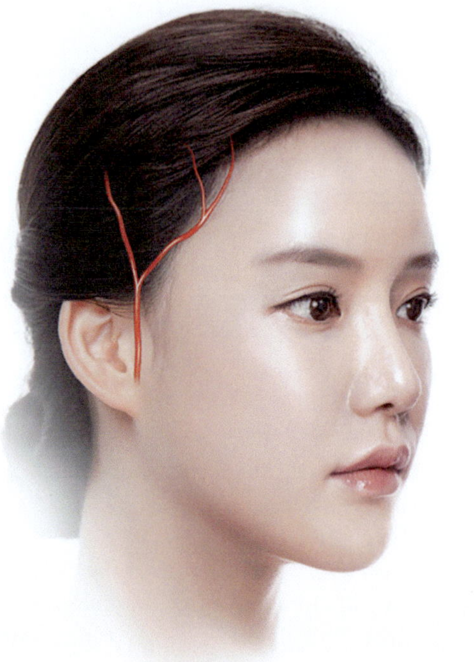

Fig. 8.29 Blood vessels to be cautious in designing the fascia anchoring method—STA (superficial temporal artery)

Summary Hairline Preparation and Draping (Fig. 8.30)

Hairline preparation

Either cut few pieces of hair with scissors or shave using a shaver. In preparing the hairline, all hair in the opposite area to the progression direction as well as the progression direction must be prepared. Preparing the hair pieces to the minimum extent is necessary for the easy post-treatment management. Unexpected bleeding can occur severely in some cases in anchoring threads in the temporal areas. In such case, we must change the anchoring location inevitably. Considering this, it is advisable to prepare the hairline enough to allows anchoring twice.

Fixing

Prepare the nearby hairline using the Fixomer®, Tegaderm®, hairpins, rubber bands, 3 M, etc.

If procedures are performed without this step completely, it would interfere with the thread insertion a lot. Moreover, if hair gets into the entry point, it can cause folliculitis. Therefore, it is advisable to clean and prepare the hairline prior to the procedure.

Disinfection

In order to prevent foreign substances from getting on the cannula during insertion, areas which touch the cannula or all areas which can touch the cannula, including the hair, must be strictly disinfected.

8.3.2.2 Anesthesia

Anesthesia of Entry and Exit Point—Needle

It is advisable to anesthetize the entry and exit points using lidocaine (1: 100,000) which includes epinephrine. If the exit is not anesthetized, bruising can occur due to the dermal plexus bleeding.

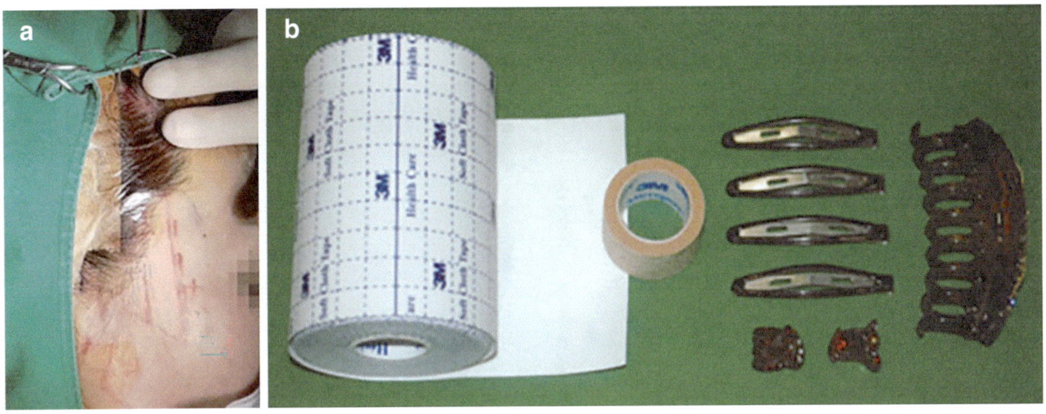

Fig. 8.30 Preparations for the fascia anchoring method—draping and preparing the hairline. A. Showing of attaching a sterile Tegaderm® B. Tools needed to prepare the hairline

Anesthesia of Thread Progression Route

1. Injection of tumescent solution or lower concentration lidocaine using a cannula.
   (a) Proper anesthesia allows smooth cannula insertion during thread lifting. Using very long and thin one can reduce pain but it is difficult to maintain consistent driving depth and easily bends during progression, an adequate thickness is recommended (diameter of 0.9~1.0 mm).
   (b) In lieu of a cannula, there is also a method of injecting anesthetic agents conveniently into various points of thread pathway using needle and dental lidocaine but has some disadvantages.
      - As anesthesia does not occur as desired, it may require additional anesthesia during the thread insertion.
      - If needles are inserted in various places, due to dermal plexus bleeding, likelihood of bruising increases.
2. Lidocaine local anesthesia using needles
   (a) In the long thread lifting procedure, the thread passes through the subcutaneous fat layer. However, as the subcutaneous fat layer is not an area where pain senses are well developed, pain is minimal in general when driving the subcutaneous fat layer except some specific area (mainly vessel crossing area).
   (b) Using this, a small amount of lidocaine is sometimes injected using a needle into the driving route to anesthetize.
      - Advantages are that less swelling occurs after the procedure, the procedure becomes simple and the depth of driving can be learned through finding out patient's pain.
      - On the other hand, compared to anesthetizing the driving route using a cannula, patients can feel pain in the interim and become anxious.

8.3.3 Entry Point and Anchoring

8.3.3.1 Tools for Entry Points

It is suggested to use an awl than a needle.

The advantages of using an awl include a low risk of bleeding due to its blunt nature, and it allows for the creation of sufficiently large holes that make advancing a cannula more convenient, avoiding the friction and difficulty that can arise from smaller holes made out of concern for bleeding.

8.3.3.2 Anchoring Tools

Needle

Temporal Ring

The advantages of using an awl include reduced chances of bleeding and the ease of creating sufficiently large holes that facilitate the insertion of a cannula (Fig. 8.31).

Depth and Direction of Anchoring Point

Various opinions exist on where to fix the thread, including the periosteum, deep temporal fascia (theoretically), superficial temporal fascia, and deep subcutaneous layer, each with its own theoretical basis.

Tip!

In some cases where SQ tissues at the anchoring point are too loose

In the process of pulling the thread after the insertion, in some cases, loose SQ tissues cannot attach and hold to the thread and the thread is dragged down from the anchoring point. Even if the SQ tissues are relatively dense, if the physician pulls the thread too strongly, the same can occur. Therefore, an assistant must press the anchoring point with fingers when the thread is pulled.

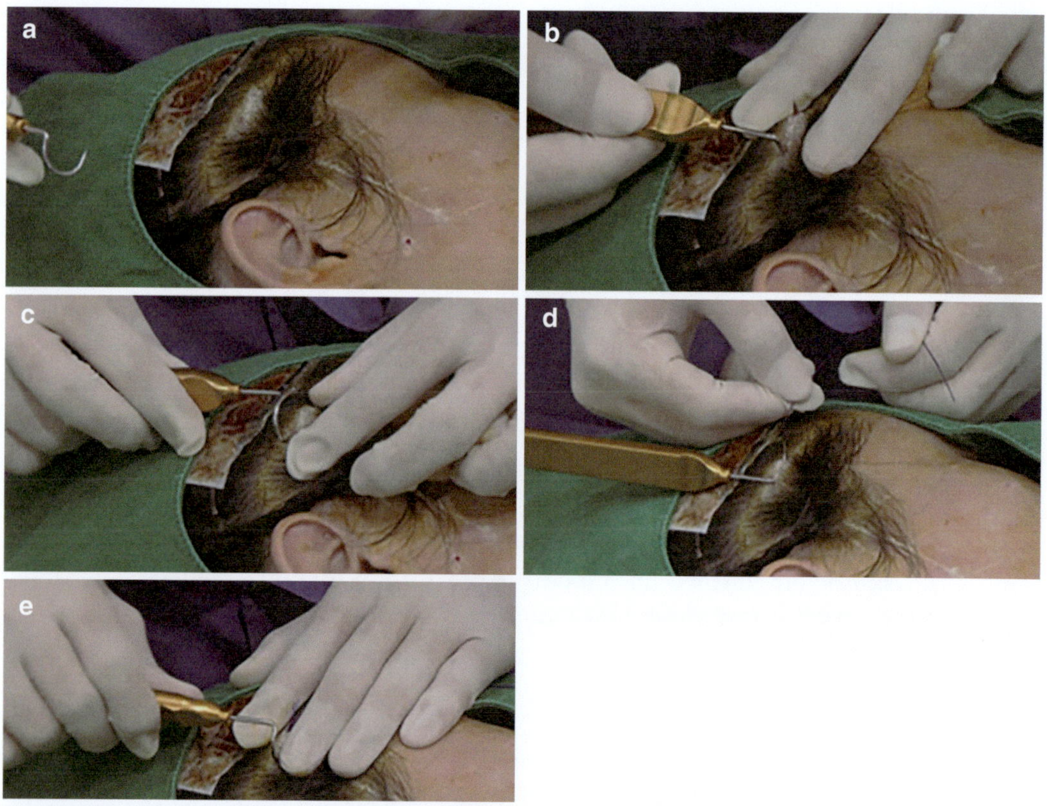

Fig. 8.31 Tools for the fascia anchoring method (temporal ring) (**a**) Hold the temporal ring (**b**) Between the two entry points, insert one side first (in this case, the two entry points can be made in advance using an awl or a needle). (**c**) After anchoring by revolving the temporal ring, exit to the opposite entry point (Cause the ring to come out partially to the extent of exposing the hole in the temporal ring). (**d**) Put the thread in the hole at the end of the ring. (**e**) Take out the temporal ring by revolving again in the direction opposite from the insertion

An entry point can be located in the line of the temporal crest (namely, much more above than the area in Fig. 8.26). In such case, there are advantages of reducing bleeding which can occur during temporal fascia anchoring and anchoring to more solid tissues (periosteum). However, differently from the structure of skull of westerners, as in many cases, Asians have triangular skull (not trigonocephaly, but the skull is more developed than the size of the face), it is not easy for a cannula to drive along the curve at a consistent depth.

Based on Michael A. Carron, etc., when anchoring is performed in the fascia area of the temporalis muscle, it has been discovered that the resistance against the pulling power is stronger in the horizontal method than in the vertical method. (1.9 vs 5.01, tearing force kg/cm) (Fig. 8.32).

Yi and Oh have conducted cadaver studies on anchoring in the zygomatic region, focusing on areas with a relatively low risk of bleeding. According to their research, there is an appropriate site for anchoring in the deep temporal fascia area, located midway between the superior and inferior temporal lines. This finding could be valuable for medical textbooks, offering a clear guide on safe anchoring points.

Summary

Strategies for addressing bleeding when performing anchoring

Bleeding after anchoring with a needle

1. Injury to small blood vessels

   Bleeding may show due to damage of small blood vessels from a sharp needle, after the passing of needle or the thread but if it stopped by pressuring, the inserted thread may continue to proceed.
2. When vessel penetration is suspected

   In some cases, almost no bleeding occurs after a needle pass, but signifi-

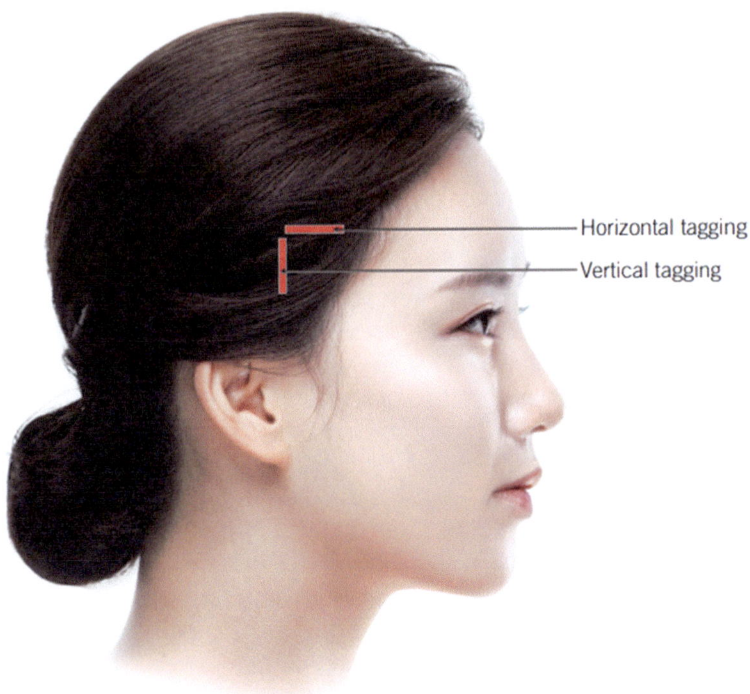

Fig. 8.32 Direction of anchoring

cant bleeding occurs after the thread is put on the needle and then anchored, resulting in swelling in the entry point area. This may be caused by passing of a sharp needle through the middle of a thick blood vessel. As it was fine when the needle passes initially, physician believes that it will stop bleeding soon. But, despite the long pressure, hemostasis is not easy. This is because vessel damage is aggravated when a thread penetrates a blood vessel. In such case, it is advisable to cut the middle of the bidirectional thread and remove it. Thereafter, pressure for a sufficient period to stop bleeding and perform the procedure again with another entry point elsewhere.

Bleeding after anchoring with a temporal ring

As the ring is thicker than a needle, even an injury occurs during anchoring process blood will not emerge at the entry point immediately. After putting the thread and passing, bleeding shows. If bleeding does not easily stop, in such case also, the thread needs to be removed and discarded.

→ Differently from a needle, a temporal ring is thicker, forming a tunnel through anchoring. After anchoring, rather than putting the thread right away, take out the temporal ring and check whether there is any bleeding in the place where it passed. If there is no bleeding, put the thread back after inserting the temporal ring again to the pre-formed tunnel. If there is bleeding, anchor to another point after hemostasis. If such method is used, the cases of removing threads due to bleeding after anchoring with a temporal ring can be reduced.

Blood vessel damage from cog

As the thread advances, vascular damage can also occur due to the cogs. However, in such cases, hemostasis is easily achieved, and the procedure can continue with the thread that has been inserted.

Complication—Prevention and Treatment of Headache

Fixing the thread to the fascia can cause headaches. It is crucial to distinguish whether the headache is due to infection or edema, or if it is simply pain. Continuous oozing at the entry point, along with a crust that persists for more than 2 weeks or exudates drying up leaving a powdery residue, indicates ongoing inflammation at the wound site or within the skin. In such cases, the use of antibiotics and anti-inflammatory drugs is recommended, typically extending the treatment for at least 5 days.

If the local swelling is severe, aspiration with a syringe can be attempted, sometimes extracting reddish exudates from the subcutaneous area. It is advisable to prescribe antibiotics and anti-inflammatory drugs after sufficiently aspiration.

While there is no need to routinely prescribe NSAIDs or Tylenol, it is wise to prescribe them preventively if the patient has a history of headaches revealed during pre-procedure history taking.

Sometimes, post-procedure headaches that do not respond to painkillers may be alleviated with Botulinum toxin injections. Botulinum toxin is FDA-approved for the preventive treatment of chronic migraines, although meta-analysis by Jeffery L. Jackson and others indicates it is ineffective for chronic tension-type headaches. The mechanism behind headaches caused by temporal tagging is unknown. Some cases of headaches after temporal tagging procedures, unresponsive to NSAIDs, respond to Botulinum toxin treatment, suggesting a vascular component might be involved. Further research and clear treatment guidelines are needed.

In patients with temporal muscle hypertrophy, Botulinum toxin injections for headache relief can also slim the appearance of a broad-looking head as an additional benefit.

8.3.4 Adequate Cannula for Long Thread Insertion (17G)

It consists of two components, internal needle and external sheath and is approximately 15–20 cm in length (Fig. 8.33).

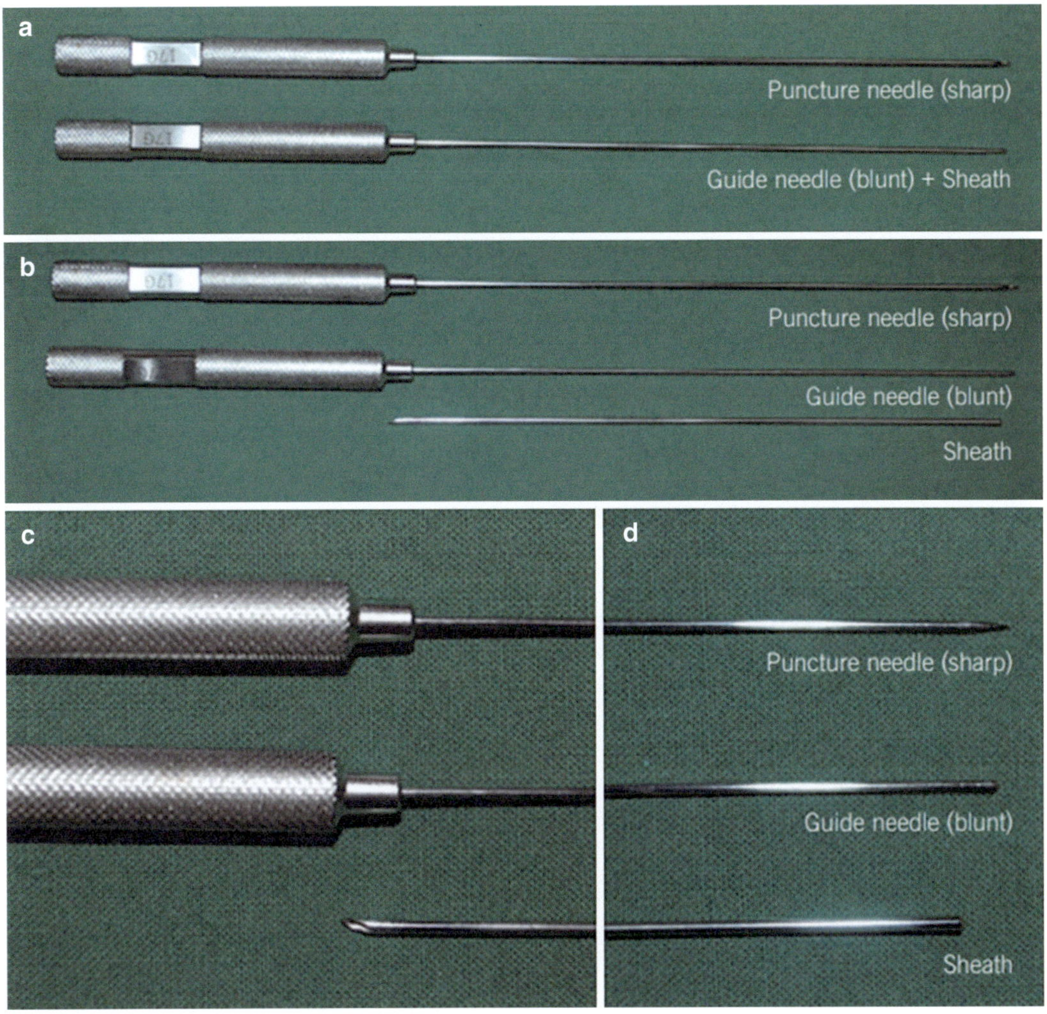

Fig. 8.33 Tools for the fascia tagging technique include: (**a**) A guide needle (blunt) combined with a sheath, (**b**) A guide needle (blunt) separated from the sheath, (**c**) (Enlargement of the handle part) The end of the sheath connected to the handle has a bevel. (**d**) (Enlargement of the opposite end) The guide needle and sheath are combined for entry, causing minimal tissue damage. The exit point skin penetration is performed with the sheath and puncture needle combined

8.3.5 Cutting and Finishing

After the thread insertion is complete, cutting is not done immediately. Instead, the treatment area is further lifted before cutting.

8.3.5.1 Finishing (Tightening)

Hold both ends of the thread with one hand around the exit point and use the other hand to push the skin upward, moving the cog/cone one notch further than its original position and then anchoring the skin (tissue) onto the cog/cone (i.e., the skin is pushed up toward the entry point, while the thread remains in its original position). Repeat this process 2–3 times. An assistant must press down on the anchoring point with their fingers during this process, gathering the pulled tissue around the anchoring point.

8.3.5.2 Cutting

Hold the thread and use scissors in the other hand to push the skin up by 4–5 mm and then cut the thread. Immediately after cutting, a dimple may appear due to the last cog; this needs to be released. Placing a thumb under the exit and pulling the skin downward with a snapping motion easily releases it. The thread end must be buried more than 4–5 mm inside the skin from the exit point to avoid complications like dimples or infections.

8.3.5.3 Changes in the Skin around the Entry Point (Dimple)

After the procedure, it is normal for the skin around the entry point to bulge upward slightly.

8.3.5.4 Fine Wrinkles around the Eyes and Zygomatic Area (Skin Distortion)

In cases of significant skin laxity (typically in middle-aged and older individuals), fine wrinkles may appear around the eyes and zygomatic area after the procedure, occurring perpendicular to the direction of the thread (Fig. 8.34). However, these usually disappear within a few days as the skin slightly reverts due to gravity, and they do not typically cause discomfort. Therefore, there is no need to push the skin back in the opposite direction of the lifting to address this issue.

Tip!

How to distinguish procedures which are within a normal range from abnormal ones.

After inserting a thread in a U-shape and both ends of the thread are pulled,

- If there is no sinking in the skin near the two entry point holes, it is normal.
- If the skin near one or two entry point(s) is concaved inward.
  - → Cause (see Causes and Preventions of Entry Point Dimples)
  - → Treatment: Dissection must be performed using scissors or other tools
  - → Prevention: Form a tunnel using an awl or use a temporal ring instead of a needle

After creating a vertical hole, it is important to properly establish a bidirectional pathway (Fig. 8.35).

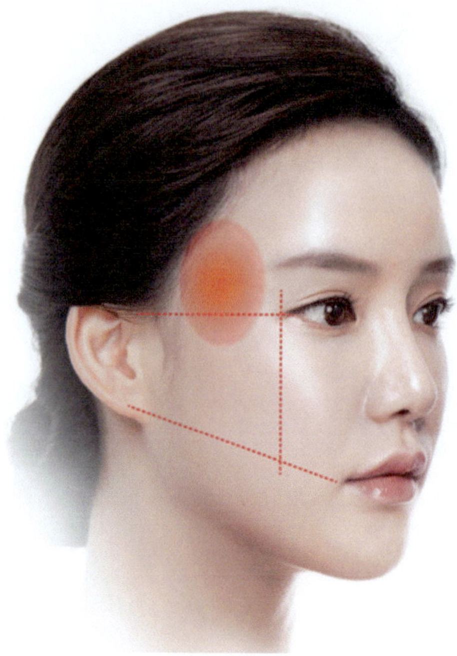

Fig. 8.34 Areas where fine wrinkles may occur after the fascia tagging technique

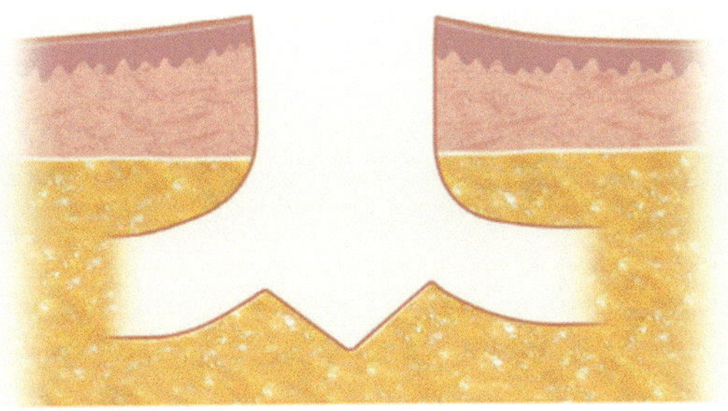

Fig. 8.35 Well-made entry point

In older individuals with thin skin, undergoing the fascia tagging technique may result in very fine wrinkles around the eyes and zygomatic area, resembling the pattern of a broom. Typically, these will improve on their own within 2–3 days without treatment.

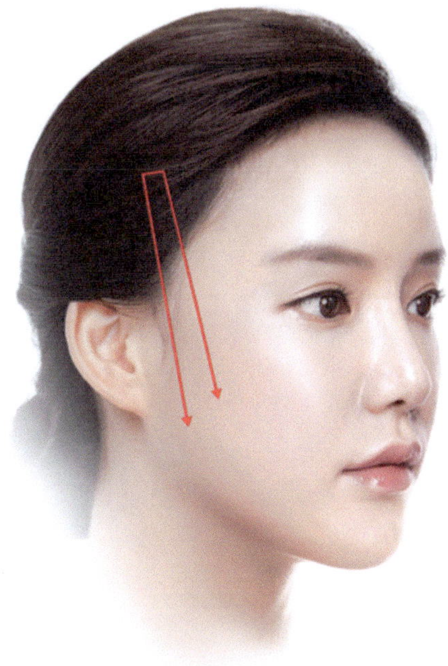

Fig. 8.36 Examples of designs using the fascia tagging technique

8.3.6 Differences in the Procedure According to the Number of Threads

8.3.6.1 One Thread per One Side of the Face (Figs. 8.36, 8.37 and 8.38)

8.3.6.2 Two Threads per One Side of the Face (Figs. 8.39, 8.40 and 8.41)

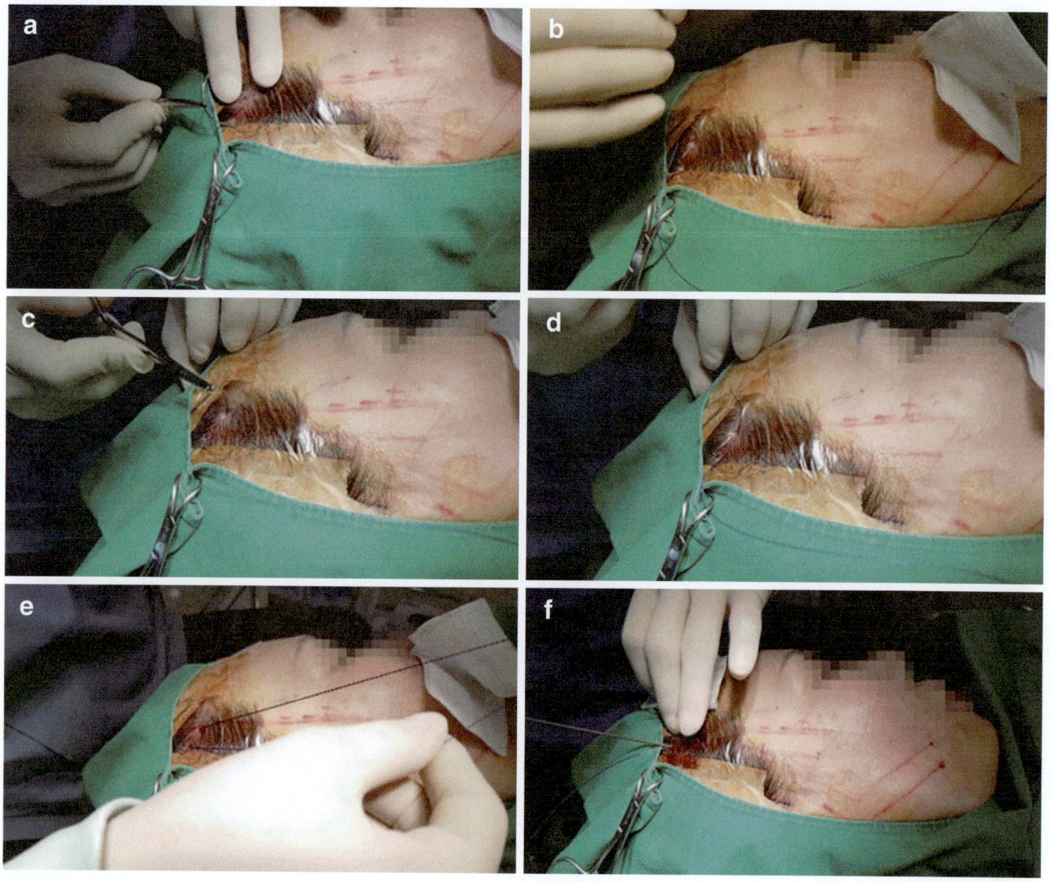

Fig. 8.37 Temporal fixation (long thread—41 cm)—U-pattern. (**a**) To insert the long thread, first anchor it in the zygomatic area using a long needle. (**b**) Connect the thread to the hole at the end of the needle. (**c**) Use a needle holder to guide the entire needle through to the opposite side's entry point. (**d**) Once the needle has passed through, detach the needle from the thread. (**e**) Pull the thread into a "U" shape, with half of it spanning each of the two entry points. (**f**) Insert a long cannula (Fig. 8.33. A blunt guide needle + sheath) into the first entry point and proceed at a uniform depth within the SubQ layer. (**g**) Make an exit by piercing through toward the exit point. (First, separate the blunt guide needle from the sheath and remove it, then insert the puncture needle into the sheath. Next, support the exit with forceps in the opposite hand and break through the skin with force in the right hand, see (**g**, **h**) for reference). (**h**) Once the puncture needle is removed from the sheath, there is only the sheath between the entry and exit points. (**i**) Insert the thread through one hole of the sheath (entry point) and guide it out through the opposite hole (exit), ensuring only the front part of the thread without cogs emerges. (**j**) Pull the sheath from the opposite side. (**k**) This action causes the thread to be pulled out toward the exit. (**l**) By inserting the remaining half of the thread in the same way, one long thread is hung in a "U" shape. (**m**) Gently lift the skin upward with the opposite hand and anchor the skin onto the cog. (**n**) Finally, cut the thread (push the skin with sterile scissors and cut above 1–2 inserted cogs)

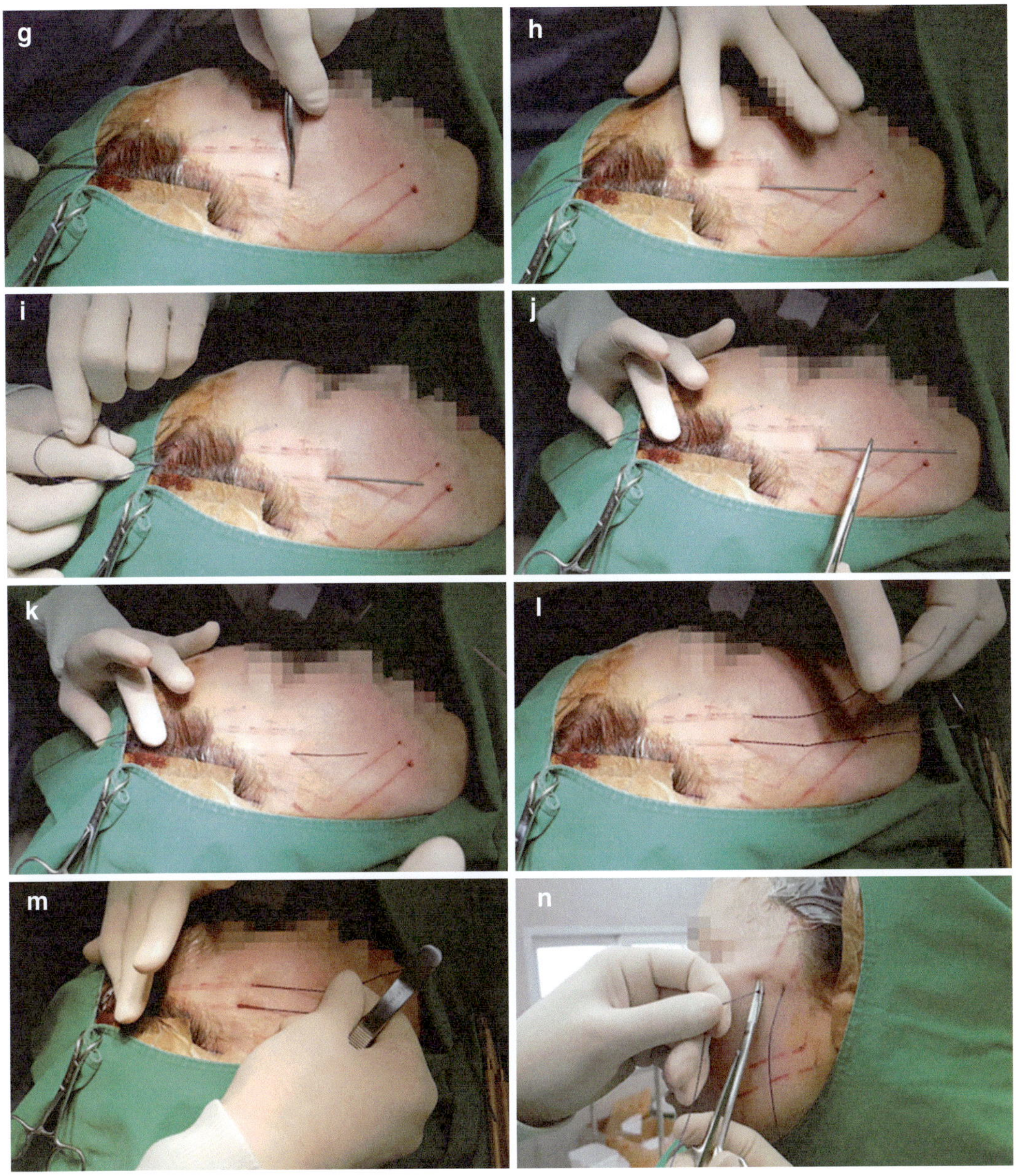

Fig. 8.37 (continued)

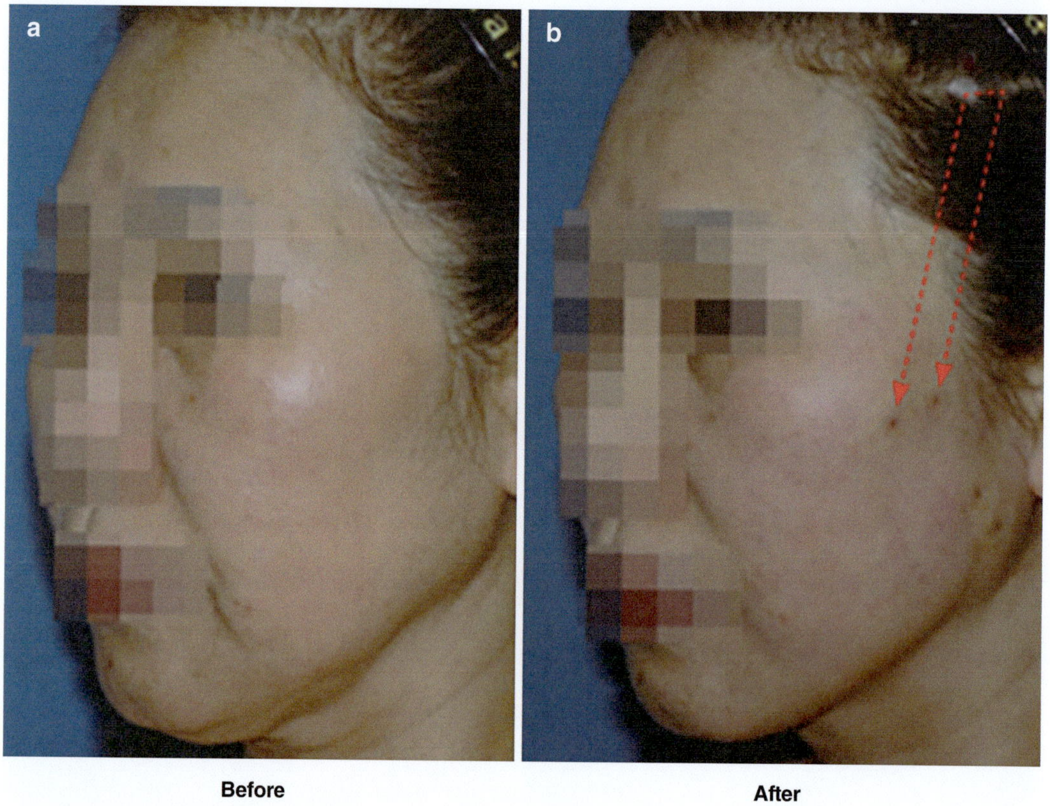

Fig. 8.38 Before and after photos of the fascia tagging technique, one line per one side of the face

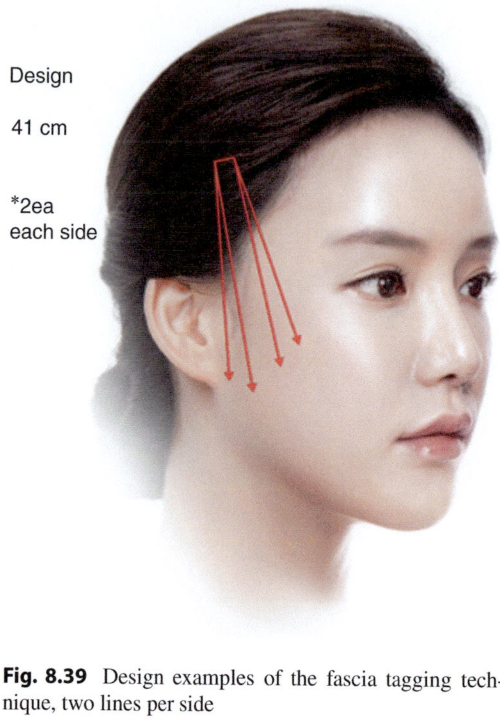

Fig. 8.39 Design examples of the fascia tagging technique, two lines per side

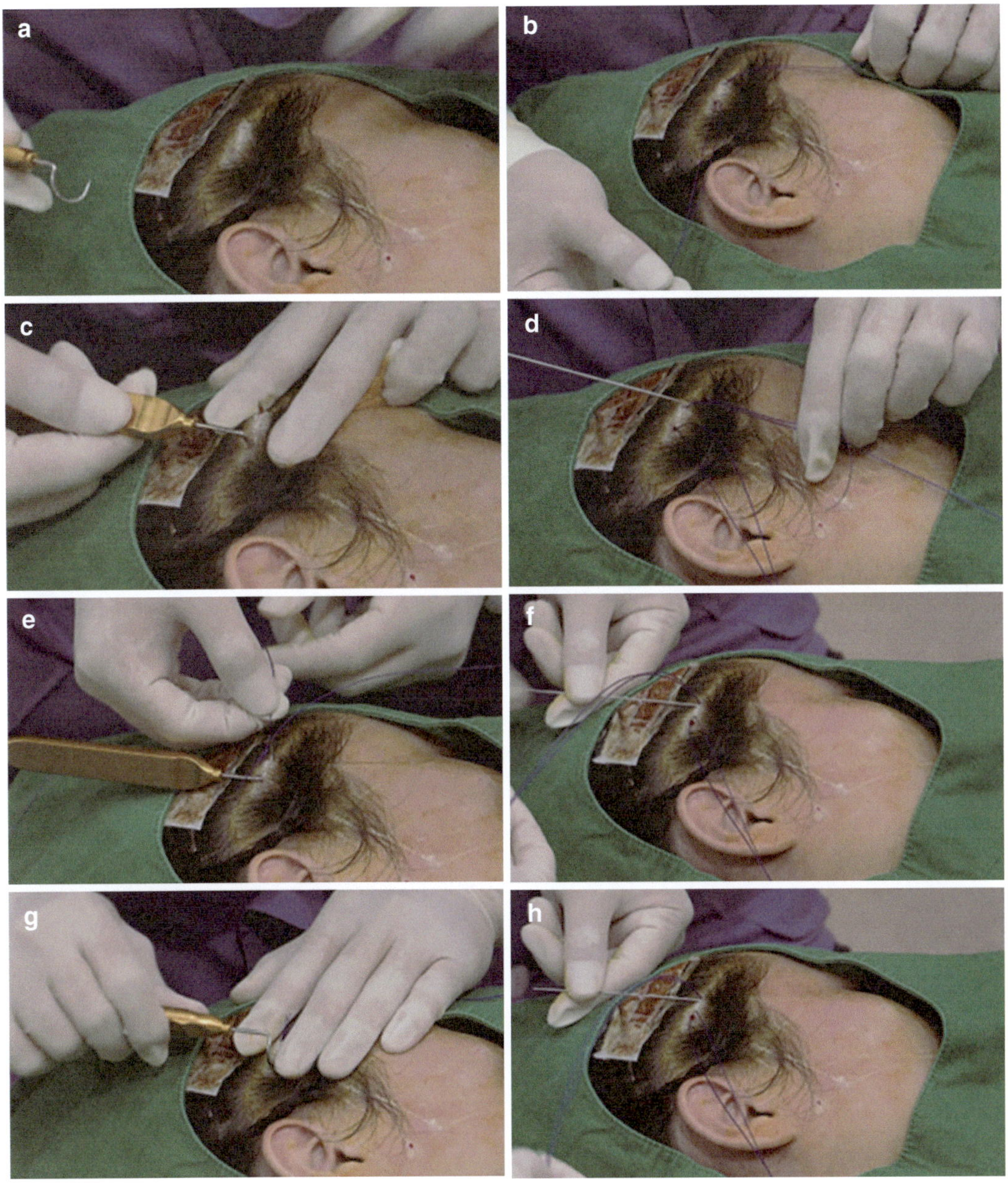

Fig. 8.40 Temporal fixation (long thread—41 cm)—U-pattern: Using a temporal ring, two lines per side. (**a**) Grasp the temporal ring that has an end shaped like a half-ring. (**b**) Insert first through one entry point, anchor by rotating the temporal ring, and then come out through the opposite entry point. (**c**) Fit each thread into the two holes at the end of the ring (if the tool has two holes, inserting two threads at once can save treatment time). (**d**) Remove the temporal ring by rotating it back in the opposite direction of insertion. (**e**) Detach the temporal ring from the thread, and pull the thread into a "U" shape with half of it spanning each of the two entry points. (**f**) Insert a long cannula (Fig 8.33a, blunt guide needle + sheath) into the first entry point and proceed at a uniform depth within the SubQ layer, going up to just before the exit. (**g**) Remove the blunt guide needle from the sheath. (**h**) Only the sheath remains in place. Insert the puncture needle from Fig 8.33a into the sheath. (**i**) Hold forceps in the opposite hand to support the exit point and use force in the right hand to pierce through the skin. (**j**) Once the puncture needle is removed from the sheath, only the sheath spans between the entry and exit points. (**k**) Insert the thread through one hole of the sheath (entry point) and guide it out through the opposite hole (exit). The subsequent steps are the same as Fig. 8.37**j**–**n**

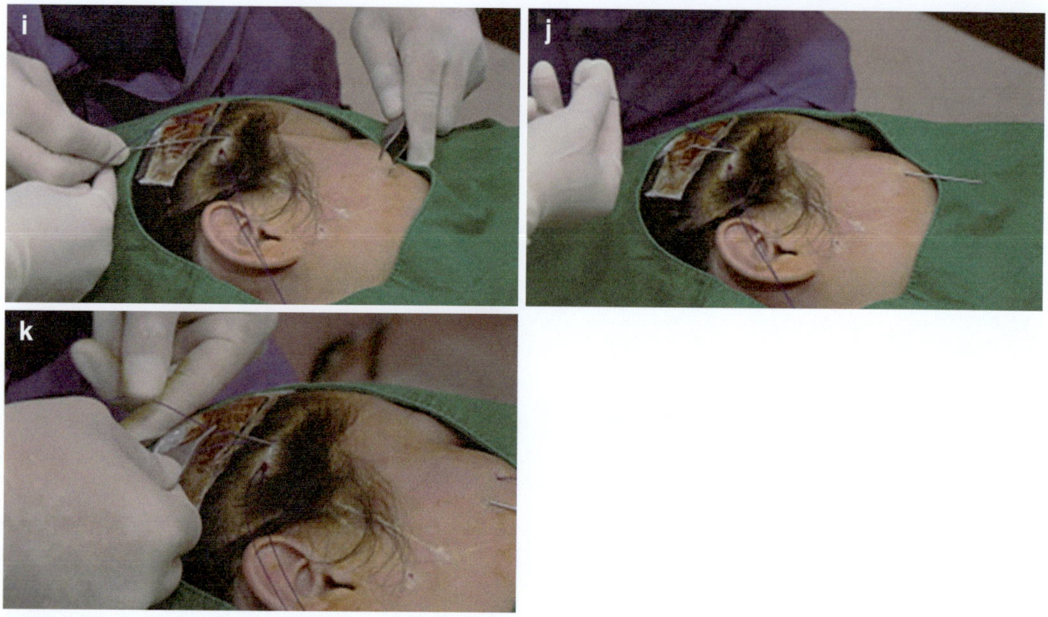

Fig. 8.40 (continued)

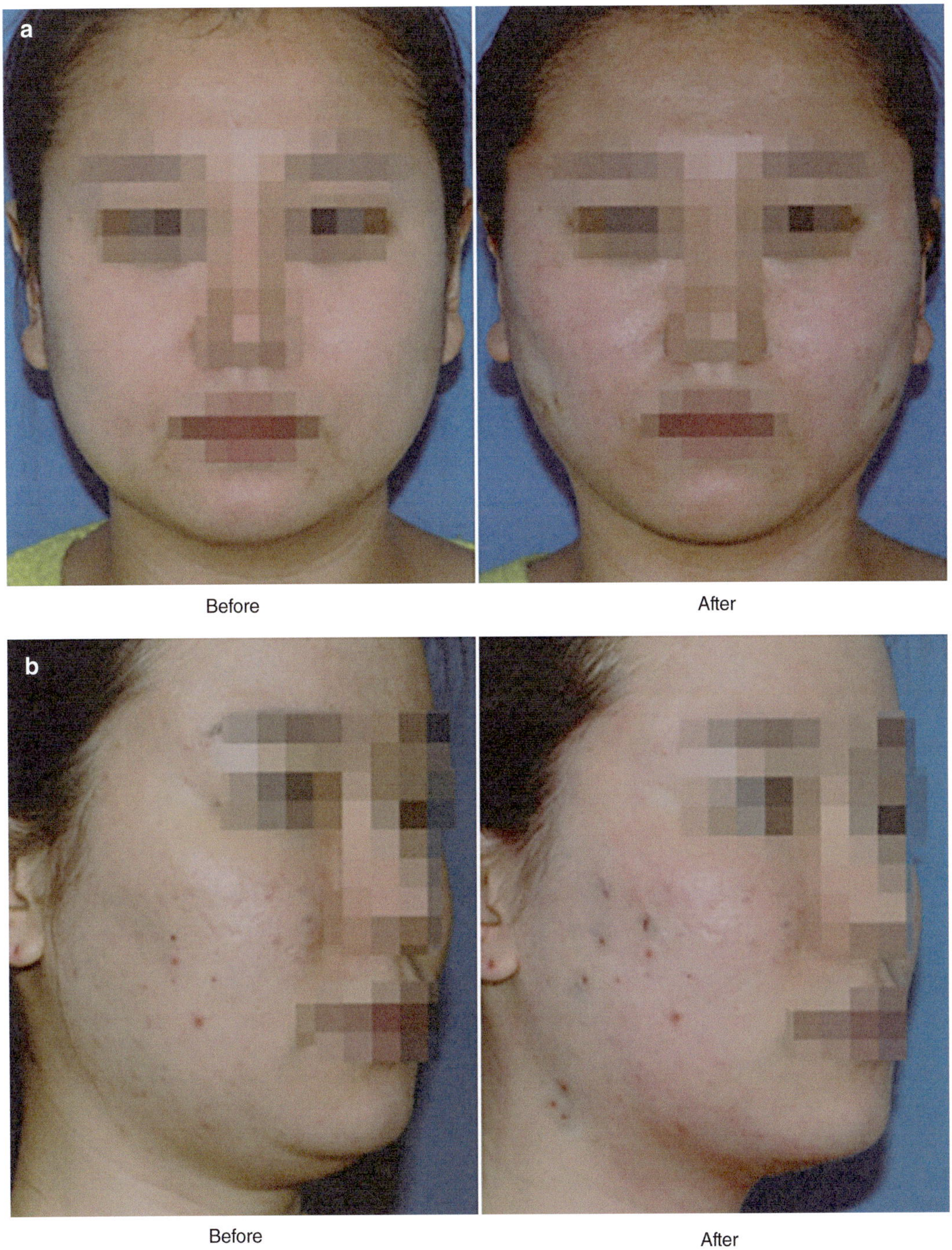

Fig. 8.41 Temporal fixation (long thread—41 cm)—U-pattern: insert two lines per one side using a temporal ring

8.4 Techniques Using the Bidirectional Needle Cogged Thread (I-THREAD Magic Plus)

8.4.1 Principle

The bidirectional needle thread, created by attaching a needle to the end of a bidirectional cog thread, is user-friendly. It allows for a procedure without the need for a cannula, and it is possible to carry out the procedure without creating a separate entry point.

The principle of using a bidirectional needle thread is mainly divided into two categories, which create differences in procedural design. The first method gathers tissue from both sides toward the center. This method is commonly used for neck and double chin lifting, where an entry point is created in the middle, and the thread runs to both sides, gathering tissue toward the entry point (Fig. 8.42).

There is a method that involves creating an angle in the middle part of the thread, pushing tissue together in a slightly modified form (Fig. 8.19).

The second method is the U-pattern technique (Fig. 8.43).

8.4.2 Bidirectional Needle Cogged Thread Introduction

The thread has needles attached to both ends, and there is a section in the middle of the thread without cogs. The cogs on both sides are oriented in one direction (Fig. 8.44).

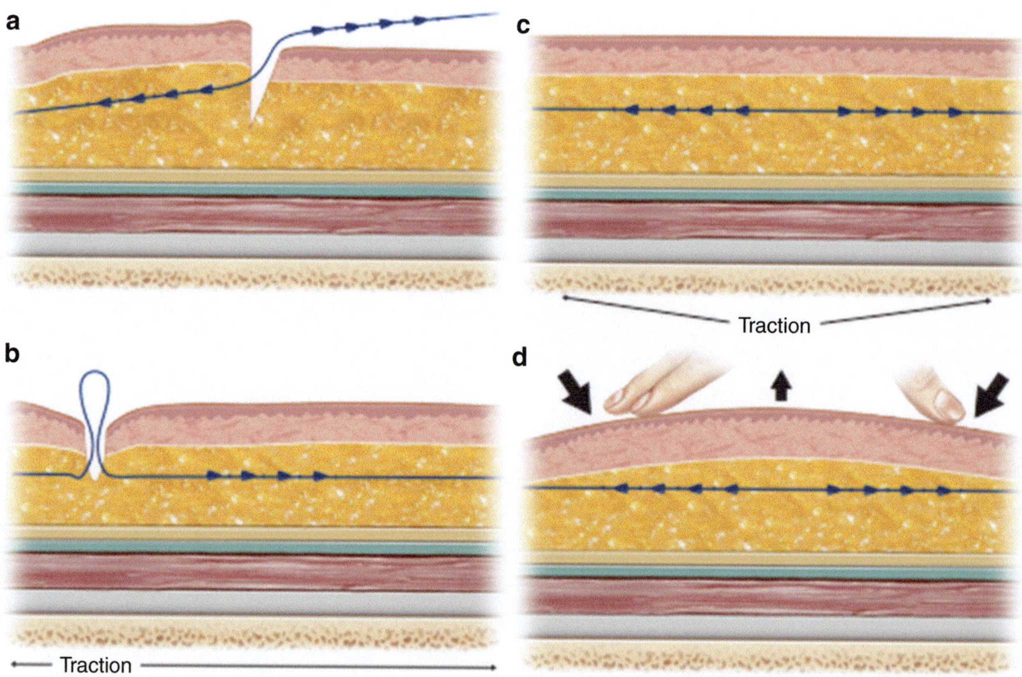

Fig. 8.42 Principle of bidirectional needle thread—straight pattern. (**a**) Insert one end of the thread through the entry point. (**b**) Insert the other end of the thread through the same entry point. (**c**) Bury the thread completely inside the tissue, with the opposite end exiting through the exit point. (**d**) When pulling the end of the thread that has been exited, the tissue gathers toward the middle part of the thread

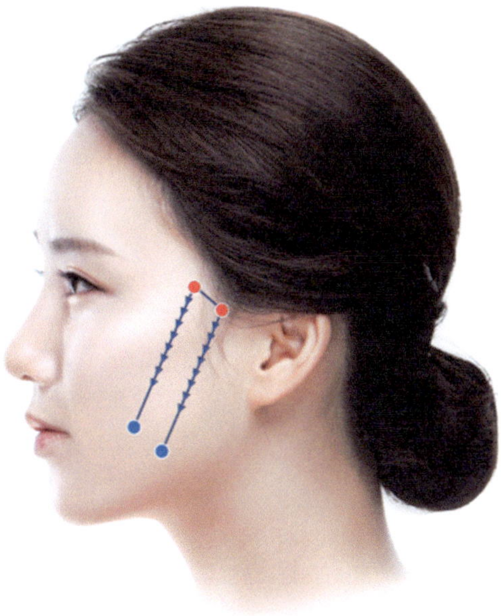

Fig. 8.43 Principle of bidirectional needle thread—U-pattern

8.4.3 Procedure Method

8.4.3.1 Design

Straight Pattern

The fundamental principle of the straight pattern technique is to gather tissue in the central area. An entry point is marked at the desired central area to be gathered, followed by marking exit points on both sides. The distance from the entry point to the exit points is designed to be similar to the length of the needle.

For the i-THREAD Magic Plus, it has a design with bidirectional needles attached to the ends of a bidirectional thread. As shown in the above Fig. 8.45, there are few restrictions in setting the length corresponding to a. Even if the length of the tissue corresponding to a. is longer than the length of the needle b., the procedure can still be performed smoothly as long as the

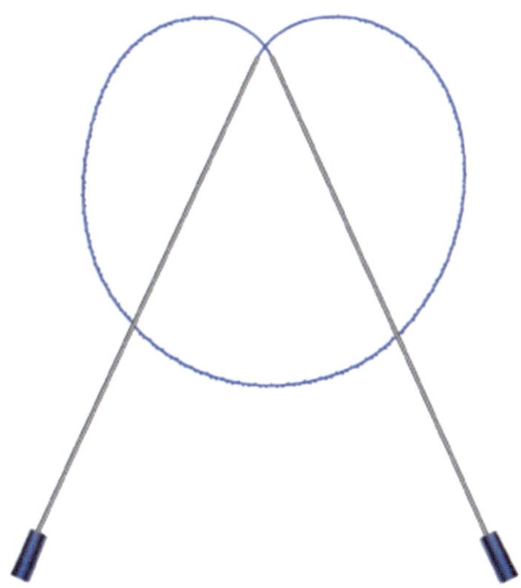

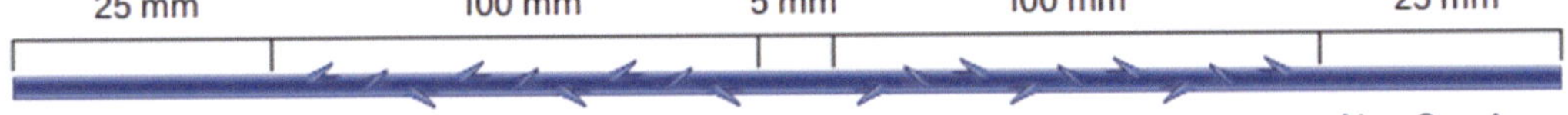

Needle gauge	Needle length (nm)	Thread length (nm)	Thread thickness (USP)
21 G	107 mm	255 mm	0–0

Fig. 8.44 Bidirectional needle cogged thread (HEALUX, i-THREAD Magic Plus)

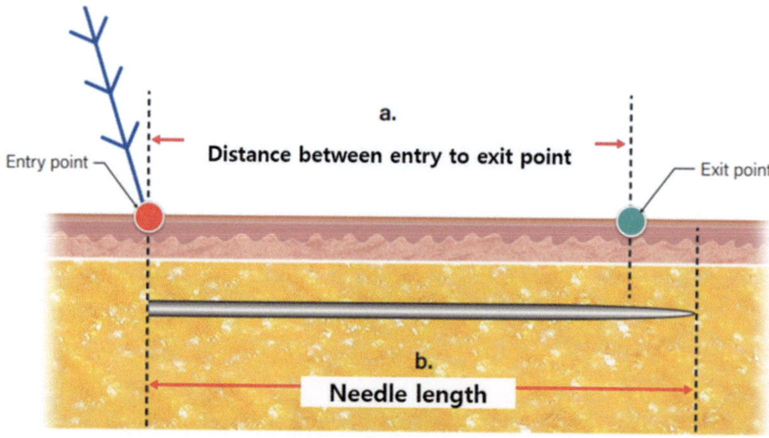

Fig. 8.45 Comparison of the needle's length and the designed length of the thread. The procedure becomes easier when the length of the needle, b, is similar to the length of the thread, a, that is buried subcutaneously

difference in lengths is not significant. This is considered an advantage of the i-THREAD Magic Plus.

You can see some basic designs in Fig. 8.46.

U-Pattern

The U-pattern is a thread lifting method that utilizes the midpoint of the thread as a fixed point, pulling the ends of the thread toward the middle part. It is crucial to create a strong fixation point, as having firm tissue at the fixation site can yield good results (Fig. 8.47).

Another technique that is good for using i-THREAD Magic Plus is PMA (post-mandibular anchoring) technique (Fig. 8.48).

PMA technique is a type of U-pattern and is a good method to use for jawline or marionette line sagging. When there is a sagging of jawline or marionette line, consideration should be given to the vector directed behind the ear (mentalis-mandible angle) and the vector directed upward (mandible body-zygoma-temple).

When the angle between the mandible body and the horizontal line is large (more than 30 degrees), the above-mentioned two vectors work at the same time, so a sufficient effect can be achieved only by pulling to the back of the ear. On the other hand, if the angle between the mandible body and the horizontal line is small (less than 20 degrees), or if the square jaw is developed a lot, the pulling force mainly appears toward the vector toward the back of the ear. As a result, the thread lifting is less effective (Fig. 8.49).

8.4.3.2 Anesthesia

The anesthetic solution typically used is dental lidocaine (lidocaine 1% with epinephrine 1:100,000). To reduce pain, I create and use a tumescent solution. The addition of bicarbonate solution neutralizes the hydrochloric acid in the lidocaine, eliminating pain during injection (Fig. 8.50).

The injection sites are generally only at the entry and exit points. It is not always necessary to anesthetize the entire path of the thread, but in the following cases, full-path anesthesia might be performed additionally:

- In patients who are very concerned about pain.
- if the patient complains of pain during the procedure, an injection is given directly to the painful area.
- When the subcutaneous tissue is too thin or there are adhesions making it difficult for the needle to pass through.

A 30G long needle is commonly used to minimize injection points while anesthetizing the path. Care is taken to avoid bleeding and nerve damage while considering the paths of nerves and blood vessels. Generally, injecting the anesthetic into the subcutaneous fat layer does not lead to serious complications.

8.4.3.3 Entry Point

Making an entry point also requires technique (Fig. 8.51). When making a hole with an 18 G needle, pinch the skin with the opposite hand,

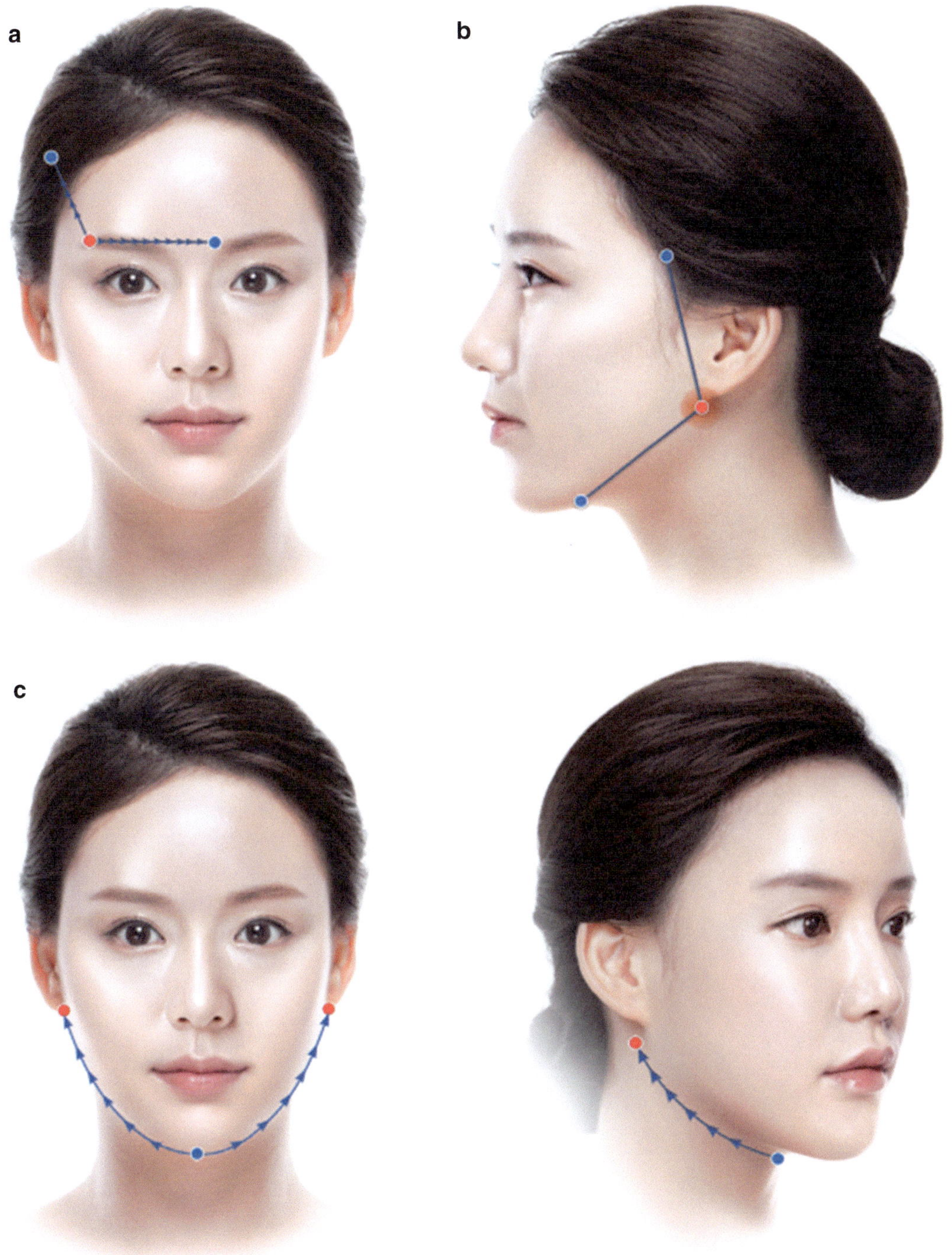

Fig. 8.46 Basic designs

insert the needle vertically, and then slightly stir (rotate) it to separate the dermis and SubQ tissue beneath the entry point. It is possible to reduce the likelihood of dimpling after the procedure. The needle should be inserted to a depth of about 5 mm (Fig. 8.52).

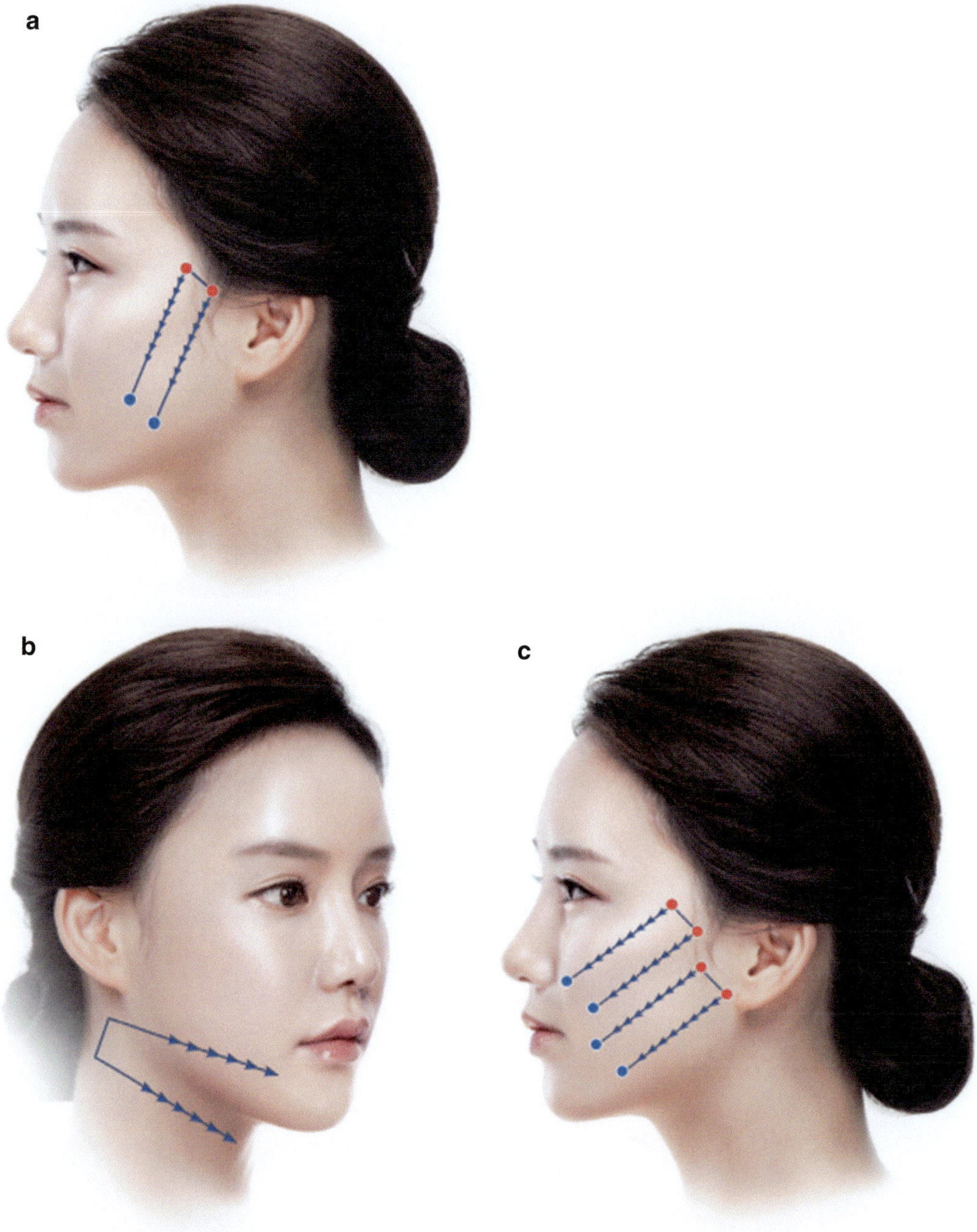

Fig. 8.47 Basic form of the U-pattern

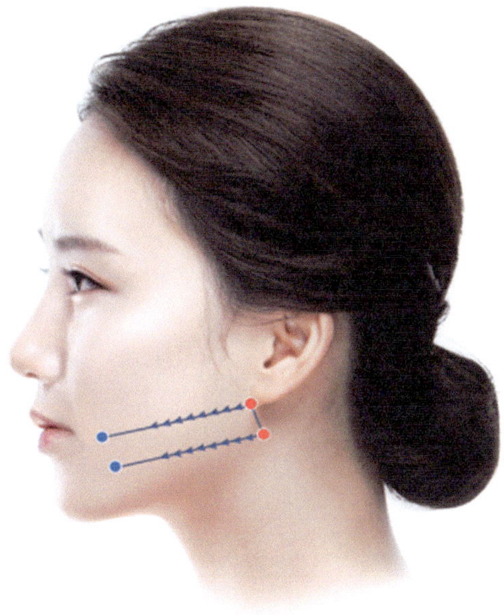

Fig. 8.48 PMA technique

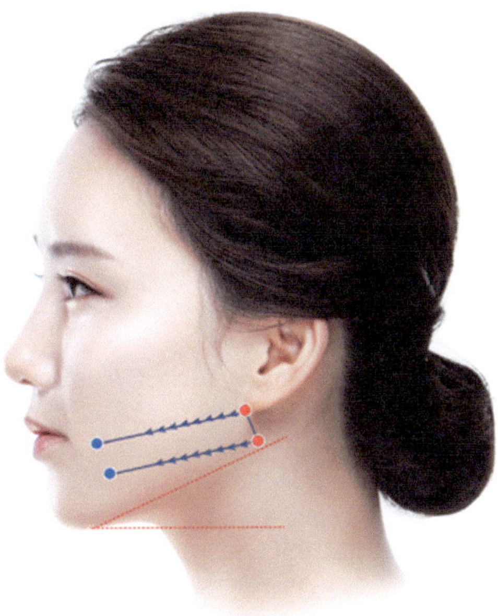

Fig. 8.49 Angle formed between the mandibular body and the horizontal line

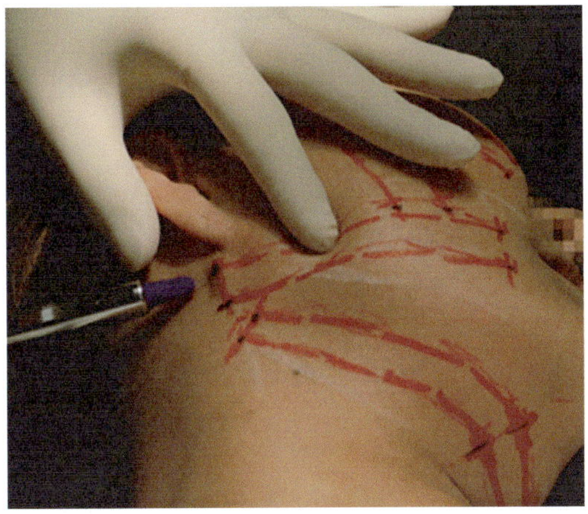

Fig. 8.50 Anesthesia with dental lidocaine

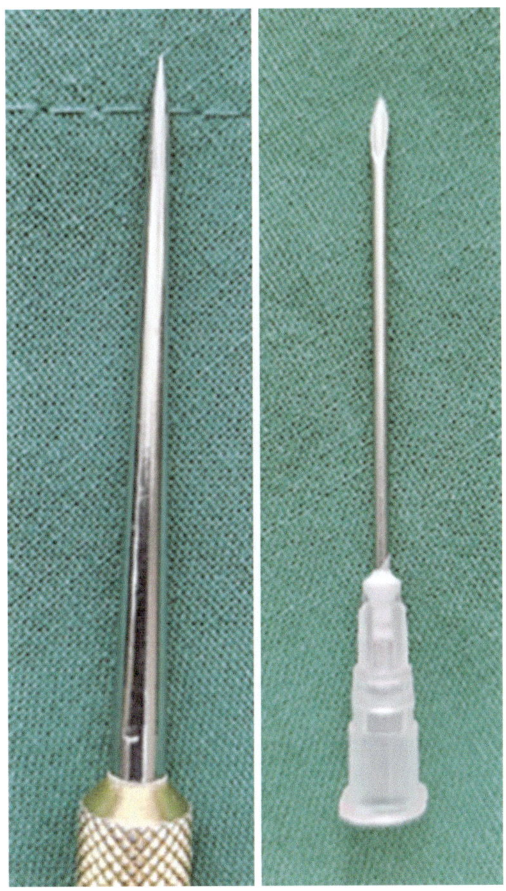

Fig. 8.51 Tools for making an entry point

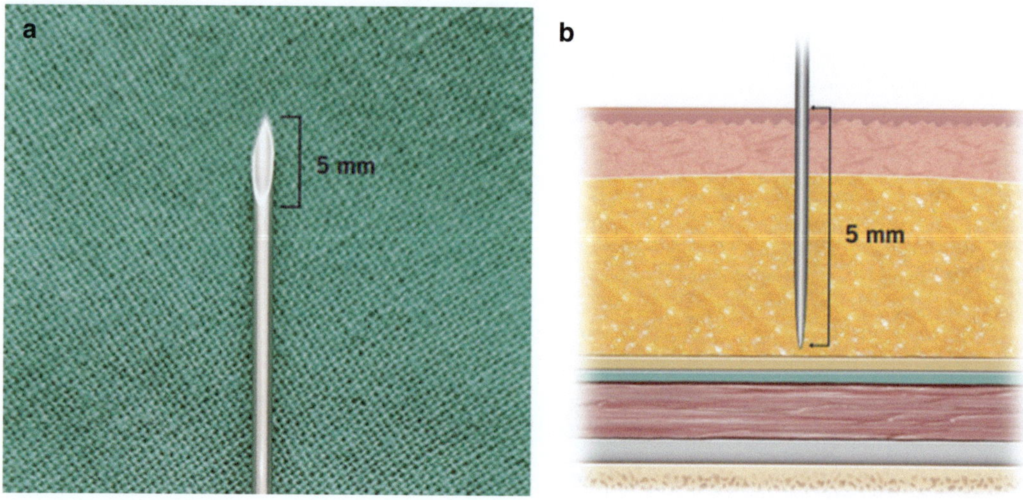

Fig. 8.52 Why the depth of the entry point is about 5 mm. (**a**) The length of 18 G needle bevel (**b**) The meaning of a depth of 5 mm

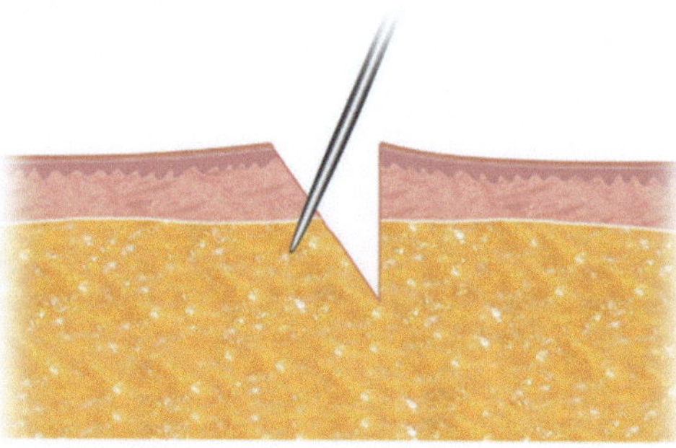

Fig. 8.53 Appearance of a needle being inserted into the subcutaneous fat while tagging the lower part of the dermis

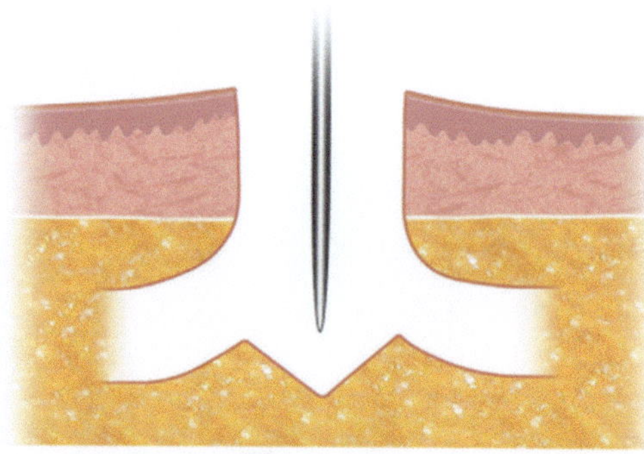

Fig. 8.54 Appearance of a needle correctly inserted

It is the most important part of the bidirectional needle cog thread. This is because dimples easily occur at the entry point. For this, it is necessary to understand the structure and principle of the bidirectional needle cog thread. The key to the entry point is to prevent dimples from occurring.

The principle of dimple formation is as follows (Fig. 8.53).

When the needle enters through the entry point and catches a part of the dermis, a dimple is formed. Therefore, the entry point should be made in such a way that the needle can enter the subcutaneous fat without catching the dermis in one go (Fig. 8.54).

Especially, the insertion of the second needle is crucial.

After the first needle is inserted, the direction of the entry point tends to be slightly inclined as the thread follows it (Fig. 8.55). If the second needle is inserted vertically or in the intended direction at this point, it will also catch the lower part of the dermis as it enters. In this case, a dimple is formed as well.

Therefore, when inserting the second needle, as shown in Fig. 8.56, it is necessary to inject the needle obliquely in the direction in which the first needle was inserted.

Then, change the direction of the needle and insert it toward where you want it to go.

There is a method to create not just one, but two entry points. This is also done using an 18G needle. The method involves bending the 18G

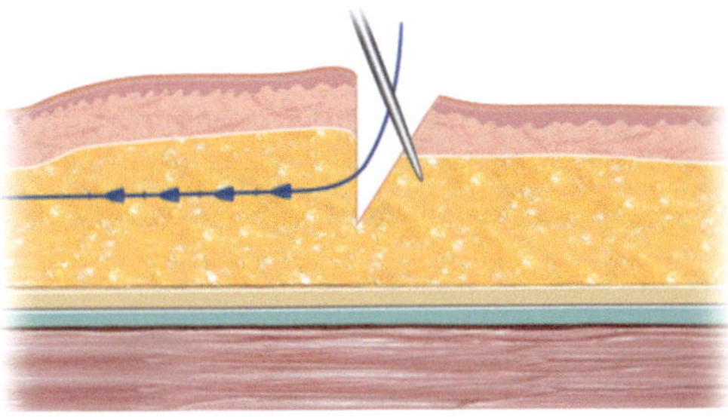

Fig. 8.55 Incorrect direction of the second needle insertion

needle or using it as is to pierce the skin, then passing the needle attached to the thread through, followed by removing the 18G needle (Fig. 8.57).

8.4.3.4 Needle Insertion

Hold on the needle to the shortest as possible closely to the entry point (If the needle is held long, it bends well during insertion). Then hold with the thumb and the index finger (Fig. 8.58).

At this time, it is very important to insert the needle at a consistent depth. This is to prevent

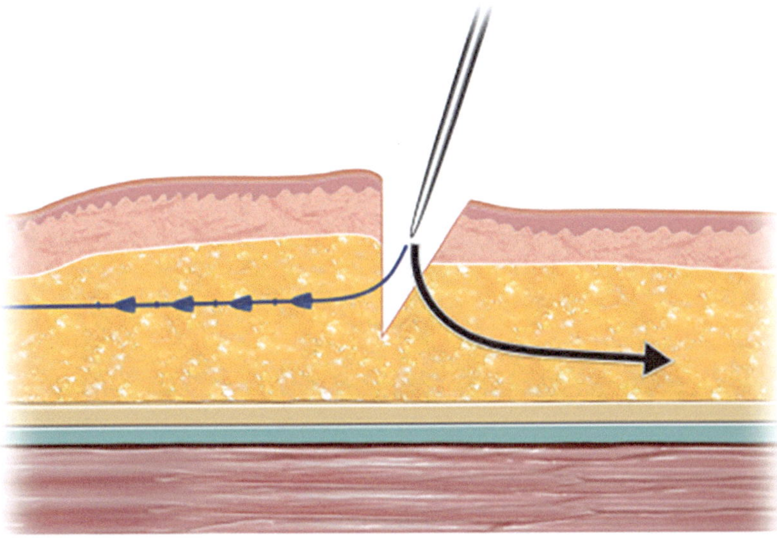

Fig. 8.56 Correct direction for the second needle insertion

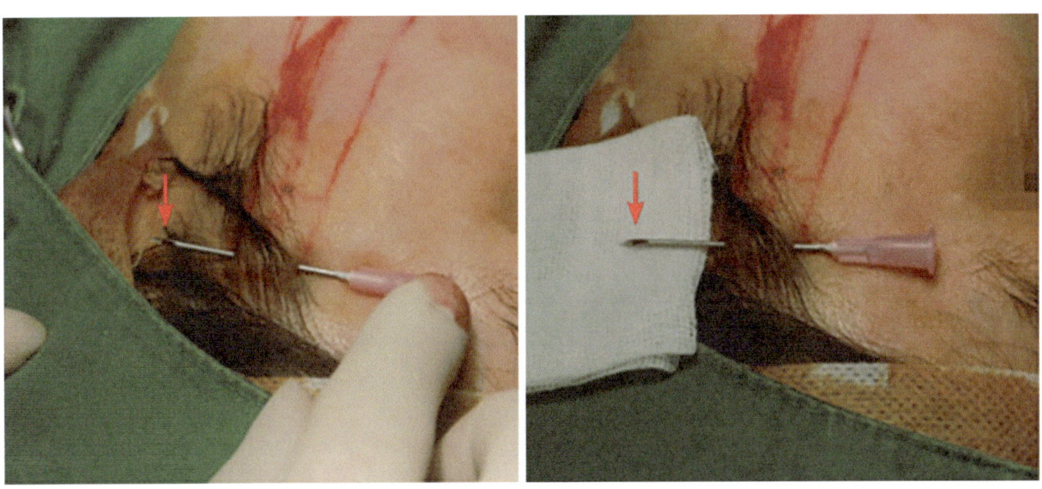

Fig. 8.57 Method for creating two entry points

dimples (Fig. 8.59). At this time, various PINCH techniques are used, such as finger pinch, V-pinch, and press.

Finger pinching is necessary when creating an entry point and when proceeding to the first 1/3 of the way after insertion. V-pinch is useful when driving in the midsection, especially around the neck. The press operation is useful when passing the last third, using the second, third, and fourth finger tips. It is useful in the curved area/thick skin area under the cheek, and when passing through the curved surface of the cheek, it can be made easier by pressing while holding the needle in a slightly curved state (Figs. 8.60 and 8.61).

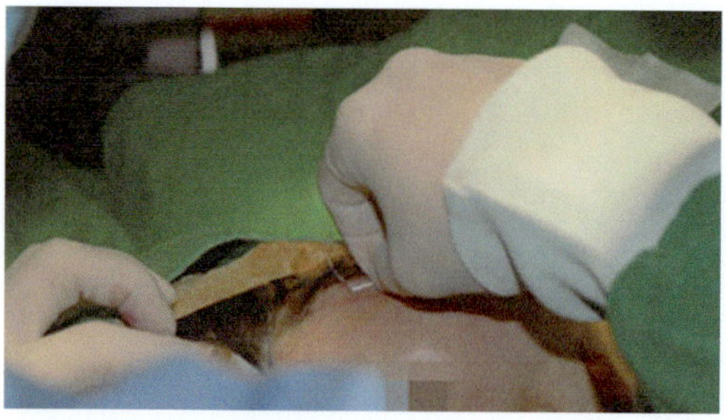

Fig. 8.58 Needle holding

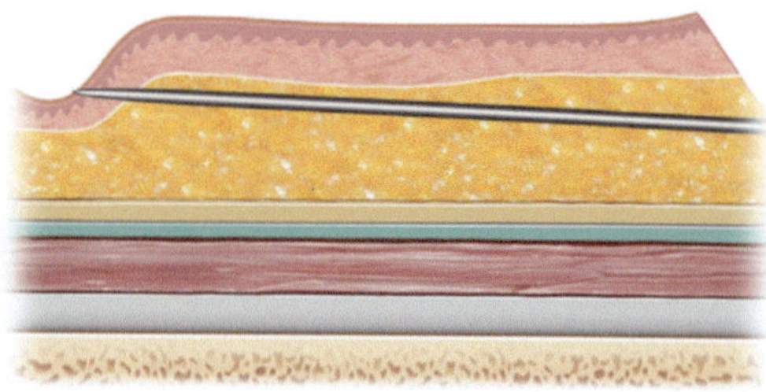

Fig. 8.59 Movement of the needle

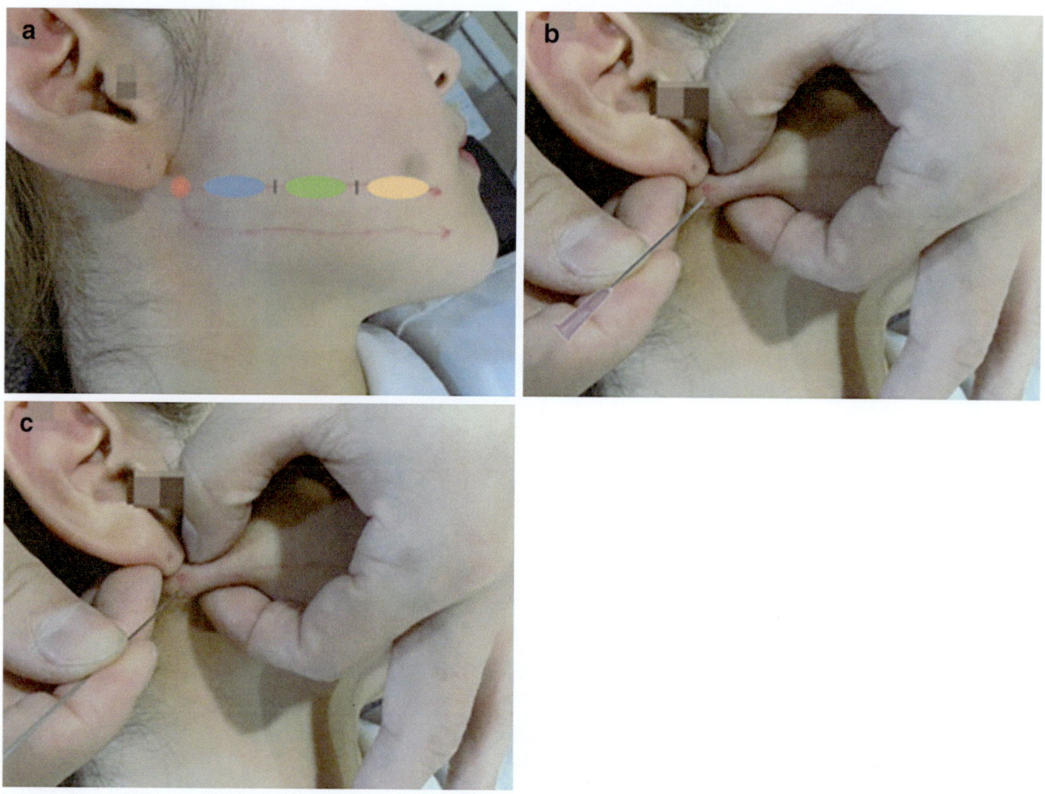

Fig. 8.60 Pinch technique as above. (**a**) Shows the design when injected from the angle of the mandible toward the corner of the mouth. From the left, the entry point, proximal 1/3, middle 1/3, and distal 1/3 are indicated, respectively. (**b**) Point-pinch (hard): When creating an entry point using a puncture needle, hold it with the tip of your finger. You have to pull the skin tissue to avoid vessel and muscle damage, so hold it firmly. (**c**) Point-pinch (soft): When the i-THREAD needle enters the entry point, hold it with the tip of your finger. If you hold it too tightly, the entry point will not be secured well and there is a high possibility of dimples, so hold it weakly so that the entry point is slightly visible

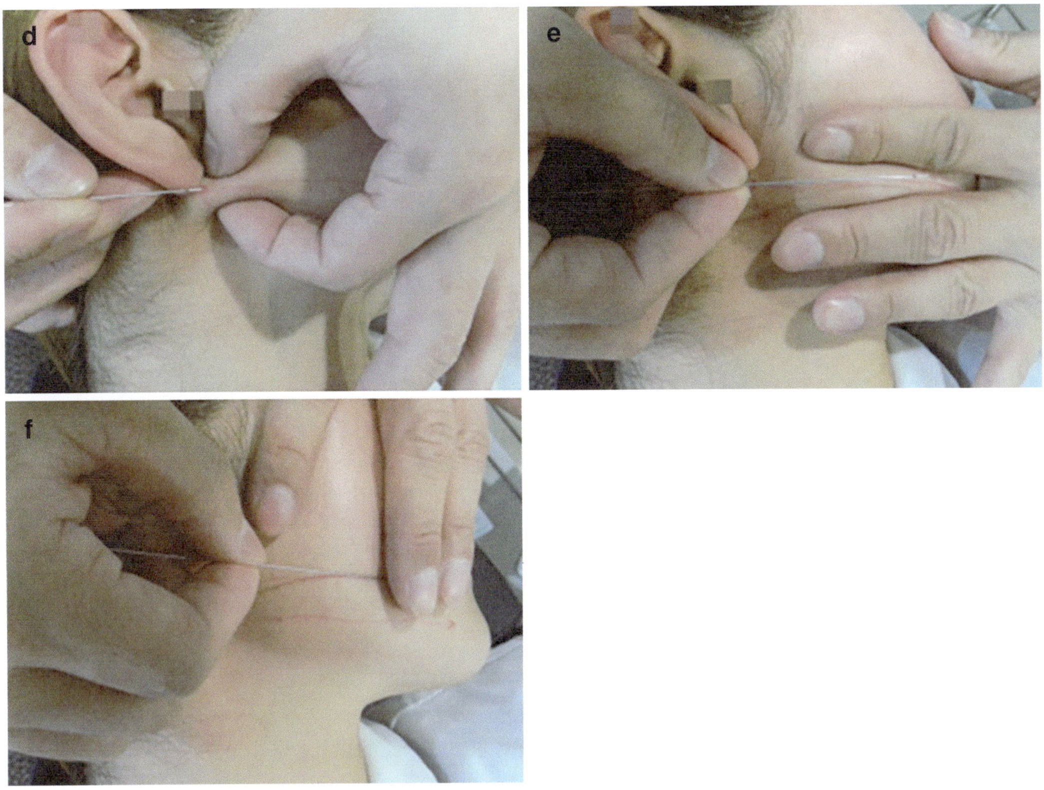

Fig. 8.61 Various pinch techniques. (**d**) Block-pinch: After inserting into the entry point, when it passes proximal 1/3, hold it with a large finger and insert it at a certain depth within SubQ. (**e**) V-pinch: middle 1/3 SubQ fat is very soft. The procedure is easy if you pinch in a "V" shape using your second and third fingers and then insert. (**f**) Press: SubQ fat of distal 1/3 is very dense. It is advantageous to insert while lightly pressing the tissue from above to allow the needle to pass at a uniform depth

While driving after needle injection, you must check the driving depth.

This can be confirmed through tenting operation. After advancing the needle from the entry point to the exit point, rather than immediately removing the needle, hold the tip of the needle with both fingers and bend it toward the top of the skin to lift the tissue (Fig. 8.62). At the same time, check whether the needle runs at a certain depth within SubQ.

If the thickness of the lifted SubQ is not constant and there is a thin part in the middle, it is best to retract the needle and run again. If the needle is inserted while the depth of SubQ is not constant, the thread will naturally run at an uneven depth and skin folds or dimples are likely to occur.

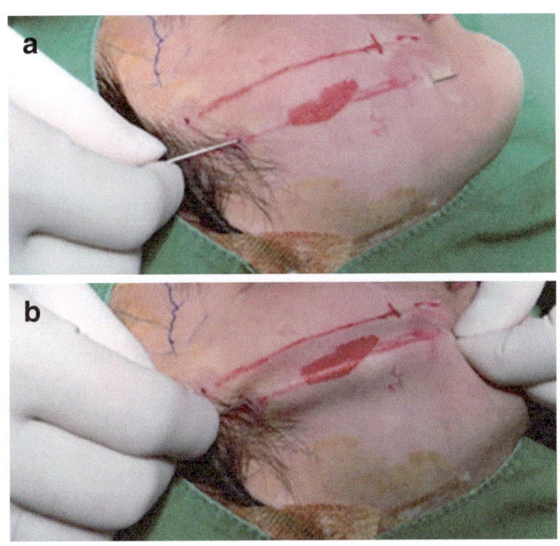

Fig. 8.62 Tenting and bending for checking the depth of needle

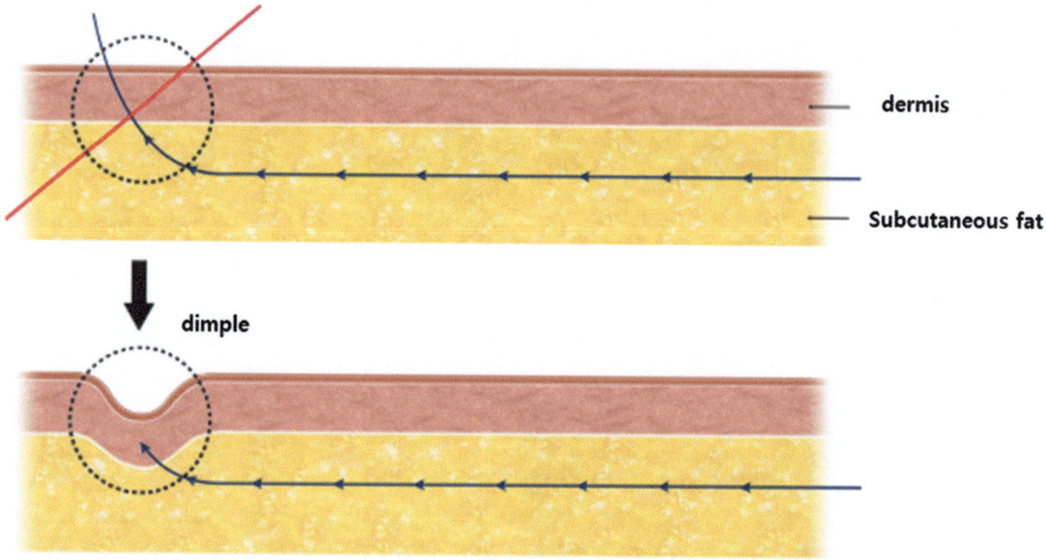

Fig. 8.63 An example of a dimple that occurs when the thread is not sufficiently buried into the skin at the exit point and the end of the thread is located near the dermis

8.4.3.5 Cutting and Finishing (Traction: Pulling Threads)

After confirming that the thread and needle run at a uniform depth through the bending operation, cut between the thread and needle.

Afterward, traction is performed. When using a U-pattern, it is necessary to press the entry point to prevent the thread hanging from the anchoring point from coming down during traction. After pulling as much as desired, check that there are no skin folds or dimples, and then remove the thread by cutting (Fig. 8.63).

When cutting, rather than pulling the thread, use curved scissors to push the skin and cut the thread. This is because an additional lifting effect occurs through folding of the skin during the final cutting process, and the tissue being lifted should never be gathered around the exit point. The lifted tissue must be gathered around the entry point so that a proper lifting effect occurs and skin folds or dimples are not visible.

When you push up the tissue with a curved scissor and cut the thread, the tissue gathers at the exit point and must be pulled to release it. Therefore, the tissue at the exit point must be spread out flat. At this time, the end of the cut thread is buried in the skin, leaving a certain distance from the exit point. This is essential to prevent dimples at the exit point area.

8.5 Considerations for Skilled Thread Lifting Procedures

8.5.1 Temporal Muscle Hypertrophy (or Trigonocephaly)

If the horizontal width of the temporal area is wide due to the development of temporal muscles or the shape of the skull due to trigonocephaly, it may be difficult to advance a long cannula. In other words, after the cannula enters the entry point, it should proceed to a certain depth of the SQ, but in this case, as the cannula tilts, it tends to go deeper or shallower than intended.

In order to prevent these side effects, when designing, the path of the thread should be made as straight as possible. If temporal muscle hypertrophy is severe enough to make it difficult to avoid a curved path in the area where the fixation point is to be created, it is helpful to reduce the curved path of the head by injecting a large amount of anesthetic solution into the area of the fixation point to swell the tissue.

8.5.2 Temporal Hollowness

Problems also arise when the temple area is caved in.

In this area, the cannula passes more superficially than it should, and in the zygoma area, it tends to pass deeper into the muscle. In particular, if the cheekbones are developed, the procedure becomes more difficult.

In this case, if tumescent solution or lidocaine is sufficiently injected into the SubQ layer using a cannula to fill the depression, the depression will be temporarily corrected and passage through the cannula will become easier. Alternatively, if the temple depression is first corrected using filler, passing the cannula becomes easier.

8.5.3 Zygomatic Prominence

Developed cheekbones are especially common in Asian faces. In this case, when the cannula or needle that has passed through the temple tries to advance through the zygomatic prominence to the anterior cheek, it must pass through a sharp curved surface, making it difficult to pass at a certain depth. In addition, because this part has less fat and is denser, more force is required for the cannula or needle to pass through.

In this case, a good method is to temporarily inflate the depressed area above and below the protruding zygomatic arch using a tumescent solution. Because a relatively straight path can be created, progression of the cannula or needle becomes easier (Fig. 8.64).

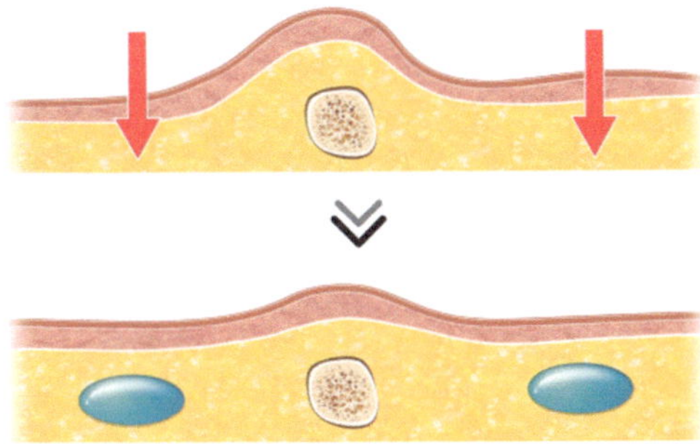

Fig. 8.64 When there is a zygomatic arch prominence, the prominence is reduced and a straight path is created after tumescent injection above and below the arch

8.5.4 Sunken Cheek

A depression on the side of the cheek occurs in everyone as they age. To Westerners, the side cheek depression actually highlights the Ogee Curve and makes it look attractive, but Asians do not like it. Therefore, side cheek depressions are sometimes corrected with filler. In the case of thread lifting, which is effective, correction of this depressed part is sometimes performed along with jowl lifting. This part needs to be carefully examined anatomically. It is a structure made up of the zygomatico-cutaneous ligament and the masseteric cutaneous ligament and is shaped like a diamond or triangle.

The vector of facial sagging is usually directed downward (inferior) or toward the center of the face (medial), but the vector of the area where the side cheek depression occurs is not toward the lower center but rather toward the deep skin (inner vector). This area is the densest tissue during facial thread lifting procedures. Therefore, it is difficult to control the depth when passing, and it requires a lot of force. This is a part that cannot be easily lifted by pinching with your fingers. When the thread penetrates the exact center of this area, dimples or skin distortion (abnormal jamming due to cog) often occur.

When designing, avoid passing through this part through the exact center (depending on the type of thread, a skilled practitioner may be able to avoid causing side effects even if it passes through the exact center, but it is better for beginners to avoid it when designing).

Also, when designing, if you pass through the sides of the diamond, it will be easier to pass and reduce the possibility of side effects. However, if you avoid this area altogether and perform the treatment, you may feel disappointed because the rest of the area is lifted well and this area is not. In this case, inserting 1–2 short cog threads that extend only to the middle of the sunken cheek at the end of the procedure can improve the effect and prevent dimples.

Since it is difficult to pinch this part, it is better to press it with your fingers instead. You can use your second and third fingers, or use your second, third, and fourth fingers to press this part and pass the cannula or needle.

When treating a patient with this type of case, it is best to look in the mirror before the procedure and make the patient aware that there is a dent in the side of the cheek. In some cases, although the face has been lifted after the procedure, there are cases where patients complain that there is a depression on the side of the cheek that was not there originally.

8.5.5 OP Scar (Bone Surgery, Face Lifting Surgery, Etc.)

If traces or scars from surgery are in the path of the thread, it is difficult for the cannula or needle to pass through. Sometimes, the needle does not pass through well and the skin is pushed in the direction of progress. Not only must you check the medical history before the procedure, but you must also carefully check for scars when designing. This is because patients sometimes hide their previous surgical history. In addition to visible surgical scars, it is also necessary to check whether the movement of the subcutaneous tissue is more fixed than normal.

Therefore, the operator must design to avoid this part. When the cannula or needle does not pass easily, you should use the second and third fingers to press the tissue or alternate pinch operations to find a path which the needle or cannula can pass.

8.5.6 Liposuction/Accusculpt

In patients who have undergone this surgery, the fat in the facial area has a lot of fibrotic changes, making it difficult to pass a cannula or needle.

At this time, proceed by pressing the tissue using the second and third fingers or using a pinch operation to carefully find an area where the cannula or needle can easily pass. At the same time, when holding the cannula, it is easier to control the force by holding it close to the entry point.

8.5.7 Acne Scar

Among the types of acne scars, in patients who have developed rolling scars or boxcars, the lower part of the scar is often connected to the subcutaneous fat tissue like fibrous tissue. When passing through this part, it is not easy to pass because it affects the movement of the cannula or needle.

In this case, use your second and third fingers to press the tissue and delicately find an area that allows easy passage.

8.5.8 Previous Lifting Procedure History

When a patient who has received thread lifting comes back for the procedure a year later, the area through which the threads passed is bound to have fibrotic changes compared to when they first received it. Passing this part may affect the movement of the cannula or needle, making it more difficult than the first procedure.

And even when a patient who received HIFU undergoes thread lifting several months later, the operator can feel that the facial fat has become fibrotic overall.

When the cannula or needle does not pass easily like this, you can use your second or third finger to press the tissue or repeat the pinch operation to find an area that can pass easily and proceed carefully.

Summary—Differences in Density of Fat Tissue Depending on the Facial Area

- The fat from temple to zygoma is non-fibrous.
- When passing through zygoma, it is fibrous.
- Sunken cheek area is the most fibrous and dense.

- After passing through the sunken cheek, the fat tissue that appears next is soft.
- It becomes more fibrous toward the medial side of cheek.

8.5.9 Points to Check with the Patient Before the Procedure

8.5.9.1 Lateral Canthus Lifting

When inserting a thread from the lower cheek through the cheekbone toward the temple (mandible-zygoma-temple), if the innermost (medial) thread is close to the corner of the eye, the eyebrow raising phenomenon may occur. Most patients do not want their eye corners to rise after a thread lifting procedure. Because it can look fierce.

Sometimes, among young patients, there are people who want the corners of their eyes to be raised. In this case, the desired result can be achieved by moving the innermost thread further inward than originally designed. Since most patients do not want this, it is necessary to check in the mirror before the procedure.

8.5.9.2 Show Simulation of Treatment Results

Representative vectors during thread lifting include the vector from the marionette line toward the earlobe/the vector from the lower cheek through the cheekbone toward the temple/the vector from the nasolabial fold through the cheekbone toward the hairline.

Before the procedure, do a simulation using your hands while looking in the mirror and determine the optimal vector. When pulling the skin with your fingers, sometimes it is easier for the patient to understand if you use different numbers of fingers and explain the difference in the type and number of threads. This process is necessary because the vector imagined by the operator and the result desired by the patient may be different.

8.5.9.3 Entry Point Downtime/Hairline Shaving

The entry point of the thread can be broadly divided into three types.

The entry point on the side of the face (hairline or behind the ear) is not well exposed, so there is less discomfort for the patient and disinfection and preparation before the procedure are easy.

The location visible from the front of the face (medial than the hairline) is easy to disinfect and prepare before the procedure, but if the entry point hole is large, it may be uncomfortable because it is easily exposed.

The temple area (lateral to the hairline when located on the scalp) has the advantage of not being exposed when the entry point is located on the scalp, but the disinfection and preparation process before the procedure is complicated. At this time, cutting the hair is inevitable.

If you prepare by cutting about 3–5 hairs at the entry point (minimizing the number of hairs cut off), there will be no discomfort to the patient, but hair located next to the entry point may become an obstacle to the procedure. Therefore, tools that securely hold the hair are essential. In some cases, the hair around the entry point is shaving loosely to prevent it from becoming tangled. It is convenient for the operator because the obstructions are eliminated during the procedure, but the patient must be explained and consent is obtained before the procedure.

8.5.9.4 Asymmetry Check

Everyone has some facial asymmetry. Patients tend to be aware of asymmetry when they look in the mirror. If you take this into consideration during the procedure and pull more on the sagging side, it will be corrected to some extent.

However, sometimes the procedure is performed without the patient being aware of the left-right asymmetry, and sometimes, the patient complains of left-right asymmetry after the procedure. In these cases, even if it is explained that there was original asymmetry, patients may not accept it well. Therefore, it is necessary to check left and right asymmetry when designing.

Sometimes, there are patients who want complete correction of severely asymmetric cheeks or jaw lines. At this time, it is best for the practitioner to show the expected results in a mirror and explain them honestly. Also, when performing the procedure, it is necessary to pay attention to lifting on the relevant side.

8.5.10 Prognostic Factor

8.5.10.1 Masseter Muscle Hypertrophy

For patients with severe square jaw due to masseter muscle hypertrophy, the lifting effect does not appear well even if the operator simulates lifting by hand before the procedure.

In this case, pretreatment with botulinum toxin is necessary to correct the square jaw. It is most effective to perform the lifting procedure 1 month after the toxin treatment, when the masseter muscle shrinking effect appears, but it is generally performed together with the thread lifting procedure. Also, when comparing and explaining the effects before and after the procedure, be sure to show the front and side views and confirm to the patient that the jaw line, jowl, and marionette lines have been corrected.

8.5.10.2 Thickness of Facial Fat Tissue

If the overall amount of fat in the cheeks is large, the effect may be reduced because a lot of pulling force is required. Therefore, the problem is solved by using long threads rather than short threads or increasing the number of short threads. At the same time, consider performing a fat reduction procedure in parallel.

8.5.10.3 Degree of Sagging in the Marionette Line or Jowl

The lifting effect is good when the marionette line or jowl is slightly sagged. It is easy to show the expected results by looking in the mirror and doing a simulation before the procedure.

8.5.10.4 Degree of Submandibular Fat Sagging

In cases where there is a lot of fat under the chin or a double chin has developed, good results can be expected by using a bidirectional needle cogged thread. It is possible to obtain results similar to those obtained from liposuction in the past with a simple thread lifting procedure. When performing a face lifting procedure, if you also lift the skin under the chin, your jaw line will become more defined.

8.5.10.5 Elasticity of Tissues in the Front of the Face

In the case of patients with poor elasticity in the front of the face, lifting may not be sufficient or the maintenance period is short. When examining a patient, it is very important to measure the elasticity of the tissue and try to predict the outcome of the procedure. It is necessary to get into the habit of checking the patient's skin elasticity status—especially the elasticity of the front part of the face—by pinching and pressing the skin tissue or simulating a lifting procedure.

Procedural Methods of Cogged Thread Lifting by Target Site

9

Contents

S. M. Oh et al., *The Art and Science of Thread Lifting Based on Pinch Anatomy and Moving Plane*,
https://doi.org/10.1007/978-981-97-5516-5_9

When explaining cogged thread lifting for different facial areas, I would like to emphasize the following points. First, an explanation of the "moving plane" is essential. During the thread lifting procedure, it is crucial to identify which plane is primarily involved in movement to achieve effective results. Clinicians need to be well-informed about this aspect to ensure the procedure's success. Secondly, the topic of "fixing points" is important. Fixing points are critical for effectively pulling the tissue and creating directionality.

9.1 Eyebrow Lifting

9.1.1 Considerations for Forehead-Eyebrow Lifting

The forehead area has a limited amount of soft tissue, and wrinkles are formed by the expressions of the forehead muscles. From the perspective of the moving plane, the layer 4, which is the loose connective tissue beneath the frontalis muscle, moves well (Fig. 9.1).

Additionally, the movement at the lower part of the forehead is greater than at the upper part. Therefore, when bidirectional cog threads are inserted and pulled, the tissue is drawn toward the upper forehead, which moves less. In other words, the fixing point would be the upper forehead, and the tension point would be the lower forehead.

Furthermore, paralyzing the muscles that pull the forehead downward using botulinum toxin can maximize the effect of the thread lift.

For patients with sunken foreheads, using fillers to add volume can be beneficial.

9.1.2 Simulation of Eyebrow Lifting (Frontalis Pulling/Traction Test)

Perform simulation by showing a mirror to the patient prior to the procedure and the degree of the effect must be understood. When the frontalis muscle is pulled upward pressing near the hairline, people whose eyebrows lift have the anatomical structure in which the frontalis muscle reacts in constant direction from the hairline to below the eyebrow.

Lifting eyebrow lines and lifting drooped double eyelid lines should be considered separately. Until the mid-40s, when the eyebrows are lifted, the double eyelid lines elevate together, but if there is a skin laxity for those in the 50s or older, even the eyebrows are lifted, changes to the

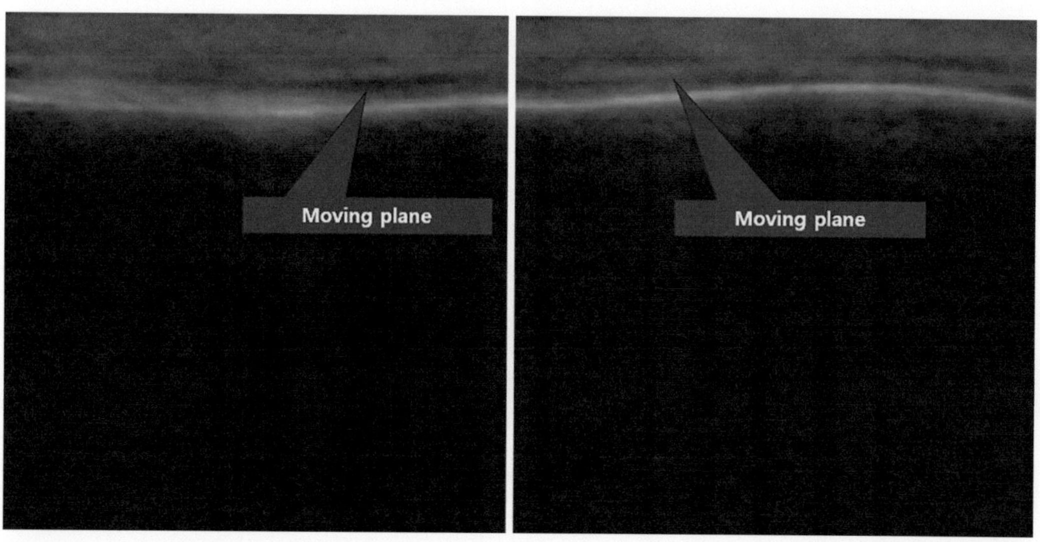

Fig. 9.1 Moving plane of the forehead

double eyelid lines may be minimal, which needs to be confirmed to the patient as well.

9.1.3 Simple Fixing Method

The method of thread insertion can be from bottom to top, or from top to bottom. Lifting the forehead using the simple fixing method is insufficient. To produce a good effect, supplemental procedures are required (Fig. 9.2).

After dissecting the loose connective tissue layer below the muscles of the forehead, pull upward using cog threads.

9.1.3.1 Cog Thread Tie or X-Cross Technique

Create multiple entry points at the upper part of the forehead, then insert bidirectional cog threads and either tie them or insert the remaining cogs in the opposite direction (Fig. 9.3).

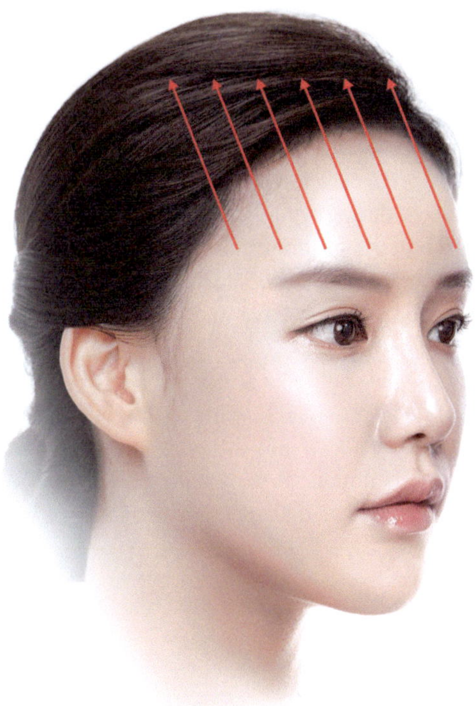

Fig. 9.2 Eyebrow lifting—simple fixing method: entry points and the number of threads to be inserted differ depending on the patients

After inserting and pulling the thread, the finishing method can be categorized into either the tie method or the X-cross method, depending on how it is completed (Figs. 9.4 and 9.5).

9.1.3.2 Anchoring Method

The anchoring method involves creating fixing points using the periosteum at the upper part of the forehead (Fig. 9.6). Because the soft tissue is thin and the periosteum itself is also thin in this area, actually anchoring the thread to the periosteum is not easy. However, since the upper part of

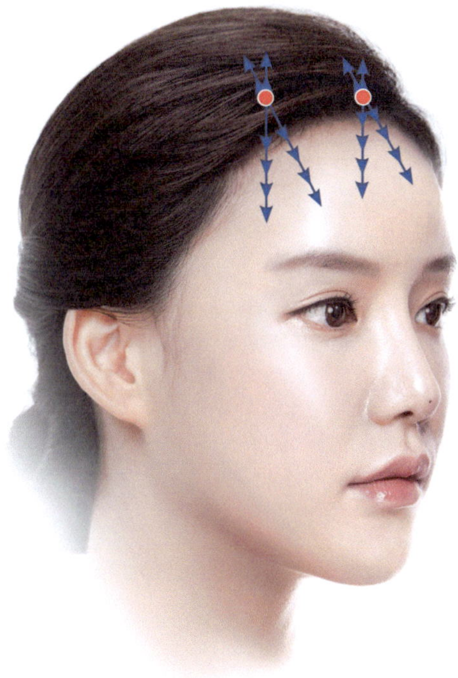

Fig. 9.3 Design of X-cross technique

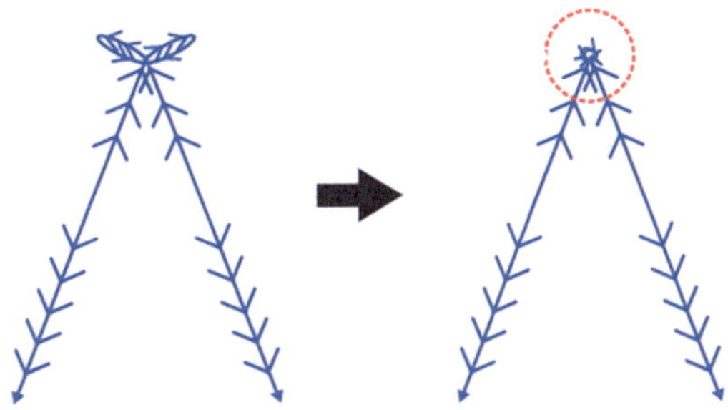

Fig. 9.4 Tie technique

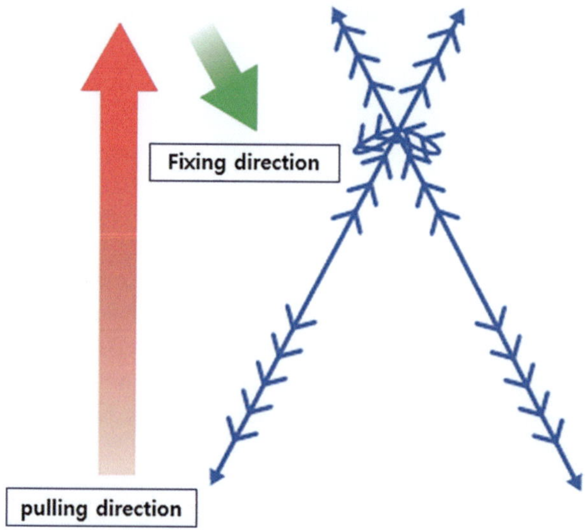

Fig. 9.5 X-cross technique

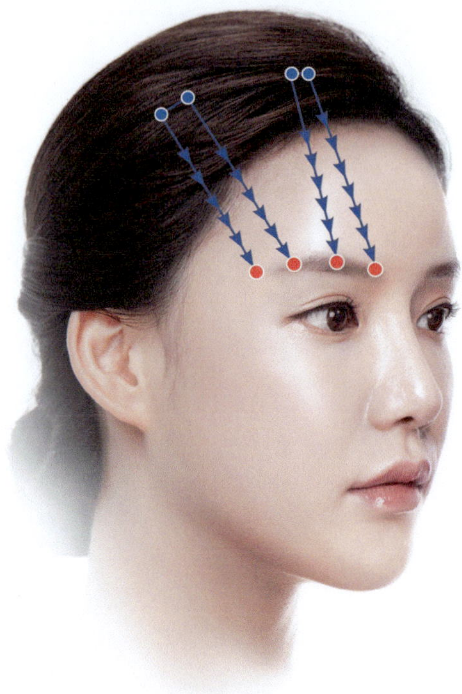

Fig. 9.6 Anchoring method

the forehead has relatively less movable than lower part, a fixing point is well established (Fig. 9.6).

This lifting method often requires tagging inside the hairline. It is generally a convenient procedure for using threads with needles attached to both ends (e.g., i-THREAD Magic Plus).

9.1.4 Anatomical Considerations

When performing procedures in the central forehead area, care must be taken not to damage the supra-trochlear artery and supra-orbital artery at the exit point. In treatments on the outer forehead, attention should be paid to the sentinel vein, superficial temporal artery, and superficial temporal vein. Especially, since the larger veins can be somewhat visible when lying down, they should be carefully checked to avoid vascular damage during tagging.

The path of the needle or cannula, as well as the thread, utilizes the deeper layers beneath the frontalis muscle, passing below the major vessels.

It is advisable to keep the thread's path as straight as possible. Finding a straight path on the outer forehead is not difficult. However, in this area, it is important to visually check the course of the vessels and take care to avoid major vessel damage.

9.1.5 Design

Always consider the curvature around the frontal bone to design a cannula or needle insertion path that minimizes the curve, and determine the entry and exit points accordingly. If the curvature complicates the design, adjust the entry and exit points to aim for a design as close to a straight line as possible.

If the patient usually exposes their forehead, create the entry point above the hairline to avoid exposure of the entry point. The end of the thread at the exit point should be draped over the corrugator muscle or muscle fibers for optimal effect. The number of threads can vary depending on the degree of forehead sagging.

When lifting the forehead using the anchoring method, it is crucial to understand the tissue changes in the forehead area due to aging. Typically, the skin around the eyes and eyebrows tends to sag more severely, making the lifting of the lateral part important. Also, since the forehead soft tissue is thin, it is essential to insert the thread deeply to avoid the thread being palpable or creating an uneven surface. Since nerve pathways mostly run in the superficial layers where threads are inserted, deeper layer is safer. However, during lateral part procedures, damage to the facial n. zygomatic branch can result in eyebrow ptosis.

9.2 Lateral Canthus and Temporal Hairline Lifting

The area around the eyes experiences significant stretching of the skin and soft tissues. The first thing to determine in treating the lateral eye area is whether the patient is a suitable candidate for the treatment. Lifting with absorbable threads is fundamentally not a surgery, so it does not involve the removal of skin or soft tissues. Therefore, one cannot expect the same effects as surgery.

Compared to other facial areas, considering surgical treatment options for eye area lifting might be necessary. This is because the skin, soft tissues, and eyelids around the eyes sag much more severely than the outer forehead. This area has the greatest difference between upper and lower part movements. So, pulling on the soft tissue on the outer part of the forehead may not result in significant movement around the eyes, as the soft tissue on the outer forehead is relatively firm and less mobile. Therefore, surgical treatment that directly removes the most severely sagged areas is often necessary.

In the area around the eyes, the primary moving plane is the layer 4 corresponding to the innominate fascia, which is beneath the superficial temporal fascia. This is due to the loose connective tissues between the superficial temporal fascia and the deep temporal fascia.

9.2.1 Anatomy of Eye Area

When performing absorbable thread lifting to lift the area around the eyes, it is advisable to insert the threads in the supra-periosteal plane in the frontalis muscle area, and in the subcutaneous fat layer in the temporalis muscle area. Due to the potential for damaging the superficial temporal vessels, gentle manipulation and the use of the pinch technique should be appropriately employed to minimize bleeding (Fig. 9.7).

The frontal branches of the facial nerve form numerous branches, so significant clinical nerve damage is unlikely unless damaged all at once. However, to avoid the side effects of nerve damage, it is always necessary to clearly understand

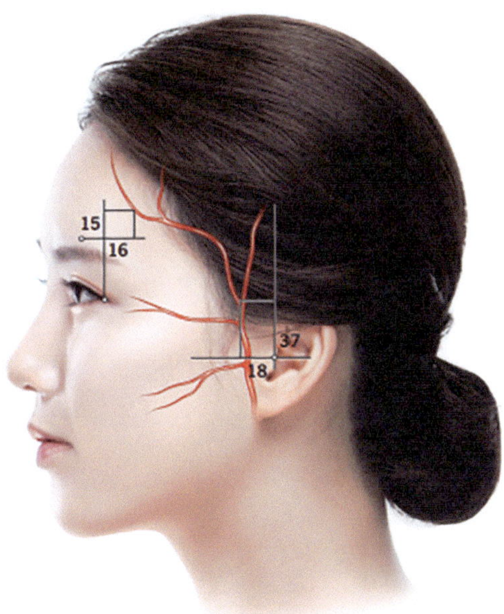

Fig. 9.7 Pathway of superficial temporal artery

the entry layer and perform gentle manipulation (Fig. 9.8).

9.2.1.1 Techniques That Can Be Used Around the Eyes

There is a thread lifting technique by tumescent dissection that is applicable only to some specific areas.

The approach to lifting using threads can be viewed from two perspectives.

The first approach involves directly pulling the tissue. This method is applied to all areas and is the basic model. The second method involves dissecting a specific layer of tissue, pulling the tissue along the dissected plane, and then fixing it in place with a thread. Even before inserting the thread, a natural lifting effect occurs due to the dissection and pulling. However, if the pulled tissue is not secured, the effect immediately disappears. In other words, it involves dissecting a specific layer using tumescent, and then inserting and securing a cog thread in that area.

This facilitates the insertion of threads, reduces pain, and leads to less bleeding, which are significant advantages. The author uses a method where a specific layer of the face is dissected using a tumescent solution, then the solution is manually squeezed out before inserting the thread. In this case, the anesthetic effect is maintained, resulting in less swelling after the procedure.

9.2.1.2 Creating Fixing Points Around the Eyes

In the area around the eyes, the tie method or the X-cross method is often used (Figs. 9.9 and 9.10). For the area around the eyes, the higher the fixing point is made above the head and the lower the hanging point is made, the better the lifting effect. To prevent the appearance of a fierce expression caused by only lateral eyes being lifted, it is recommended to perform a wide hydrodissection including the upper lateral part of eyes before pulling. The layer for hydrodissection is beneath the frontalis muscle in the upper forehead area and between the deep temporal fascia and superficial temporal fascia layers or in the subcutaneous fat layer in the temple area. After dissection, inserting and pulling the thread is much more

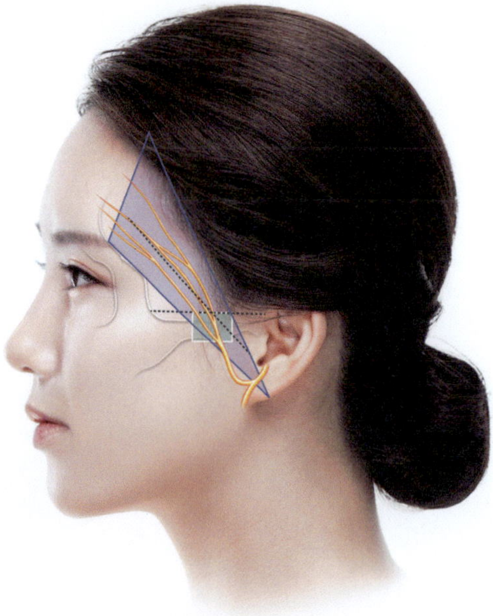

Fig. 9.8 Pathway of facial nerve temporal branch

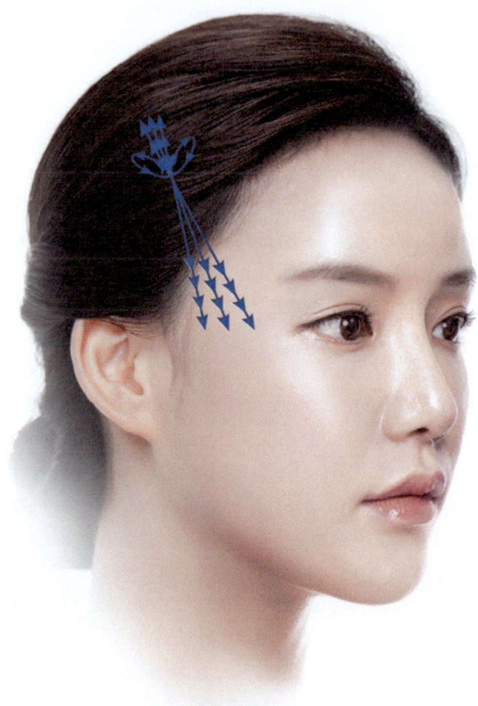

Fig. 9.9 Tie method of eye lifting

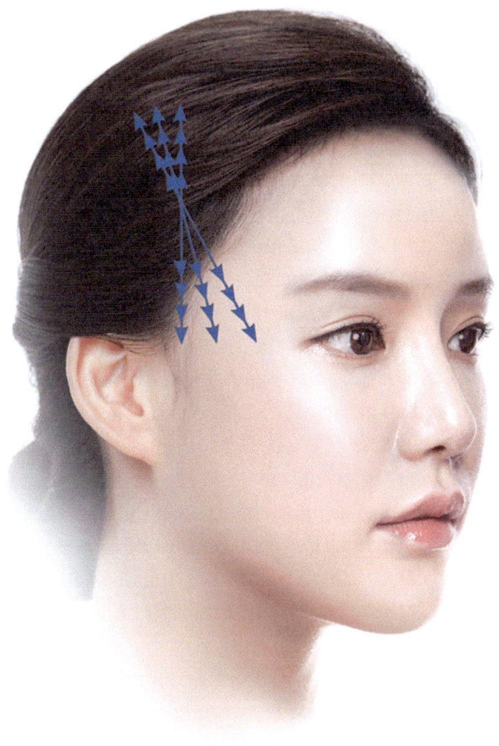

Fig. 9.10 X-cross method of eye lifting

effective in drawing the tissue compared to pulling without dissection. Afterward, supplementing with a fixing type of thread (zigzag-type cog thread) helps with securing.

Similar to the tie method, after tying the cog, instead of removing all of the remaining opposite cogs, some are left and then inserted upward. It is expected that the lifting effect will be stronger and last longer due to the function of the opposite direction cogs. Typically, the remaining cog thread is reinserted into the cannula, and when the cannula is inserted in the opposite direction, the remaining cogs are inserted and fixed on the other side (Fig. 9.10).

9.2.2 Precautions

The area around the eyes involves lifting both the lateral part of the forehead and the temple area simultaneously. Therefore, the procedure is performed on two anatomically different areas. It is safe to perform the procedure only after understanding the anatomical structures of both sides—the course and depth of blood vessels, and nerves. At the same time, a combination treatment with botulinum toxin for the hyperactivity of the muscles that cause sagging in that area is also necessary. However, above all, the most important thing is not to waste resources by unnecessarily recommending thread lifting to patients who need surgical treatment.

9.3 Anterior Malar Lifting for Ogee Curve

9.3.1 Anatomical Considerations

With aging, the deep layer of the malar fat pad, which makes the apple cheek, is depressed and the supporting of superficial layer is poor, and resultantly, the tissues below are drooped and bulging.

In this case, the muscles that make wrinkles around eye can be weakened with botulinum toxin, and the sunken of tissues around eyes is filled with filler or fat graft. In addition, when the wrinkles are settled and seem like fine cracks, the crack can be filled with soft consistent filler. However, when the soft tissues that have been bulging up are not pulled up, it is basically impossible to solve the problem, so we need to lift the tissues upward by using the cogged threads. Also, when inserting non-cogged volumizing threads underneath the depressed tissues, the skin texture can be firm by collagen regeneration and maximize the effect of the filler and fat graft.

Ultimately, you may see the effect of pulling up the infraorbital skin and tissues, resultantly making the skin firm, and lessening the folds. So then, we will discuss the age-dependent changes of important anatomical structures in infraorbital area that need to be noticed before thread lifting.

As the age increases, the medial cheek volume deficiency, together with sagging, reverses the central cheek triangle and creates an oblique midcheek groove that extends outwardly and entirely in those with weak nasojugal grooves. In this case, the fat tissue and the skin located on the upper side of the depressed groove appear malar bag which seems relatively bulging. This requires lifting with cogged threads in order to correct the bulging malar bag without surgery (Fig. 9.11).

When the correction is not made, the above symptoms become worse over time, especially volume of the deep fat layer located under the arcus marginalis (SOOF) and deep medial cheek fat, which is the deep fat supporting the central cheek decrease. In addition, when the elasticity of the skin is decreased, it is accompanied with the sagging of the skin and soft tissues of the anterior cheek and infraorbital hollowness that shows the wide depression of infraorbital region (Fig. 9.12).

The structure of the anterior cheek area for the successful procedure is as follows: The layer from the upper part of the cheek is composed of the skin, superficial malar fat pad, orbicularis muscle, deep malar fat pad including suborbicularis oculi fat (SOOF), and muscle for facial expression, including zygomaticus muscle, periosteal fat, and periosteum. There is a zygomatico-cutaneous ligament in the anterior cheek region which starts from the deepest part of the bone layer and runs obliquely from the medial side to the outer side down to the skin. When this ligament develops, the midcheek groove or furrow mentioned above can be seen in the anteromedial cheek region.

Midcheek groove refers to the band-like fibrosis along the zygomatico-cutaneous ligament at the cheek. The malar fat pad is divided above and below this ligament. When the pulling force of the ligament is strong, two upper and lower parts may appear bulging around the middle band. The deep medial cheek fat at the lower part of the ligament, which occupies a relatively large area as the patient ages, is reduced and becomes shallow. The nasolabial fat and medial cheek fat are loosened downward as the volume of the supporting layer is reduced.

On the other hand, malar fat, including SOOF on the upper side of the ligament, is held by the tear trough ligament and orbicularis retaining ligament that surrounds the orbital bone, so that the difference between the upper and lower boundaries becomes evident. In addition, when laughing or making facial expression, the skin of the groove where the skins are pulled inside is not moved easily due to the fibrotic bands of the ligament, so that the groove tends to be seen more easily (Fig. 9.13).

When performing anterior malar lifting using cogged threads and volumizing non-cogged threads, the position and role of these ligamentous structures that support the skin and soft tissues of the anterior cheek area and maintain their shape should be taken into consideration to restore the volume of the face by pulling the droopy tissues.

The main vessel below the eye includes infraorbital artery that comes out of the infraorbital foramen that is 8–10 mm below the orbital margin based on the medial pupillary line, and zygomaticofacial artery that emerges from the

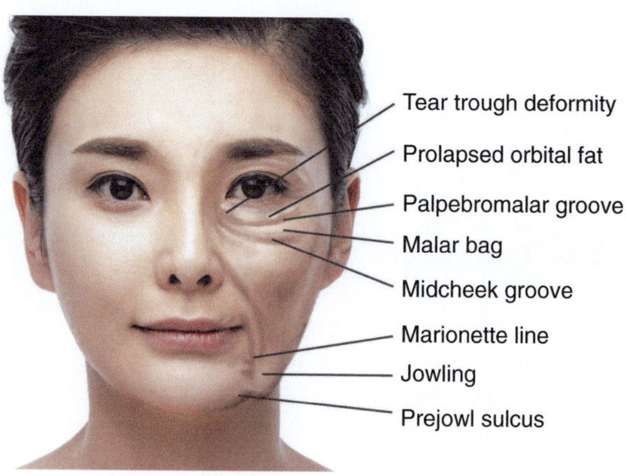

Fig. 9.11 Midcheek groove with malar bag

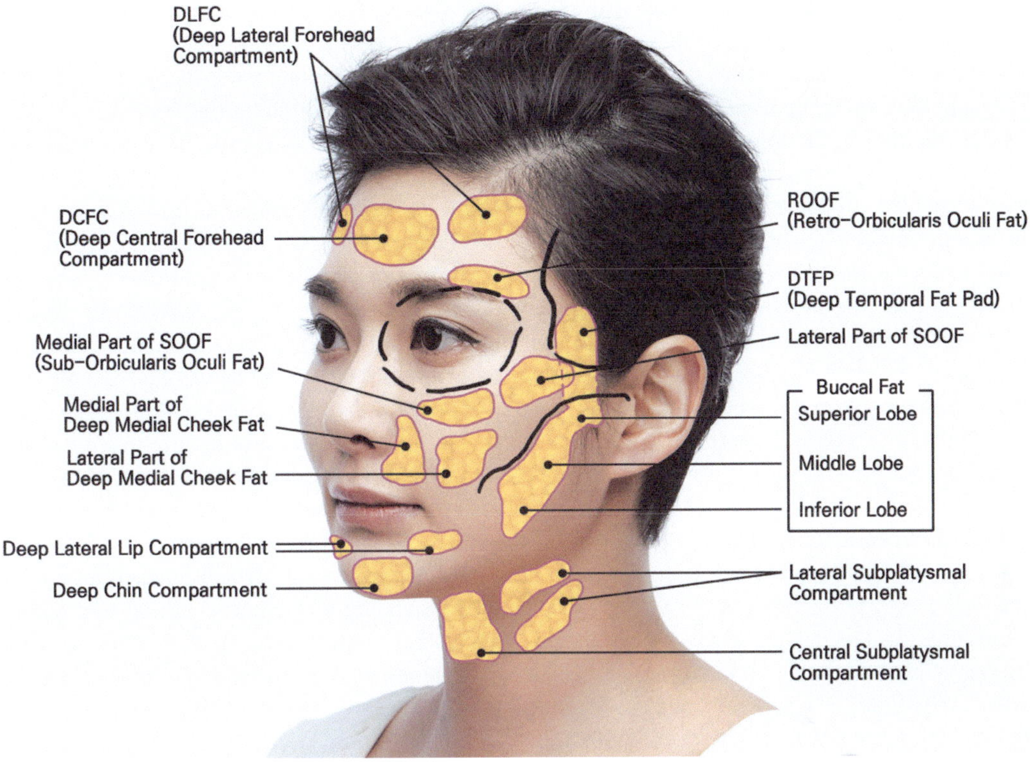

Fig. 9.12 Location of SOOF and deep medial cheek fat

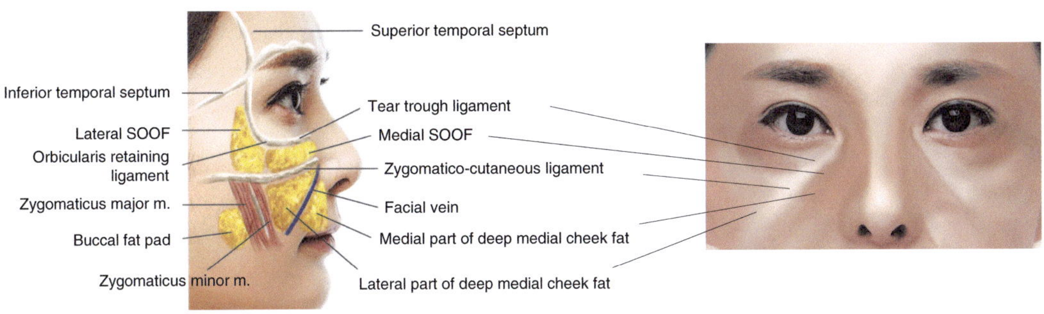

Fig. 9.13 Infraorbital hollowness with loss of deep fat layer

zygomaticofacial foramen that is below the lateral margin of lateral orbital rim (usually 10–15 mm below the horizontal line of lateral canthus). In more than 30% of Koreans, there is an infraorbital trunk of the duplex-type facial artery called the detoured branch of the facial artery that passes into the medial and lower eyelids of the inferior orbit along the nasojugal groove which is connected to the medial part of the midcheek groove, and also, the angular vein that runs deeper than the angular artery is always seen. The infraorbital trunk of the duplex-type facial artery and angular vein runs along the medial border of the SOOF which is the infraorbital deep fat and the lateral part of the deep medial cheek fat. Therefore, care should be taken when performing on this site. Also, as the medial branch of the infraorbital artery travels along the nasojugal groove, and it comes out to the surface layer from the point where the nasojugal groove and the tear trough come into contact with each other, the special care should be needed when performing the procedure in this point (Fig. 9.14).

In addition, when we want to use non-cogged volumizing threads to improve the infraorbital areas that are depressed, it should be considered that veins that are developed under the eyes, including inferior palpebral vein, are difficult to avoid when the needles are used. Therefore, it is good to use the needle when lightly treating the border of the tear troughs, but it is better to use the thread inserted into the cannula to avoid severe vascular damage when performing the procedures in the entire infraorbital region.

9.3.2 Procedural Design and Techniques

With aging, the tear trough gets worsened due to the loss of elasticity and sagging of the midfacial tissues, the orbital fat protrusion, and the volume loss of soft tissue around the eyes. With this symptom of depression, the area under the tear trough is retained by the skin attachment of the ligamentous tissues and is transformed into a hanging shape with the weakening of ligamentous tissues. If these symptoms are accompanied by tissue loss, an additional thread lifting procedure is required along with filler procedures that volumize the region for correction.

The position and shape of the apple cheek preferred by Westerners and Asians are different when performing the thread lifting which pulls up and gathers the sagging and flattened structure of the anteromedial cheek and tightens it by collagen regeneration effect. Westerners like to make a protruding part on the side or upper part of an anterior cheek, but since Asian people have a wider face than Westerners and often have protruded malar eminence in nature, making a protruding part in the middle of anterior cheek may make the face more concentrated and visually softens the side lines of the face.

Usually, when the vertical line is drawn at the outer boundary of the lateral orbital rim, mainly the medial soft tissues based on this line are made to be augmented. Rather than pulling the sagging tissue forcibly as much as possible, it is appropriate to make the fat pad look as soft and round as it is pulled up by the movement of the muscles when laughing.

It is advisable to lift nasolabial fat that runs along the nasolabial crease above the medial part

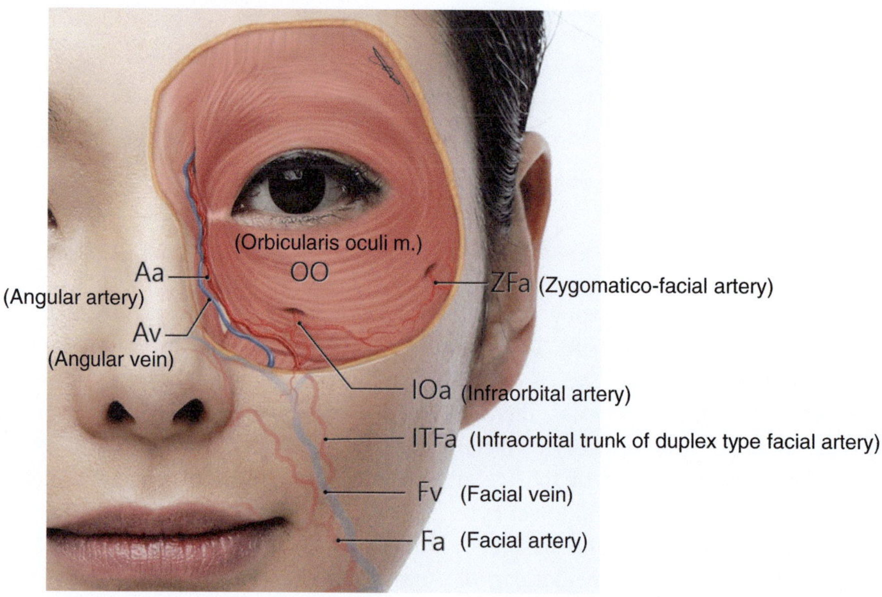

Fig. 9.14 Main vessels of infraorbital region

of deep medial cheek fat, which wraps tissues around nose under the orbicularis oculi muscle, to volumize the medial part of anteromedial cheek, depending on the shape of the face and the maxillary bone. Also, it is good to perform procedure, examining whether the procedure is not interfering upper lip elevator muscles including zygomatic muscles to make the smooth shape of anteromedial cheek by lifting the soft tissues on anterior malar area.

For the design of the cogged thread lifting that pulls the sagging tissues around the eyes, a puncture site for cannula insertion around the orbital rim is made and a threaded cannula is inserted to allow the cogs of threads hold the sagging tissues. For designing the procedure, the patient is made to open the eyes in a seated position and then the puncture site and the direction of the thread are marked. In order to reduce the bruising on the needle puncture, the vein should be avoided as much as possible.

When designing the entry point into which the cogged thread is inserted, care must be taken to avoid damage to the infraorbital artery and nerve and the zygomaticofacial artery and nerve coming from the orbital bone. When the patient is laid down and hands are put under the patient's eyes for the procedure, the soft tissues under the eyes, which are sagging downward, can easily be seen to lean toward the head. When puncturing a needle for insertion of a cannula, care should be taken to puncture the skin only since it may cause severe bleeding if the vessels are punctured. The plane for insertion of a cannula for thread lifting procedure should be deep enough to penetrate the underlying orbicularis oculi muscle and pass through the ligamentous tissue around the eye because the skin is thin and there is little space between the skin and the orbicularis muscle (Fig. 9.15).

If you want to augment the central part of the anterior malar region, draw a vertical line from the lateral limbus as shown in Fig. 9.16 and make an entry point at the point where this line meets the orbital rim. Through one entry point, three or four cogged threads in the fanning shape are inserted from upper part to lower part to pull the stretched fat layers around the eyes. As with other areas, the intensity of lifting can be determined as making the patient lying down with his/her chin lifted to let the skin and tissues under the eyes lean toward the head. After insertion of the

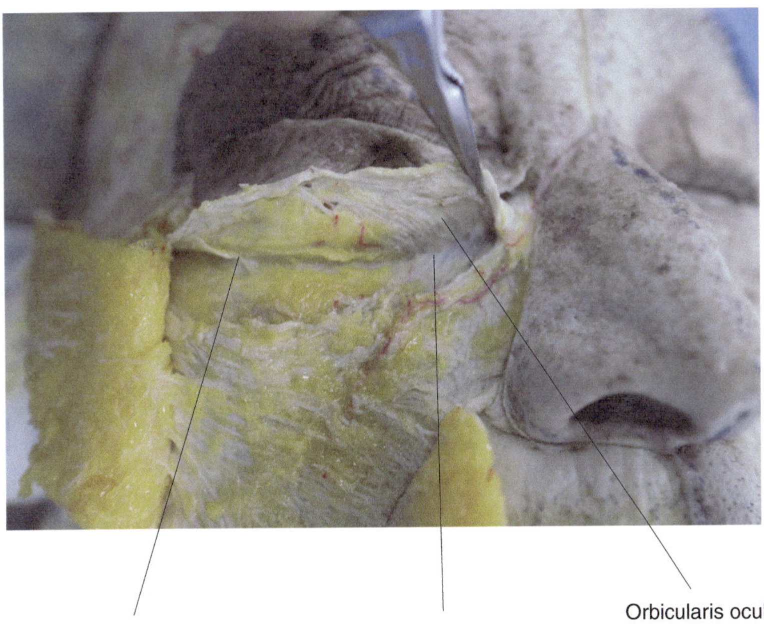

Fig. 9.15 Infraorbital ligamentous tissue

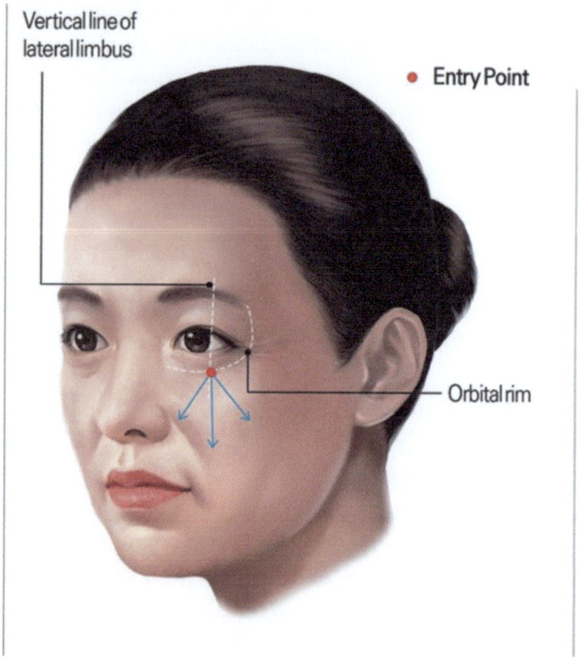

Fig. 9.16 Entry point and direction of cogged threads for anterior malar lifting (middle part)

cogged thread cannula under the orbicularis oculi muscle through the entry point, the fat pad of the area to be pulled by the untreated hand is grasped and then gently massage the skin and soft tissues of anterior malar region toward the eye. Turn it upward and slowly advance the cannula down to the desired position along the pre-designed direction of the cogged thread (Fig. 9.16).

Sometimes, there is a midcheek groove formed by the zygomatico-cutaneous ligament of the anterior malar region, and a sagging nasolabial fat beneath it. In this case, the tissue should be pulled in the vertical direction of the nasolabial fold on the nose, so the entry point and lifting vector of the cogged thread should be changed.

It would be the most proper position to insert the cogged thread making an angle to the lateral orbital thickening (LOT), which is made up of the tough ligament tissues around the eye can be used as a fixation point for cogged thread lifting. It would be the most proper to insert cogged threads obliquely at this entry point and to lift the medial parts of fat around orbicularis muscle (Fig. 9.17).

In the procedural design, as shown in Fig. 9.18, the entry point is made at the area where the horizontal line of the lateral canthus meets the lateral orbital rim or the orbital rim margin slightly below. If the cogged thread is inserted through the thin skin inside the rim that is not supported by the bones, it may irritate eye movement after the procedure and the end of the thread tends to be pushed out. Therefore, the entry point should always be on the skins that are supported by orbital bones. To know the depth of the tissue through which the thread should pass, the shallow pinch can lift up only the thin skin tissue loosely, but if you pull the deep tissue tightly, you can feel that there is a stiff tissue under the skin. After thinly puncturing the entry point with needle, the cannula is inserted to penetrate the tight fascia tissue under the skin, and then, the cannula can be advanced to the area of the drooped fat layer adjacent to the nose (Fig. 9.18).

You can do two kinds of tests beforehand to find out how much improvement of infraorbital area can be achieved. A smiling test to check the level of the protrusion of the infraorbital fat is a

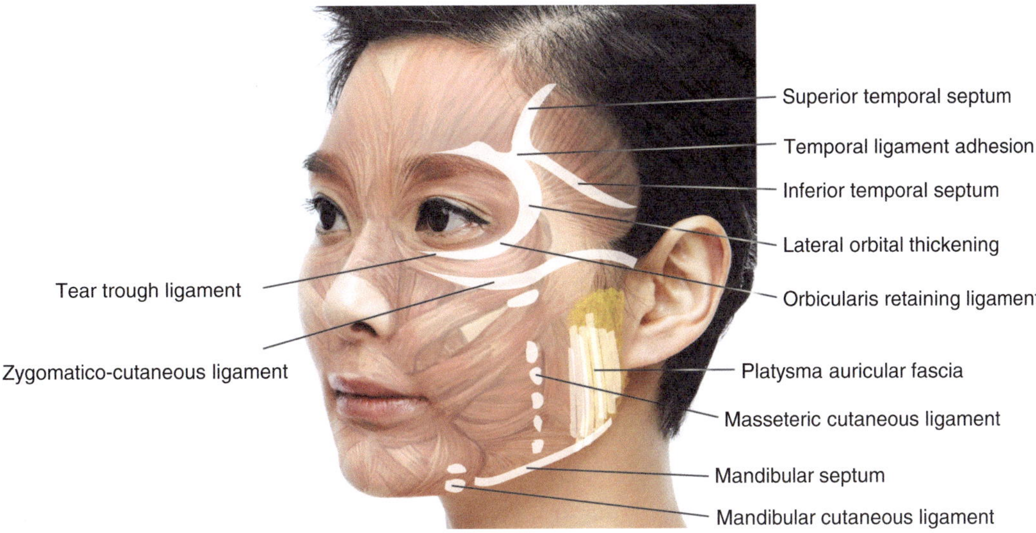

Fig. 9.17 Periorbital tight ligamentous tissue

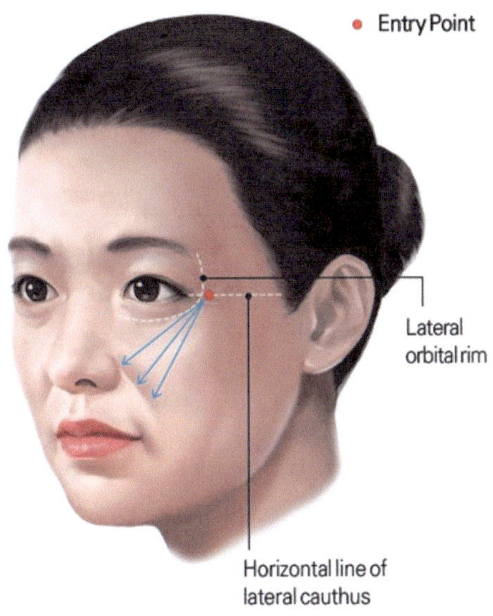

Fig. 9.18 Entry point and direction of cogged threads for anterior malar lifting (medial part)

test to see how much infraorbital fat protrudes to some extent by making the patient laugh. It is good to explain to the patient in advance that further treatment for the infraorbital region may be necessary if the infraorbital bulge is seen protruding even when the lateral orbital skin is pulled in a laugh state. The pushing test to know the extent of skin sagging is a test to see how much excess skin is left when the skin under eye is pressed by the fingertip and pulled laterally. If the skin excessively gathered when pulling the skin toward the eye is more than 1 cm, there would be a limit to the lifting the skin only by procedure other than surgery. Therefore, it is good to show and explain the test results to the patient. These tests may explain to the patient the effects and limitations of the thread lifting procedure and naturally suggest if additional procedure is required.

With aging, as the skin under the eyes gets thinner and the volume of subcutaneous fat reduces with adding of pseudo-herniation of the orbital fat, dark circles may appear due to lighting conditions. Dark circles are also improved after the thread lifting procedure in cases caused by changes in structures other than skin pigment problems or blood vessels fundamentally viewed.

In order to have the above-mentioned effects through the thread lifting procedure, it is necessary to distinguish the patient suitable for the thread lifting. Patients with prominent orbital fat protrusions, patients with severe drooping of infraorbital skin and tissues, patients with severe allergic or edema around the eyes with skin damage, and patients with scar tissue on infraorbital region due to previous lower eyelid surgery or for other reasons need careful examination before the procedure, since the above effects may not appear sufficiently during the procedure.

9.4 Lateral and Buccal Cheek Lifting for Oval Shape

In lifting this area, the primary moving plane is the subcutaneous layer. This is because the SMAS is relatively firmly attached to the layer below it. The formation of fixation points is important, and depending on whether it is possible to create movement in the zygomatico-cutaneous ligament, the lifting can be divided into two types.

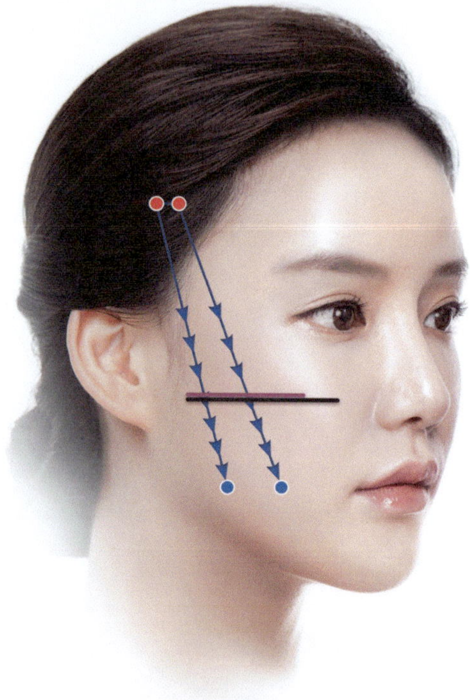

Fig. 9.19 Fascia anchoring technique

9.4.1 The Method of Inducing Movement in the Zygomatico-Cutaneous Ligament

The first method of inducing movement in the zygomatico-cutaneous ligament during lifting involves creating a strong fixing point by anchoring onto the deep temporal fascia. This technique involves pulling the zygomatico-cutaneous ligament, which is one of the strongest ligamentous structures and tends not to move much, by fixing a thread to the sturdy deep temporal fascia (Fig. 9.19). It is a method that continuously draws up the lateral face, including the lower part of the cheek.

While this is one of the most powerful and useful thread lifting techniques, it requires careful handling due to the difficulty of the procedure and the risk of vascular and nerve damage. It demands a thorough understanding of anatomical structures and attention to technique. It can be considered a true form of skin lifting. The tissues that are pulled will gather toward the tagging site inside the hairline.

9.4.2 The Method of Pulling the Sagging Tissues of the Lower Face Toward the Zygomatico-Cutaneous Ligament

In this case, movement is not created in the zygomatico-cutaneous ligament itself, but rather, lower face tissues are pulled toward that area. Short threads are typically used, inserted from below to above or from above to below, followed by pushing or pulling of tissue.

9.4.2.1 Tie Method

The lifting effect is achieved by utilizing the function of bidirectional cog threads to gather tissues toward the center (Fig. 9.20). The skin and subcutaneous fat layer converge at the midpoint of the bidirectional cogs (Fig. 9.21).

Since tissues gather at the midpoint of the thread, it is important during design to ensure that this midpoint does not align with the zygomatic arch area, as this could lead to the side effect of making the lateral cheekbones appear larger after thread lifting.

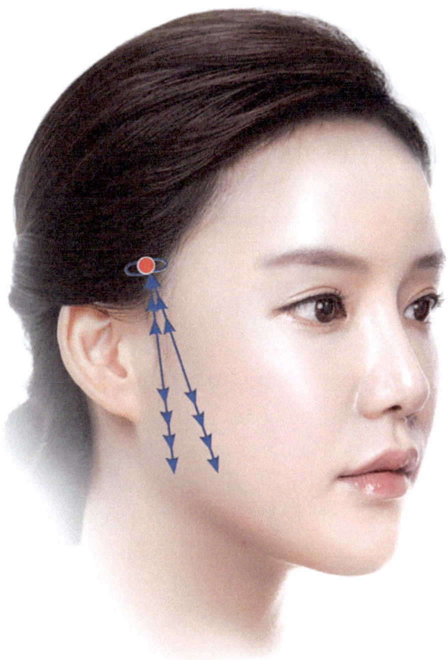

Fig. 9.20 Tie method

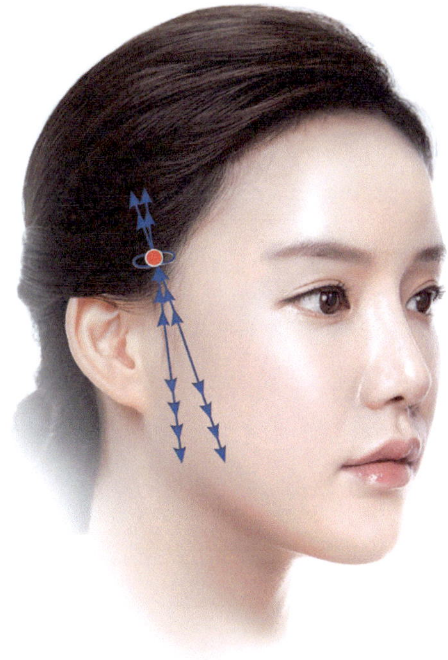

Fig. 9.22 A procedure that involves inserting the remaining cog area toward the opposite side without removing it after the tie

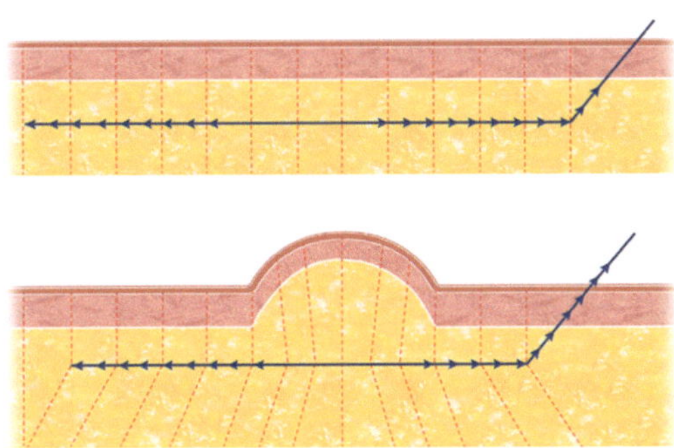

Fig. 9.21 Principle of bidirectional cog threads

Since this is not a method of creating a firm fixing point, the effect may be less pronounced in individuals with a lot of subcutaneous fat in the lower cheeks or thicker skin. The technique tends to be more effective in individuals with thin skin and less subcutaneous fat, especially those whose skin readily moves when pulled. It is necessary to insert a sufficient number of threads.

The tissues above the zygomatico-cutaneous ligament are often treated separately, leading to separate upper and lower lifts.

9.4.2.2 X-Cross Method

The X-cross method is fundamentally similar to the tie method, but it enhances the strength of the fixation cog by not discarding the remaining cog and instead pushing it toward the opposite direction (Fig. 9.22).

9.4.2.3 Reverse Technique

Instead of inserting the thread from above and pulling lower face, this method involves inserting the thread from below and pulling the facial tissues upward toward the zygomatico-cutaneous ligament. The procedure is simple and carries less risk of infection compared to when an entry point is made near the hairline (Fig. 9.23).

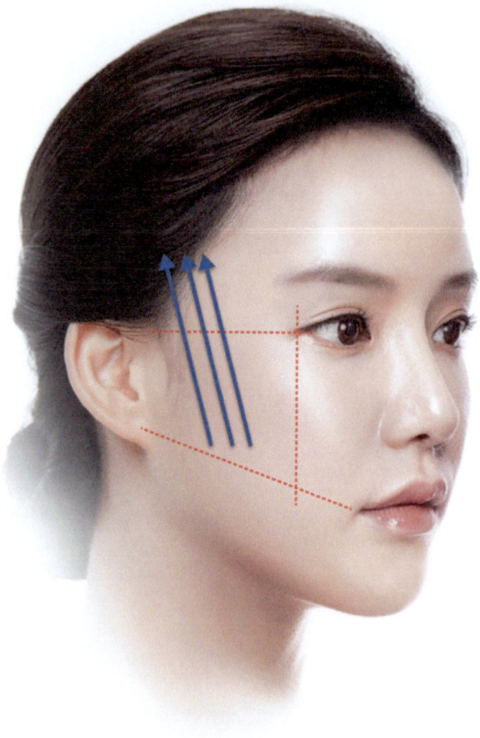

Fig. 9.23 When using the reverse technique for thread insertion, bidirectional cog threads or fixed-type threads (e.g., zigzag type) can be used. The number of threads varies depending on the degree of sagging, with typically 4-6 threads being used

9.5 Nasolabial Fold Lifting

In the past, it was common to set the entry point near the hairline and run the thread to the nasolabial fold area, but considering the potential side effects that arise from the curved route of thread lifting, as opposed to a straight path, such methods are not commonly used anymore.

Generally, a procedure that involves inserting the thread from a specific area below the lateral canthus toward the nasolabial fold and then pulling it is more widely used (Fig. 9.24a). Vertical lifting, which involves pulling the cheek tissue vertically from below the eye, is also frequently used (Fig. 9.24b).

Recently, there has been an increase in the use of thread insertion procedures that compress the nasolabial fold area using firm types of multifilament or coil threads (Fig. 9.25). Strictly speaking, it is difficult to call this a lifting procedure, but it effectively improves the indentation of the nasolabial folds by compressing the sagging tissue.

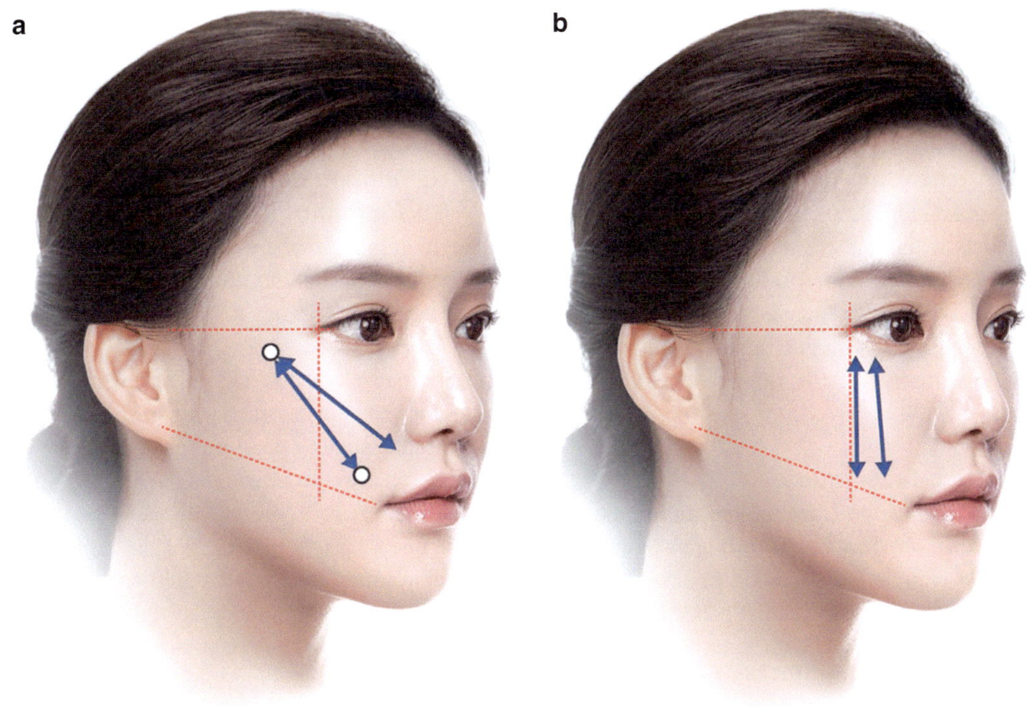

Fig. 9.24 (**a**) Lifting of the nasolabial fold area. (**b**) Vertical lifting

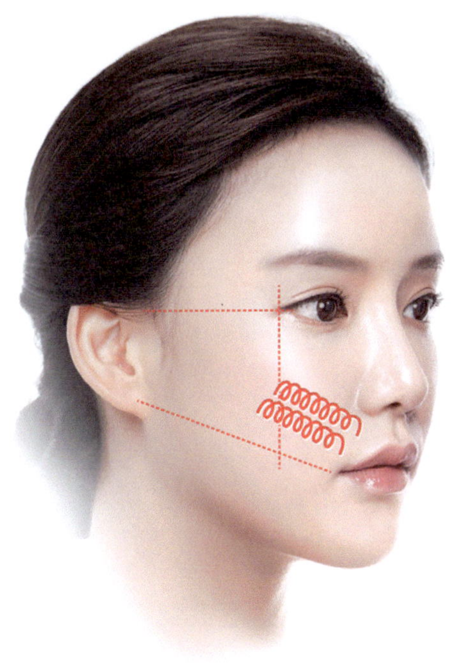

Fig. 9.25 Thread insertion in the nasolabial area—effect of compressing the nasolabial fat pad

9.6 Marionette Line and Jowl Lifting

9.6.1 Considerations for Marionette Line Lifting

When lifting marionette lines, it is essential to design the procedure in relation to the pre-jowl area. Simply injecting filler into the sunken areas to eliminate marionette lines can exacerbate facial sagging. The pre-jowl area, which contributes to the formation of marionette lines, should be pulled toward the ear. At the same time, the sagging pre-jowl area needs to be lifted upward.

The wrinkles in the marionette area fundamentally require a design that pulls toward the ear. Considering the principle of thread lifting, the tightened skin must gather somewhere.

At this time, a portion of the tightened skin gathers in front of the ear, requiring a delicate procedure to minimize the formation of wrinkles or folds as much as possible.

9.6.1.1 Angle Technique

Insert a bidirectional cog thread at the insertion point (red dot), then bend it in the middle to proceed toward the marionette line area. After reaching the hanging point, pull the thread for lifting. Then, remove any remaining thread at the insertion point (Fig. 9.26).

Due to the gathering function of the bidirectional cog inherent in the angle technique, the pulled tissue tends to move toward the inner part of the angle. By utilizing this well, one can anticipate additional benefits in improving the sunk-in areas of the cheeks.

9.6.1.2 L-Technique

In the case of the L-technique, unlike the angle technique, the thread exits through a blue-colored circular area, and the method involves removing the exiting thread. Typically, procedures are performed using threads with long needles attached to the end (e.g., i-THREAD Magic Plus). This technique provides much stronger tissue gathering and lifting effects compared to the angle technique. However, because wrinkles or sinking may occur more on the skin, delicate procedures are required (Fig. 9.27).

9.6.1.3 Tagging Method: Technique for Pulling Behind the Jaw Line

Entry points are marked at intervals of 1–1.5 cm on the firm area behind the angle. In cases where there is severe sagging of the skin in the cheek area, the effects of the angle technique or L-technique alone may be insufficient. In such cases, it may be necessary to pull beyond the mandibular angle toward the posterior aspect of the ear to lift more effectively. When tagging in this area, there is no need to tag the thread excessively deeply as the tissue here is dense. It is advisable to tag the thread shallowly in the firm tissue behind the mandibular angle to avoid potential injury to the greater auricular nerve that could occur from tagging too deeply in this area (Fig. 9.28).

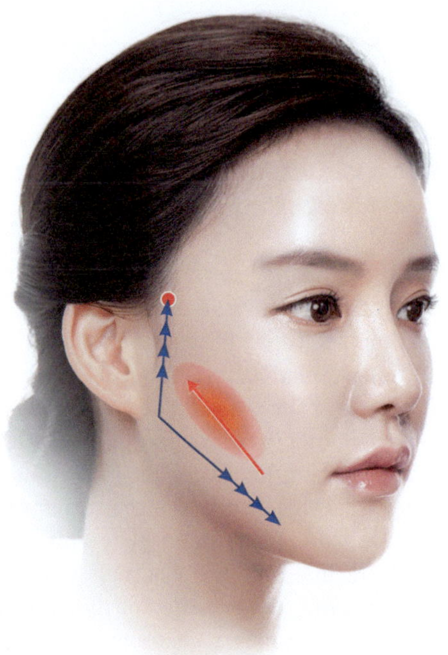

Fig. 9.26 Angle technique

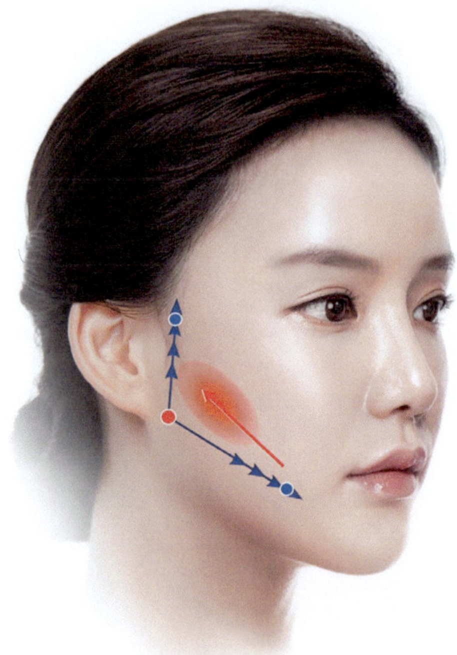

Fig. 9.27 L-technique

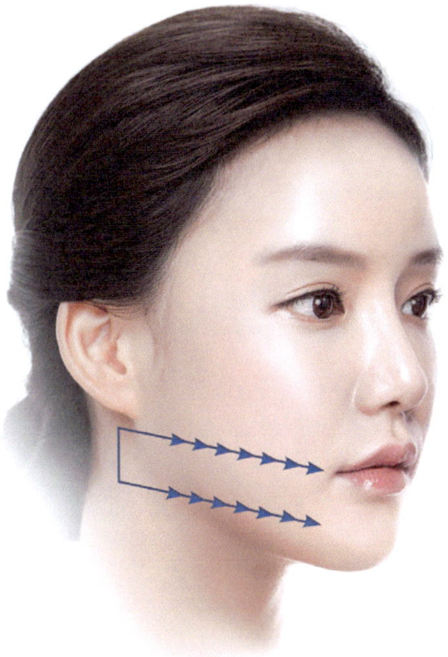

Fig. 9.28 Tagging method—technique for pulling behind the jaw line

9.7 Mandible Borderline Lifting

9.7.1 Anatomical Considerations

With aging, the skin around the jaw line is sagged and it is necessary to sharpen the blurry jaw line through the mandible border line lifting.

Basically, the cogged thread lifting on jaw line is a procedure that inserts cogged threads along the mandibular border line through the ear lobe side to lift the sagging skin and soft tissues around the jaw line, inducing a sense of tightness around the mandible border for sharp and smooth jaw line.

The entry point of the cogged thread should be made on the skin of the boundary of ear lobe and cheek located at the rear of the jaw line. At the boundary between the ear lobe and cheek, there is a platysma auricular ligament, a firm, fascial tissue that keeps the earlobes from sagging down. It is a ligament tissue of the trapezoidal shape that emerges from the deep fascia between the ear lobe and the posterior border of the platysma muscle. It is connected like a tree nest from the dermis to the deep fascia at the boundary between the lower part of the ear lobe and the cheek. Anatomically, we can see the ligamentous tissue such as a thick band when the SMAS layer under the skin is raised. It is a tissue different from platysma auricular fascia, which is located in a similar position and is widely distributed between ears and the posterior border of the platysma, although similar in name and sometimes considered to be the same tissue but anatomically different (Fig. 9.29).

By setting a fixing point of cogged thread on the ligament, the loose tissues of the chin area are pulled toward the direction of ears as the thread holds the skin and soft tissues.

When using a cannula to insert cogged threads along the jaw line, it is very unlikely that a marginal mandibular nerve, which is a branch of the facial nerve running along the direction of the cannula, is injured but care should be taken not to injure the blood vessels traversing the direction of the cogged thread. Clinicians should be careful with cannula especially around the jaw line where the facial artery and vein pass through the antegonial notch and the premasseteric branch that is branched out from the facial artery rises and passes across the jaw line to the anterior border of the masseter muscle (Fig. 9.30).

9.7.2 Procedural Design and Techniques

First, when the patient is laid down and made to put their head down, the tissues around the jaw line lean toward the ear, and the jaw line becomes more sharpened than when standing. In this state, the tissues that have moved to ears can be hold by the cogged threads and then fixed to the firm fascia tissue under ear lobe.

An entry point is made on the skin of the folded edge between the ear lobe and the cheek as shown in Fig. 9.31.

If a cannula is inserted after a needle puncture, a ligamentous tissue like a solid wooden is immediately felt, which are pulling the earlobe under the dermal tissue. After passing through the liga-

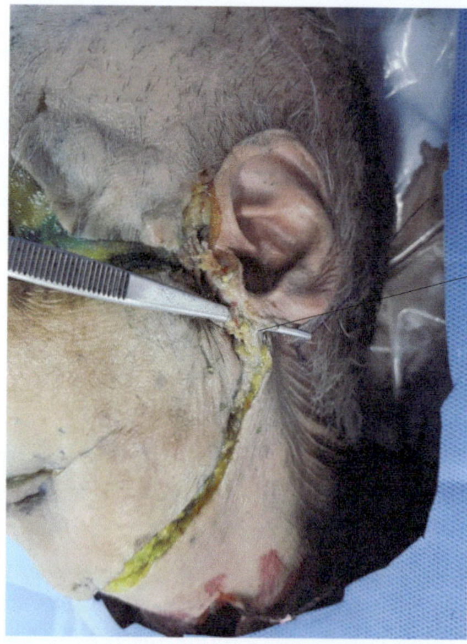

Fig. 9.29 Fixing point for mandible border line lifting

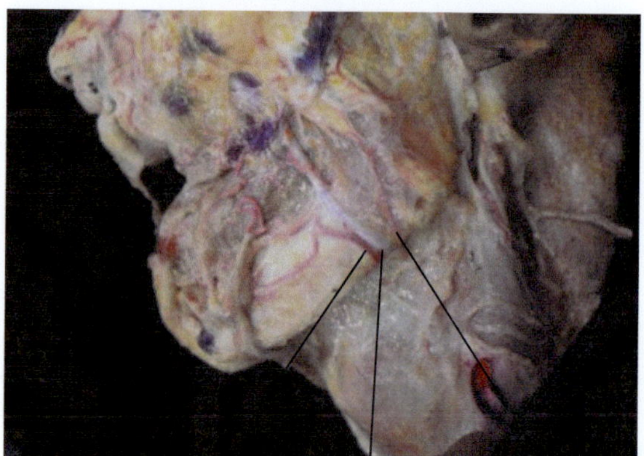

Fig. 9.30 Premasseteric branch of facial artery

ment tissue with a little more strength, we can feel the smooth progression of the cannula. It is more recommended to advance cannula after raising thick layer of tissues including SMAS using the pinch technique, not through subcutaneous fat layer near the skin, penetrating mandibular septum that runs along the jaw line with the cogged threads (Fig. 9.31).

Mandibular septum is a ligamentous tissue, also called platysma cutaneous ligaments. It is located at angle and body of mandible along the mandibular border, and as cannula passes through them, it allows the cogs of the threads to be hung to these loosened ligamentous tissues (Fig. 9.32).

As you move along the jaw line and cross the marionette line, you can feel that the mandibular ligament, which is the immobile rigid ligament under the depressor anguli oris, binds to the skin. Because the skin and tissues here do not move well, the cannula is advanced only to the skin and soft tissue outside of this ligament (Fig. 9.33).

We can insert the cogged threads on both the outer and inner parts of the jaw line. When the inserted threads are lifted to the ear, the tissues

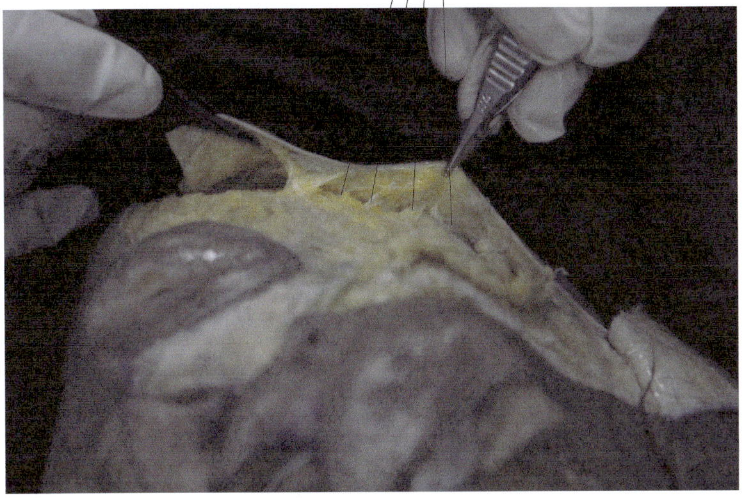

Fig. 9.31 Location of mandibular septum (platysma cutaneous ligaments)

Fig. 9.32 Location of mandibular ligament

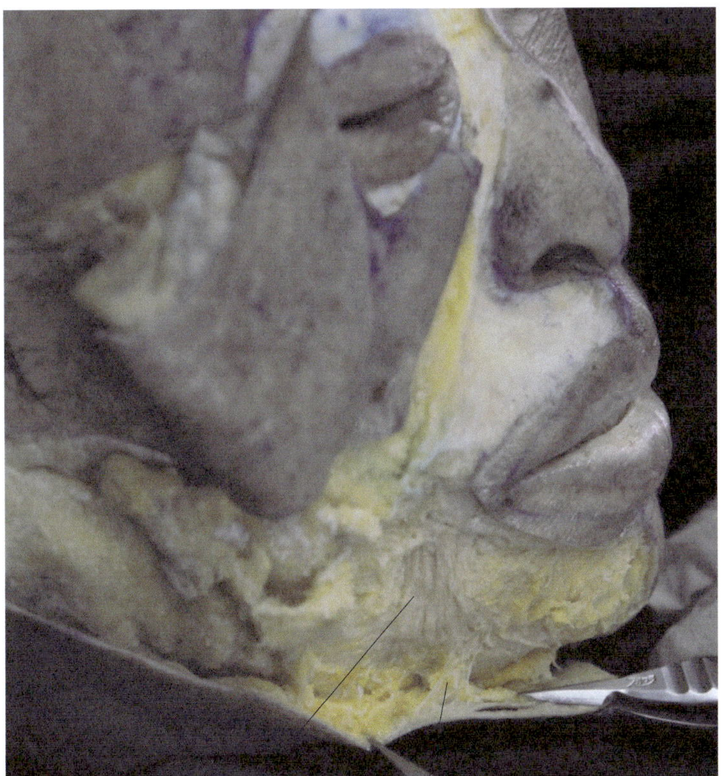

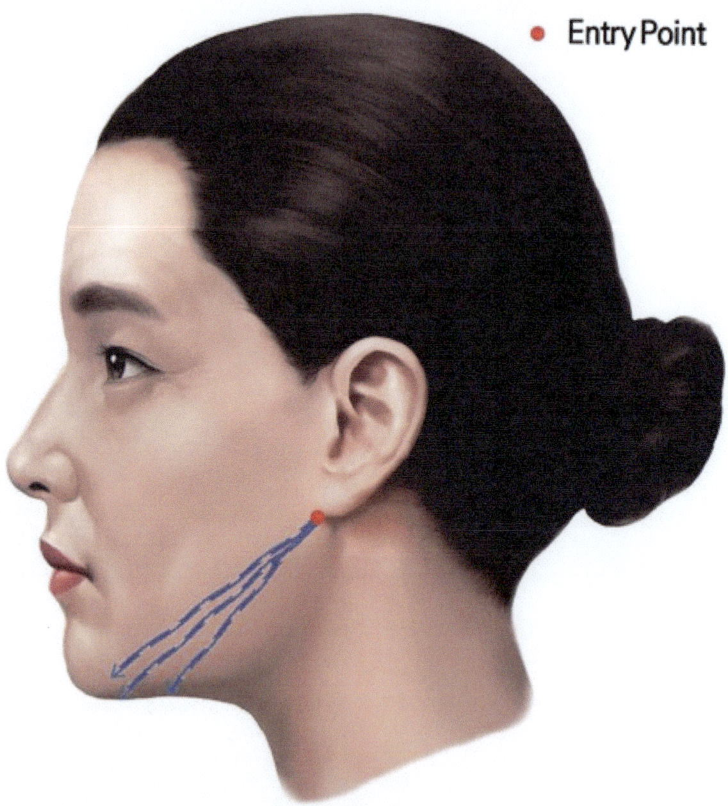

Fig. 9.33 Entry point and direction of cogged threads for mandible border line lifting

become flattened and the blurred jaw line gets sharpened as the direction of the mandibular septum is directed toward the ear, also clearing the angle between chin and neck.

I-type multidirectional cogged thread is also possible when the degree of drooping is not severe, but I-type bidirectional cogged thread is good when you want to pull the jaw line for sure, and if you use the reverse technique, you can use I-type cogged thread exclusively for the reverse technique (i-THREAD). The thickness of the thread is selected according to the thickness and severity of the loosening of the skin and soft tissue.

9.8 Double Chin Lifting

9.8.1 Considerations for Double Chin Lifting

It shows a strong effect on patients with excess subcutaneous fat while maintaining relatively good skin elasticity. However, there is a high likelihood of sinking and contraction in patients with low subcutaneous fat and poor skin elasticity. The most important skill in performing the procedure to avoid such side effects is to uniformly advance the needles at the same depth along the curve of the neck. It is necessary to proceed from the entry point to the exit point at a consistent depth, ensuring that the cog of the thread does not catch on the skin or the firm tissue at the top of the subcutaneous layer. Additionally, proper skin contraction is necessary to prevent sinking or contraction, making patient selection crucial.

Be cautious of bleeding and nerve damage, especially when moving toward the ear, by being aware of the path of the greater auricular nerve to prevent nerve injuries. When passing below the jaw line, use pinch manipulation to gauge the depth of the salivary gland and take care to avoid gland damage. During the pre-examination, determine if the cause of neck sagging is related to issues with other tissues in the neck, such as enlarged salivary glands, regardless of fat. Designing should be done while sitting, as the position of the skin and subcutaneous fat layer changes significantly between lying down and sitting. Ensure that the design of the thread path does not pass above the body of the mandible by designing in a seated position.

9.8.2 Necklace Technique

9.8.2.1 Principle

The principle of double chin lifting using the necklace technique involves pressing the centrally located fat inward to the neck while simultaneously pulling it to both sides for fat repositioning (Fig. 9.34). The entry point is placed in the center, with exits on both sides. It is the opposite concept of using two threads to pull from each side.

9.8.2.2 Design

Entry points are created at intervals of 1–1.5 cm along the centerline (Figs. 9.35 and 9.37). Exit points are positioned inside the SCM muscle. Recently, exit points are primarily made at the angular tract fascia, which is the firm fibrous tissue around the mandibular angle (Figs. 9.35 and 9.36).

9.8.2.3 Schematic Diagram

See Fig. 9.37.

9.8.2.4 Making an Entry Point

Using a needle, make the hole large enough (as it is an area where dimples form easily) (Fig. 9.38).

9.8.2.5 Insertion of Needle

During needle insertion, it is preferable for the patient to be in a slightly double chin showing position. Afterward, needles should be inserted, avoiding shallow insertion. While inserting needles, repeat the motion of lifting and lowering them intermittently, checking for excessive sinking in specific areas (Fig. 9.39).

9.8.2.6 Traction and Cutting

Once needle insertion is complete, raise the needles tentatively to ensure there are no specific areas of excessive sinking. Then, remove the needles and while pulling the threads, push the skin toward the center of the neck with the opposite fingers in a tenting sensation. It is important to adjust so that skin contraction occurs uniformly throughout the neck tissue, avoiding the formation of skin folds.

9.8.2.7 Complications: Pain, Dimpling, and Skin Fold

Immediately after the procedure or the following day, patients often complain of tightness in the neck area (feeling constricted or pressured around the neck). Particularly, the entry point area feels stiff, and dimples tend to form in this area. Typically, the pain disappears within 3–4 days.

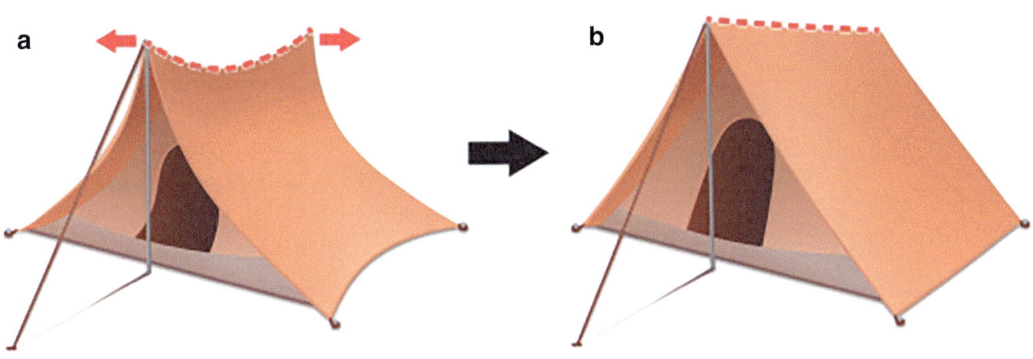

Fig. 9.34 Principle of necklace technique: It is similar to raising the roof of a tent. (**a**) Simulation of pre-procedure conditions, (**b**) simulation of post-procedure conditions

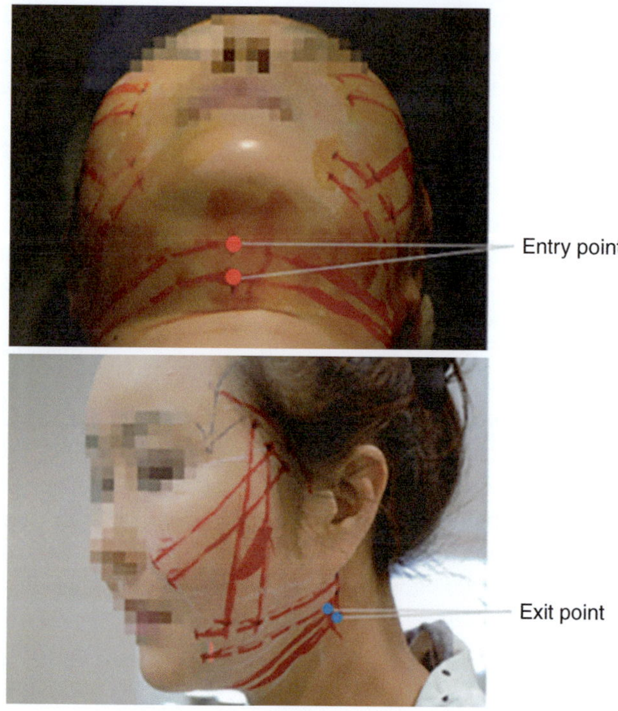

Fig. 9.35 Actual design of double chin lifting procedure

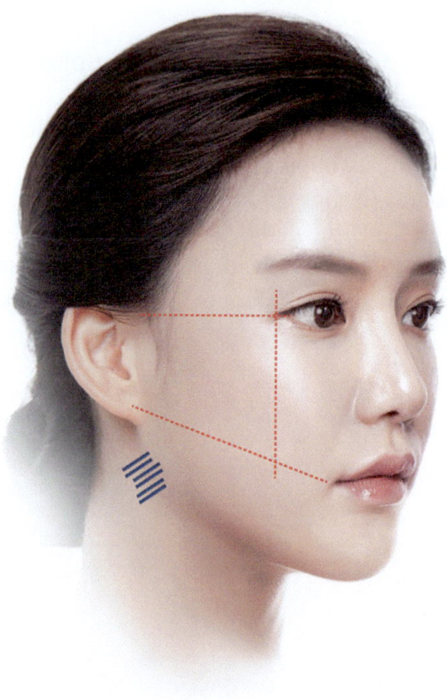

Fig. 9.36 Position of angular tract fascia

Since there is less subcutaneous fat in the entry point, which is the central area of the neck, special attention should be paid to the depth of needle insertion. Shallow insertion can lead to frequent dimpling or sinking. Therefore, after inserting at the entry point, it is advisable to perform the procedure with a sensation of inserting the needle deeply as much as possible.

Severe dimples may not improve over time, so if significant dimpling is anticipated during the procedure, it may be necessary to remove the thread immediately.

9.8.2.8 Considerations When Choosing a Patient

Indications (Favorable Outcomes Are Expected)

The effect is better when there is minimal skin laxity in the double chin area and an appropriate amount of fat. A good outcome can be expected when the thickness measures more than 1.5 cm when the double chin is pinched.

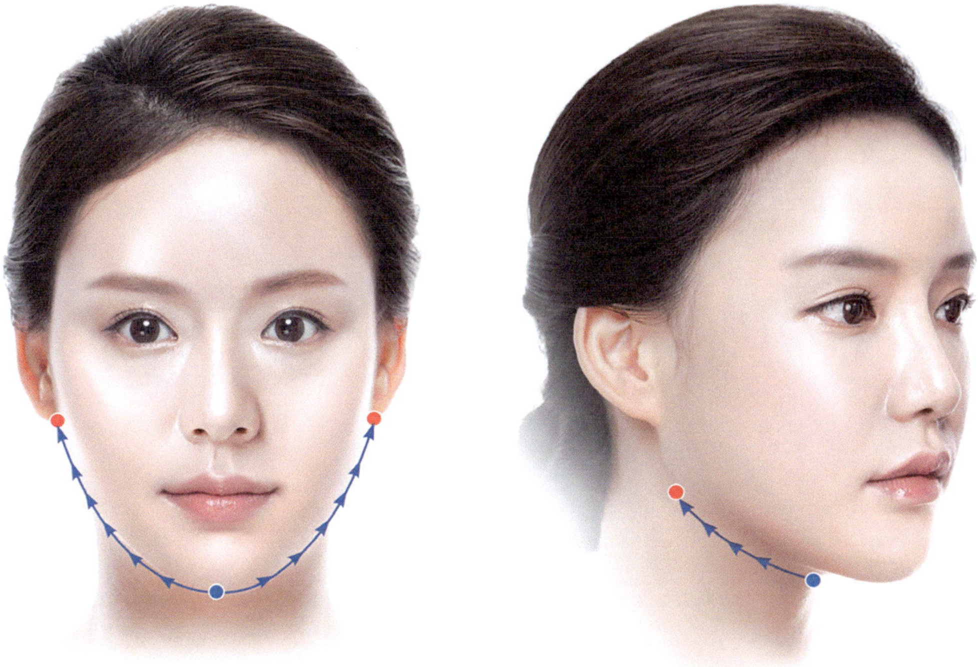

Fig. 9.37 Description of the positions of the entry point and exit point

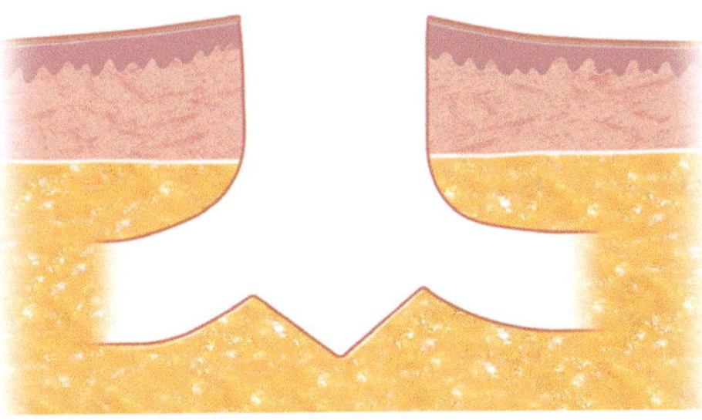

Fig. 9.38 Entry point

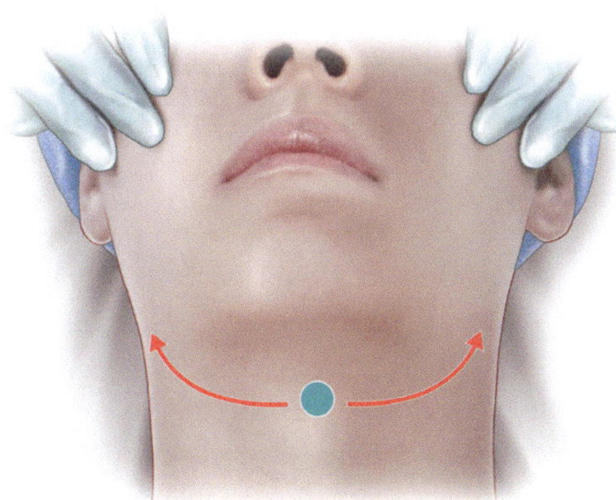

Fig. 9.39 Pathway of needle

Contraindications (Unfavorable Outcomes Are Expected)

In cases of severe skin laxity and minimal fat in the double chin area (often seen in older individuals) or in cases of severe skin sagging such as a "Turkish neck," the skin around the central neck area where the entry point is located tends not to contract as it gathers. If the skin fails to contract, the skin around the central neck area becomes wrinkled.

9.8.2.9 Factors Affecting the Results of the Procedure

When the curve connecting the entry point and the exits on both sides forms a smooth arc (Fig. 9.40 Top), and the threads are inserted deep and consistently within the subcutaneous layer,

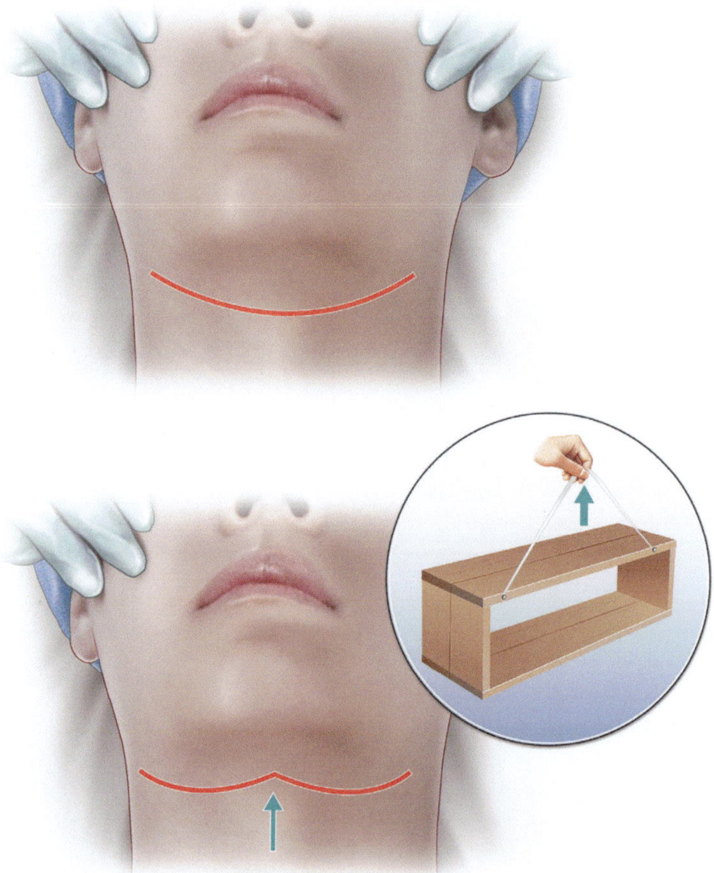

Fig. 9.40 Necklace technique top: good design, bottom: poor design

good results are achieved. On the other hand, when the curve connecting the entry point and the exits on both sides forms a W or seagull shape (Fig. 9.40 Bottom), the procedure results are not favorable. Especially when the ability to maintain a consistent depth of thread insertion is not sufficiently developed, the necklace technique should never be performed (Figs. 9.41 and 9.42).

9.8.3 Under-Ear Tagging Method

This method involves anchoring and lifting below the earlobe, near the mastoid process, or in the firm subcutaneous tissue below it. While the lifting effect is strong, severe pain may occur. Although significant skin folding may occur, it is in a less visible area (Fig. 9.43). Caution must be exercised for nerve damage, and its usage has decreased recently.

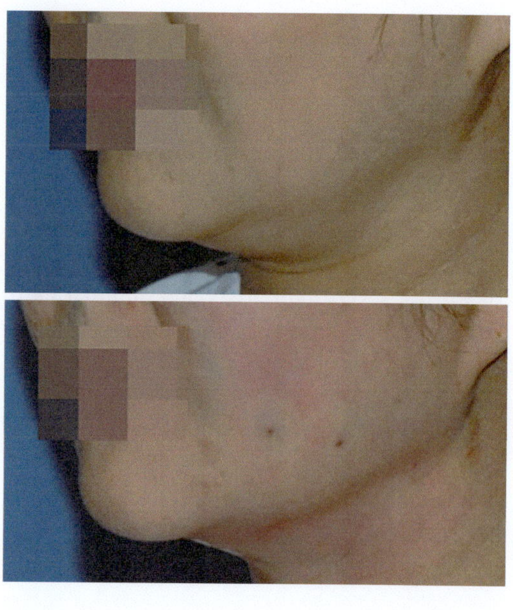

Fig. 9.41 Before and after photo of necklace technique

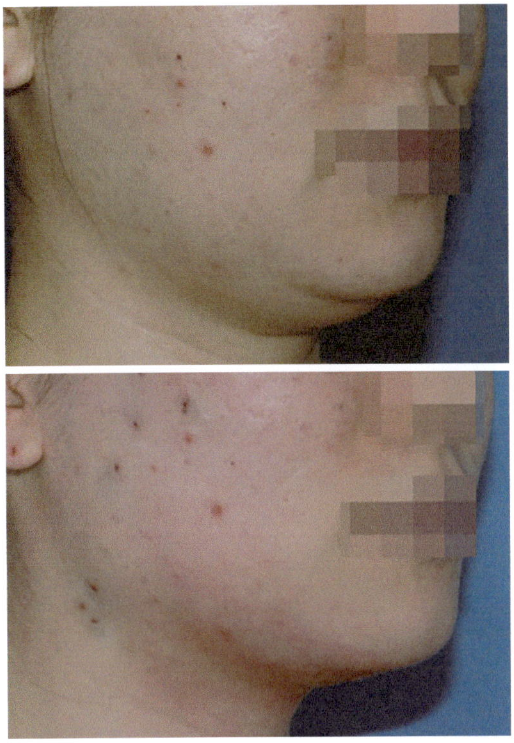

Fig. 9.42 Before and after photo of necklace technique

9.8.4 Neck-Marionette Mixed Method

When there is a need to address both the neck and marionette lines simultaneously, this method can be used. It involves using the tagging technique below the earlobe to lift both the neck and the lower jaw simultaneously. The thread used should be long enough for tagging, and the method of inserting bidirectional cog threads above and below is not commonly used. Bidirectional PDO cog threads with needles on both ends are used. The connective tissue below the earlobe is dense and has limited mobility, making it a suitable anchoring point (Fig. 9.44).

9.8.5 Tie or Simple Burying Method

This method involves using bidirectional or unidirectional cog threads to pull the sagging skin and subcutaneous fat of the neck. It works well when the skin is not too thick and there is not much subcutaneous fat. However, if there is too

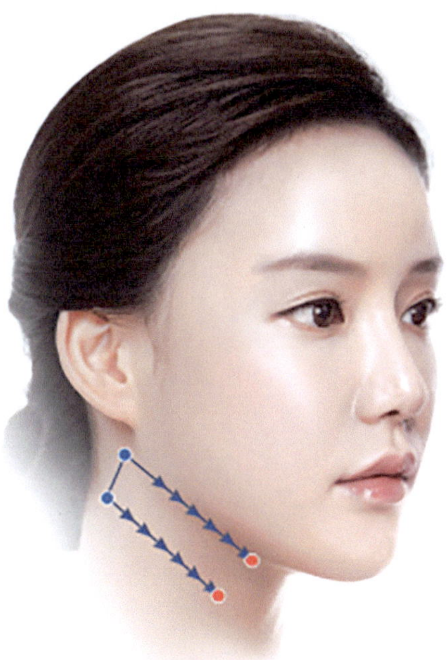

Fig. 9.43 Under-ear tagging method

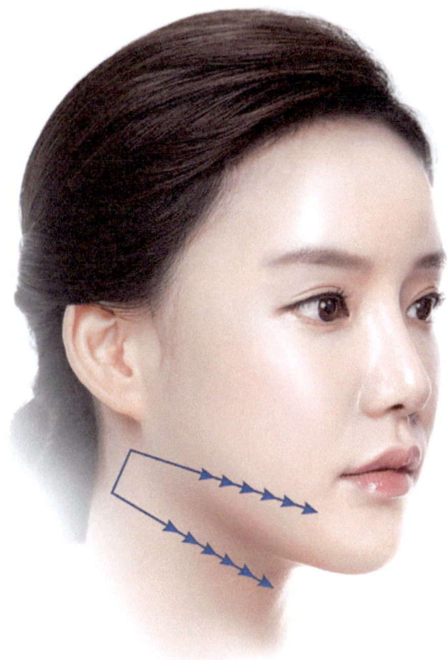

Fig. 9.44 Neck-Marionette mixed method

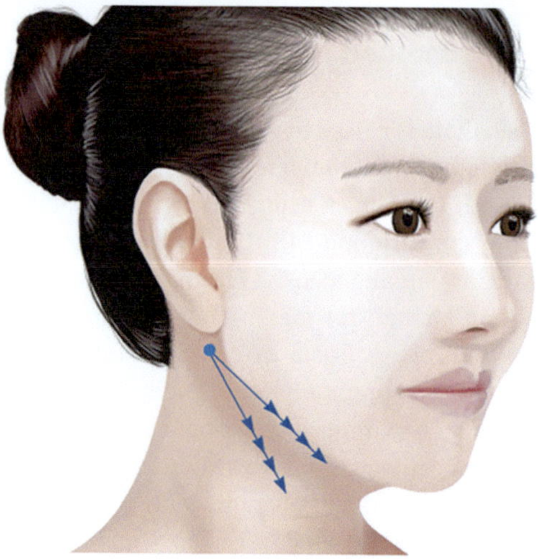

Fig. 9.45 Tie or simple burying method

much subcutaneous fat and the anchoring function is not strong, the effect may disappear quickly. Nevertheless, as PDO dissolves and disappears, it fibroses surrounding tissues, causing contraction and stimulating the dermis. Therefore, the effect may improve over time. It is necessary to design the procedure while sitting to prevent the threads from passing above the mandibular angle (Fig. 9.45).

10 Procedural Methods of Mono-Thread Lifting by Target Site for Wrinkle Improvement

Contents

10.1 Forehead and Glabellar Wrinkles

The wrinkles on the forehead can be divided into dynamic wrinkles and static wrinkles. Dynamic wrinkles are formed when the frontalis muscle is used to raise eyebrows or to widen the eyes, especially in patients with ptosis. In the end, frequent use of the forehead muscles tends to result in permanent forehead wrinkles, and for other reasons, static forehead wrinkles are formed even when the forehead skin is sagged.

Dynamic wrinkles can be mainly improved with botulinum toxin, but paralysis of the forehead muscle in a person with ptosis may cause side effects that disable keeping the eyes open. Static forehead wrinkles can be managed by pulling the skin with a forehead lift or by injecting a filler or fat grafts. However, surgery may felt as burden and volume filling procedures such as fillers and fat transplants generally have a limited effect on wrinkles that are very deeply formed.

Volumizing the dermis layer or superficial subcutaneous fat layer is effective for deep and thin wrinkles like a linear scar made by knife. However, filler is hard to be applied since the filler will pass over to the protruding parts of the wrinkles, rather than retained in the fine part of the wrinkles. It would be treated with a dilute HA filler with low G′value and a botulinum toxin, but it is more effective to volumize the subdermal layer with monofilament PDO threads.

This volume-boosting monofilament procedure is a necessary procedure for the glabella where wrinkles and deepening are found together. As one age, we can see that the wrinkled areas become depressed as the skin loses elasticity and horizontal lines formed by contraction of procerus muscle and vertical lines caused by glabellar frowning gets worse. As with the forehead lines, the superficial wrinkles caused by dermal atrophy can be relatively easily corrected with toxin. However, when the deep subcutaneous fat layer is depressed due to long-term muscle

S. M. Oh et al., *The Art and Science of Thread Lifting Based on Pinch Anatomy and Moving Plane*,
https://doi.org/10.1007/978-981-97-5516-5_10

contraction, and the wrinkles are deeply scarred, it is difficult to correct by the toxin procedure alone. In this case, if the skin is filled with a monofilament serving as support for the skin, the skin can be firm and less wrinkled even without using excessive toxin.

Deep wrinkles in the forehead and glabella are not tissue sagging, but rather a reduction in the volume of the subdermal layer including the dermis where wrinkles are generated by repeated facial expressions. Therefore, it is technically appropriate to say tightening rather than lifting because monofilament threads are inserted along the horizontal wrinkles on the forehead and vertical or oblique wrinkles on the glabellar region to fill the depressed wrinkles as shown in the picture (Fig. 10.1).

The threads that are not too thick to be seen on the surface are recommended for the procedure. Several threads of about 6-0 thickness are inserted, and the number of threads can be determined according to the degree of depression. The threads can have volume effect since several strands are inserted, and it is good to keep in shape because there is little possibility to be displaced like filler.

When performing the procedure, it is advisable to apply enough anesthetic ointment and anesthetize the entry sites of threads with lidocaine. When placing the threads in the subdermal layer, it is recommended to insert superficially as much as possible because the effect may be insignificant if it is inserted too deeply. If it is too close to the epidermis, the sense of resistance may interfere the insertion of threads. Therefore, make sure that the entry site where the thread is inserted has a hole larger than 21G with an awl or needle, so that a large resistance to the cannula is not found. If the thread is left outside, threads would be removed with pulling. Therefore, cut out only the part protruding from the end, then tape the section of the thread on the insertion site with thin forceps to prevent it from coming out.

It is better to use filler and botulinum toxin in combination than solely using the monofilament threads. It is better to inject toxin and insert the monofilament threads first and inject filler to make volumizing effect. After the procedure, there would not be any major side effect except for the needle marks on the entry sites or the bleeding caused during the procedure, so that it can be performed easily. Even if the thread protrudes occasionally, it will not be a serious problem because cutting the protruded portion will do. Depending on the situation, when there is a possibility that the thread will come out again, pulling out the entire thread as much as possible rather than cutting the end of the thread slightly can prevent the remaining threads from being pushed out and coming out again.

The monofilament PDO threads are expected to be absorbed and disappear within 6–9 months because of the thinness, but it is expected that the wrinkle improvement effect will be maintained for a certain period even after the thread absorption due to formation of tissue around the threads.

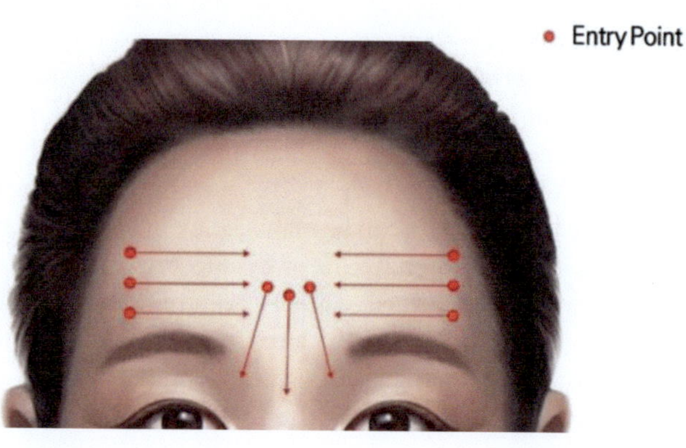

Fig. 10.1 Entry point and direction of non-cogged threads for forehead and glabellar wrinkles

10.2 Periorbital Lines (Crow's Feet)

The periorbital line that are called crow's feet due to its morphology can be divided into dynamic wrinkles caused by movement and fixed wrinkles retained even without movement like forehead and glabellar wrinkles. Dynamic wrinkles are caused by the contraction of the orbicularis oculi muscle, which occurs in almost everyone and can be somewhat alleviated by botulinum toxin. If you try not to make dynamic wrinkles beforehand, the possibility of fixed wrinkles is reduced, but when the skin around the eyes gets stretched and loses elasticity due to aging, a folding occurs unavoidably.

The way to perfectly eliminate this fixed wrinkle is a facelift, forehead lift, or sub-brow excision, which removes the skin under the eyebrows. However, if patients want a procedure other than surgery, we can use a method of filling the deep portion using the monofilament threads to improve static wrinkles that look fixed by folding the skin like a scar.

Similar to the PDO monofilament threads being inserted on the forehead and glabella to fill the deep static wrinkles, monofilament threads are inserted parallel to the wrinkles, and threads are also inserted in the vertical direction to prevent contraction of the muscles around the eyes. However, unlike wrinkles on the forehead, there are three to five short wrinkles rather than long single wrinkle, which makes it difficult to fit the threads to the length of the wrinkles. Therefore, when it is difficult to insert the thread in parallel, it is also helpful to put a thread vertical to the wrinkles around eyes to prevent the transmission of the muscle to the skin (Fig. 10.2).

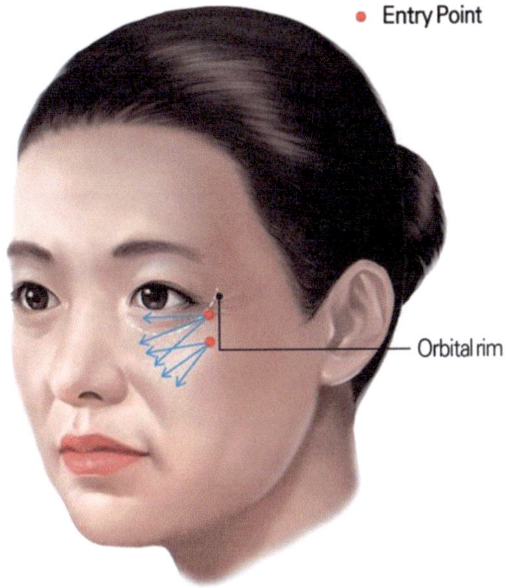

Fig. 10.2 Entry point and direction of non-cogged threads for periorbital lines

10.3 Perioral Lines (Smoker's Lines)

The wrinkles around mouth are caused by the contraction of the orbicularis oris muscle, which is similar to that of the eye, and may also be called smoker's line or cat wrinkles. As with other fine wrinkles mentioned above, there is no one definite treatment method. It is important to fill the volume with the filler together with the thread lifting since these are caused by the reduced elasticity of the skin. In addition, a very small amount of botulinum toxin can be used together since the movement of the muscle may deepen the lines. If it is permissible, a better effect can be obtained by inducing re-

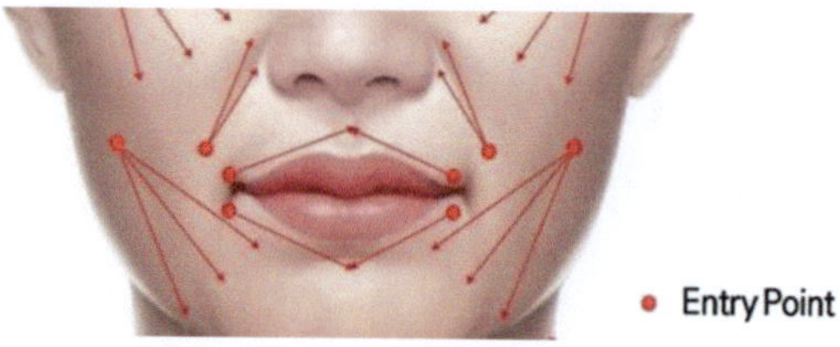

Fig. 10.3 Entry point and direction of non-cogged threads for perioral lines

epithelization through the fractional laser. Since many short lines of wrinkles appear vertically along the lips, the method of inserting the threads is to insert several monofilament threads horizontally in the vertical direction of the wrinkles, and the number of monofilament threads inserted can be determined by the degree of the wrinkle line. If the lips appear to be inverted after inserting monofilament threads for each of the upper and lower lips, fillers can be used to increase the volume of the lips to improve the inverted lips and tighten the skin more (Fig. 10.3).

Patients should be informed that after the procedure, tissues around mouth may get swollen and mouth may protrude for up to 1 week. The monofilament threads are usually inserted into the subdermal layer under the skin, and it can be easily used because it is not seen or touched even when placed a little bit superficially. However, as with the forehead, if the thread is inserted into deep dermis, which is more superficial, it is important to note that half of the thread cannot be inserted and stuck at the entrance of the entry point.

10.4 Neck Lines

For neck lines, it is necessary to consider both the stretched and thinned skin of the wrinkled area and the subcutaneous fat. Especially since the subcutaneous fat is not thick, running the threads too superficially can easily lead to protrusions or indentations.

10.4.1 Wrinkle Filling Method: Mesh-Type Thread

Strictly speaking, it is not a true lifting in the real sense. It could be referred to as a minor wrinkle correction procedure using threads.

For horizontal neck lines, it is often difficult to resolve them through thread lifting. Even with surgical methods that pull the skin, it can still be challenging to address. The cause of horizontal neck lines is the decrease in volume in the dermis and subcutaneous layers. Therefore, replenishing the volume appropriately can improve neck wrinkles. However, since the skin is thin and frequently moves, it is not easy to make it completely flat. By injecting threads that can fill in the volume along the wrinkles, improvement can be achieved. Although different from lifting in the strict sense, injecting threads in a mesh form, as shown in the figure, rather than simply injecting monofilament threads, can be expected to encourage the growth of connective tissues within, creating a filling effect. It is also worth considering various adjunctive treatments to maximize the tissue proliferation effect (Fig. 10.4).

10.4.2 Multi-filament-Type Thread Insertion

Threads can be used as a filler alternative to fill in the sunken areas of the neck. While it is possible to use mono-threads, it tends to be time-consuming and labor-intensive. Therefore, inserting multi-filament threads, which are multiple threads twisted together, into the neck wrinkles is often preferred.

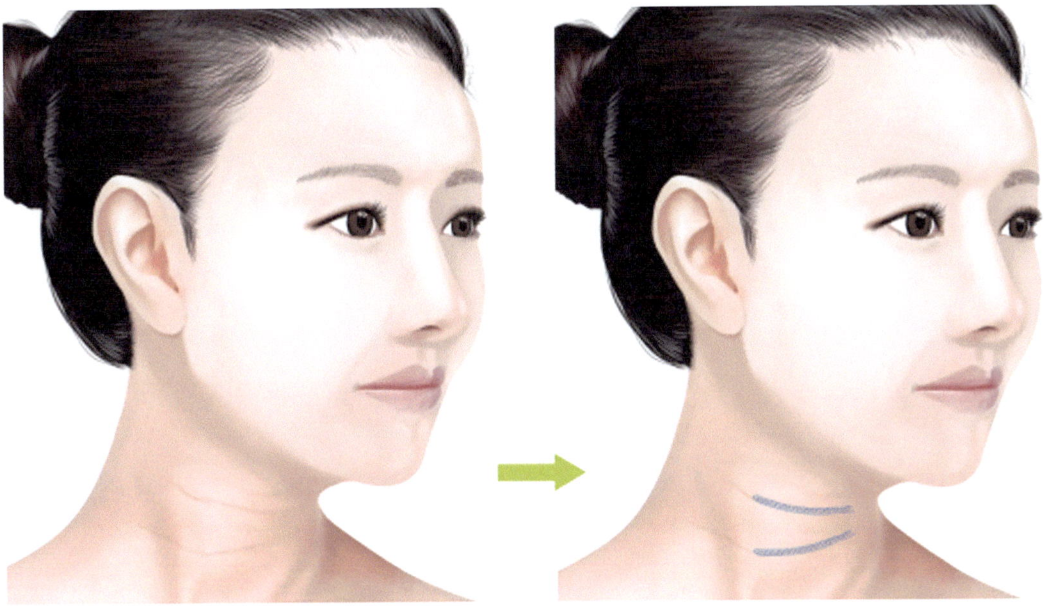

Fig. 10.4 Neck wrinkle filling method

11 PDO Volumizing Multithread Lifting

Contents

11.1 Theoretical Backgrounds

Different age groups of patients have different needs for a thread lifting technique. In general, the younger generation has less sagging and wrinkles in the skin and wants to improve the sagging and contour conditions by part or make the overall face shape narrower.

Entering their 40s or 50s, patients start to experience a sharp drop in skin elasticity and an increase in wrinkles compared with their skin conditions in their 20s or 30s. They also need improvement to their overall face shapes rather than to certain parts of the skin according to their innate build, skin, and soft tissue conditions. As people get older, the deep fat layers that maintain the volume of the face gradually disappear. In addition, ligament tissues that hold the skin and soft tissues tight in order not to sag grow loose, causing the face shape to look wide and gradually spread. Starting in their 40s, people begin to suffer less secretion of collagen, elastic fiber, and sebum, and they also have thinner skin. The deteriorated skin sags further and accelerates changes to the face shape. These face shape conditions require the physical effects of a thread life. An absorbable thread lift makes skin elasticity and tone better, improves wrinkles, and generates whitening effects by improving the blood circulation of the area where threads are inserted

S. M. Oh et al., *The Art and Science of Thread Lifting Based on Pinch Anatomy and Moving Plane*,
https://doi.org/10.1007/978-981-97-5516-5_11

thanks to the histological effects of absorbable threads.

There indeed have been attempts to give volumizing effects by inserting threads even when only fine simple PDO mono threads were available, but it was difficult to create enough volume no matter how many fine threads were used. After threads are inserted, capsules are formed around them and may add more volume, but it is difficult to have high expectations as explained above regarding the effects of absorbable threads. A doctor should prick with a needle many times to insert many threads, which will inevitably cause many bruises and considerable swelling. New threads were developed to supplement these disadvantages of mono threads and give volumizing effects.

At the early stage, volumizing threads had curls and coiled around the needle in a whirlwind form. These threads were, however, pressed by the surrounding tissues and eventually became similar to the simple PDO shape, generating no big effects. Threads were then twisted in a cylindrical form to keep the form longer, but they also lacked elasticity. Once they were inserted, they were similarly pressed by the surrounding tissues. As a supplement, volumizing threads were invented, which gathered many strands of threads so that they could go into the skin at the same time. They were made in a way so that many strands of threads were put in a single cannula simultaneously.

Another type of volumizing thread was also launched. These volumizing threads increased the elasticity of the thread itself rather than increasing the number of strands so that the thread form would not be pressed by external pressure and maintain its original shape.

Next, a cylinder-shape volumizing thread was introduced in the market. The old mesh-form threads were woven in a cylinder shape to adjust the elasticity of the volumizing thread so that its cylinder shape would not be distorted inside the skin. Its overall structure was in mesh form so that the empty spaces of the cylinder could be easily filled with fibrous tissues according to collagen regeneration.

Later, new threads were made which supplemented the disadvantage of the old whirlwind-shape threads being easily pressured in the skin tissues. The elasticity of coiling threads was enhanced so that the threads would remain firm and not stretch. These threads kept their coil form even after they were inserted into the skin, serving as a prosthesis. The threads that are made firm by adjusting the elasticity not only give volume but can also form a shape like some prosthesis inside the skin tissues. When these threads have elasticity that is too strong or the skin is thin, however, the patient can feel the threads on the surface as the threads are inserted close. The area may even look uneven, and the patient might have a foreign body sensation. When a doctor places volumizing threads that are too hard over the path of sensory nerves, they can push down the nerves and cause pain, so doctors should be careful about this. For these reasons, it is hard to say that volumizing threads of a certain strength in certain forms are better under any circumstances. It is important to select volumizing threads with proper forms and elasticity according to the goal of a procedure by understanding the types and characteristics of different volumizing threads according to their manufacturing methods (Fig. 11.1).

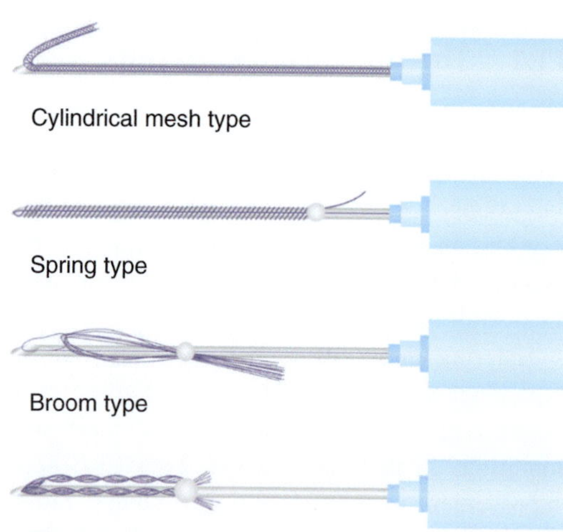

Fig. 11.1 Four types of PDO volumizing multithreads for filling effect

11.2 The Mechanism and Effect of PDO Volumizing Multithread Lifting

There are two types of effects of PDO volumizing multithread lifting according to the action mechanism appearing after the insertion of threads.

Thin mono threads are put together in as many strands as possible to maximize the effects of the old PDO mono threads, and these volumizing threads do not increase the overall thread elasticity and can thus serve as a relatively fluffy cushion. They can be used to fill the wrinkle parts that seem considerably hollow or make the uneven skin surface due to smooth wrinkles. Since their elasticity is not high, they can even be used close to the skin, which is another advantage of these threads. They are comprised of many strands of thin mono threads, which means that they will not make the skin uneven and not be touched even after they are inserted near the skin. However, the overall shape and volume created by the accumulation of threads cannot be full unless an incredible amount of mono threads are put together. It is thus difficult to use these threads to give volume to the skin or create a clear form. They are, however, useful volumizing threads to correct deep wrinkles that are hard to save only with a filler, making uneven skin smooth due to expression wrinkles, and giving a firm feel to the skin with proper volume.

It is a good idea to use volumizing threads with high elasticity to make shapes for certain parts or make the contour distinctive. Since these volumizing threads are felt for their hard form and will not be pressed down easily, the proper approach is to insert them near the subdermis or deeper rather than inserting a lot of threads too close to the skin. For wrinkle improvement, they can serve better for the parts that seem relatively depressed, such as the deep hollow paranasal parts next to the nasal ala like nasolabial folds and the prejowl sulcus that seems hollow inside the oral commissures rather than wrinkles that look like thin lines. Other effects of hard volumizing threads can be highlighted to make the contour of each facial part distinct by replacing the prosthesis. In such a case, the effects of this procedure can be maximized by adding an HA filler for a given situation (Fig. 11.2).

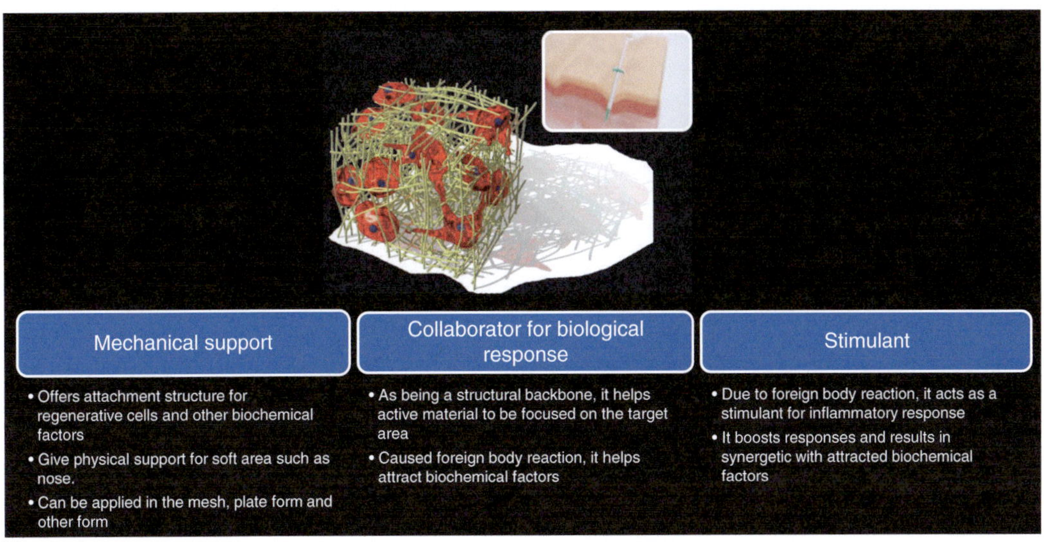

Fig. 11.2 Physical support with scaffold effect of PDO volumizing threads in combination treatment with HA fillers

11.3 Classification of PDO Volumizing Multithreads

PDO volumizing threads can be divided into two major types according to form. One has many layers of thin overlapping threads in a broom or rope form. The broom type and the braided screw or twisted coil type are good examples.

Generally, many layers of thin PDO thread of 7-0 are overlapped or twisted and then tied together. They are in a broom shape (Fig. 11.3). When they are further twisted, they are in a coil or screw shape, which is the most popular type (Fig. 11.4). These types consist of layers of thin threads. When they are inserted, they can give volume to a certain degree. Individual threads are thin, which means that they have some advantages: not being visible through the skin surface, not having a detectable form under the skin, and no feel of the thread contour with a finger. They are a bundle of thin threads in layers, not creating any shapes. They can fill a space under the skin, but they have limitations with creating a certain contour. Thus, these types of volumizing threads can serve useful purposes for deep wrinkles on the skin surface which can hardly be filled only with a filler. The scope of their utilization covers very diverse areas, including deep hollow wrinkles on a man's forehead, static lines in the glabella, around and under the eyes, nasolabial folds, above and under the lips, oral commissures, and horizontal lines on the neck.

The other type is volumizing threads in a certain form, which is usually a long and round cylinder, such as a cannula and needle. The most popular type is the spring or cylindrical mesh type. The spring-type threads that are available on the market these days are in the dual needle structure. PDO threads are coiled around a needle, which is put inside a bigger needle. After the bigger needle is pulled out of the target area, the spring-type threads and the inner needle with the threads coiled around it are left. After the inner needle is pulled out carefully, only the volumizing threads are left inside the skin. They are different from the old spring-type threads in that they have a robust spring form, are hardly pressed down after a procedure, and maintain their form wonderfully (Fig. 11.5).

There are cylindrical mesh-type volumizing threads. This type features threads coiled together in a cylindrical form. There is space inside the cylinder, and tissues can grow in it later and thus create additional volume effects. There are the effects of tissue proliferation around the cylinder as well (Fig. 11.6).

In general, spring-type volumizing threads are bigger and harder overall than cylindrical mesh-type volumizing threads. After being inserted into the skin, they can keep their form better, which can work as an advantage and disadvantage. When the threads are placed too close to the

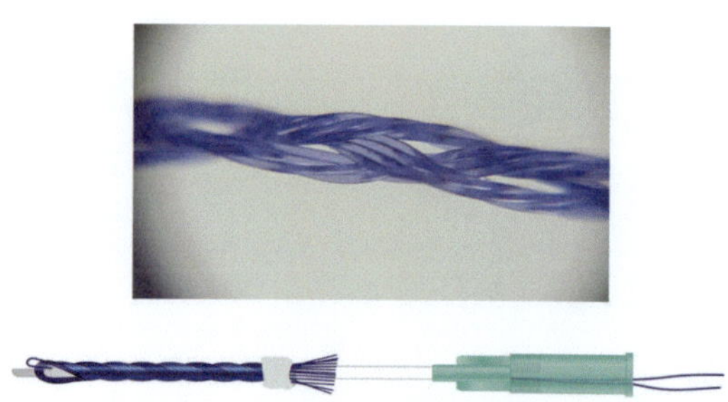

Fig. 11.4 Braided screw or twisted coil-type volumizing PDO threads (i-THREAD Scaffold, HEALUX)

Fig. 11.3 Broom-type PDO volumizing threads (i-THREAD Volume, HEALUX)

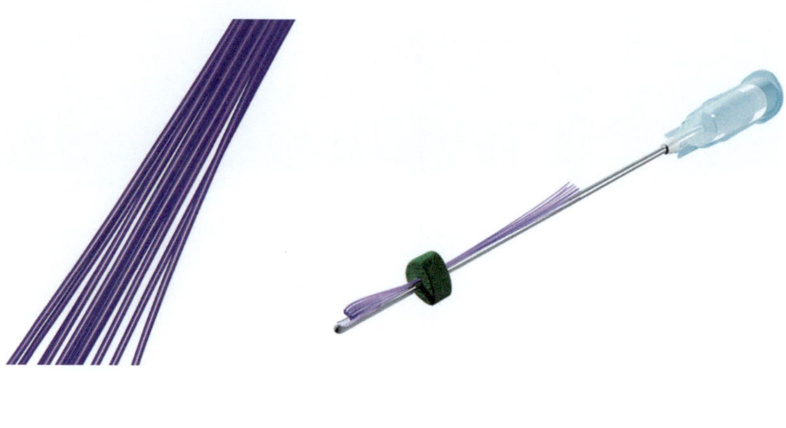

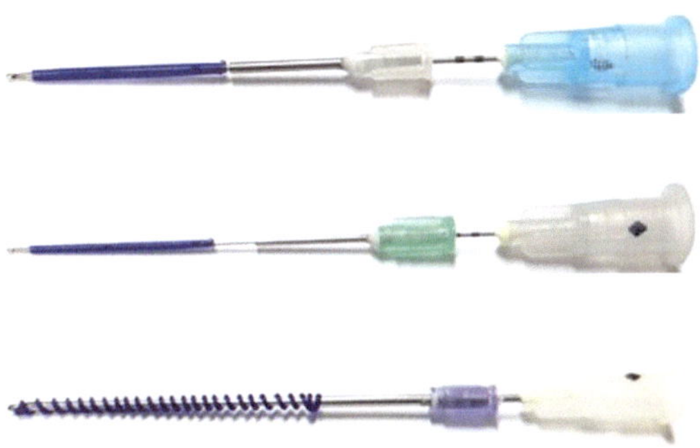

Fig. 11.5 Spring-type PDO volumizing threads

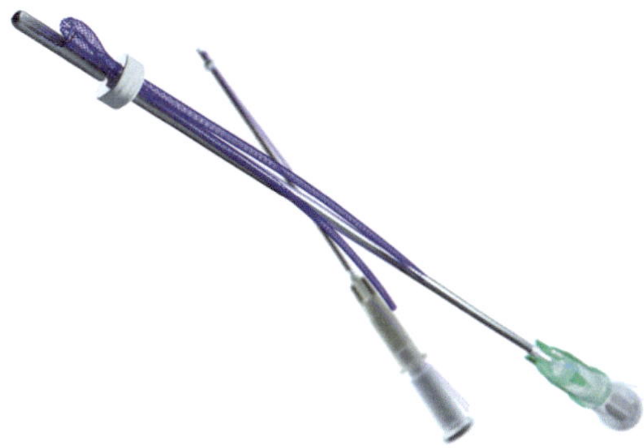

Fig. 11.6 Cylindrical mesh-type PDO volumizing thread (i-THREAD Matrix Soft & Hard, HEALUX)

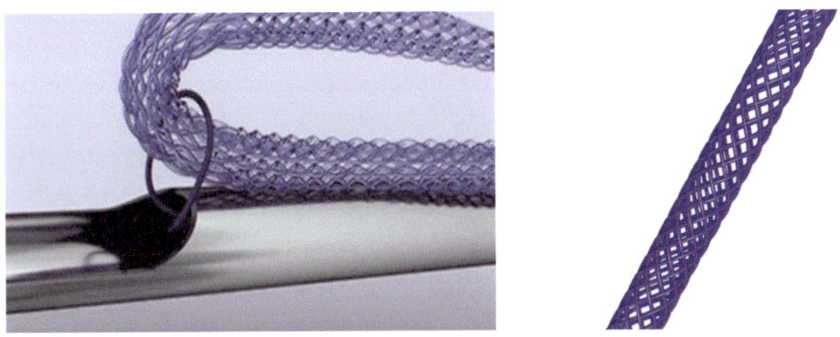

Fig. 11.7 Two types of cylindrical mesh-type PDO volumizing threads depending on the purpose of the procedure (i-THREAD Matrix Soft & Hard, HEALUX)

skin surface, the relatively hard spring form can be visible through the skin. When placed near sensory nerves, they can press the nerves and cause pain for a certain period of time. When using volumizing threads with hard elasticity, doctors need to take the shape, thickness, and hardness of threads into full consideration before a procedure and make a good choice with the insertion depth of threads according to the target area and goal of the procedure.

These days, volumizing threads of the same shape and form can be divided into ones with a soft feel and ones with a harder feel based on the adjustment of thread elasticity itself. Volumizing threads with higher elasticity can keep their shape better without being pressed down under the skin, serving as a prosthesis. There are volumizing threads designed to improve the facial contour, and their uses have begun to explode. The following section will discuss their goals and methods (Fig. 11.7).

11.4 Facial Contouring with PDO Volumizing Multithreads

In modern society, minimally invasive procedures with volumizing threads and HA fillers are used for facial contouring, including the nose, for which surgery with a prosthesis is most preferred rather than the old procedure. This type of combination treatment involves no surgeries, making a comprehensive approach available to improve the overall face shape. It can also correct an asymmetric face to a certain degree, helping to restore symmetry in the face. Since this approach does not involve a prosthesis, absorption will happen over time to some degree. As both volumizing threads and fillers are inserted, they not only increase the volume of the facial skin and soft tissues, but they also serve as the framework to keep the shape. Over time, collagen is generated around the threads and fillers, which serve as the framework, creating fibrous tissues. A few additional corrections would be enough to prevent the target area from returning to its original form while also maintaining the form and contour for some time (Fig. 11.8). A test was conducted to verify if volumizing threads inserted in the skin could serve as such a framework. After inserting volumizing threads with high elasticity in a fresh cadaver, the researchers dissected it and checked the results. They found that the threads were not pressed down and maintained their volume well. Tissues grow into the structure of volumizing threads that are maintained in this way, creating a form of fibrous tissues that will continue for a long period of time (Fig. 11.9).

Such a procedure can give optimal results when it aims to change the structure of the skin and soft tissues covering up the bones rather than the facial bone structure. The first thing to do in such a procedure is to assess asymmetry between the right and left side of the face including the target area. The next step is to think of how to improve the overall facial balance. In other words, the doctor should figure out the anatomical structures and compositions of the skin and soft tissues in the face along with the characteristics of each part of the face to consider what changes might happen according to facial expressions, life habits, or aging. The doctor also needs to figure out the unique features of each patient's face, understand the esthetic criteria according to the latest trends, and analyze the patient's face accurately before making a procedure plan. To obtain optimal results, the doctor should consider the movement of the skin and soft tissues during facial expressions rather than focusing on facial shapes and wrinkles in a static state.

The investigator is currently trying to improve asymmetry between the right and left sides of the face during a facial contouring pro-

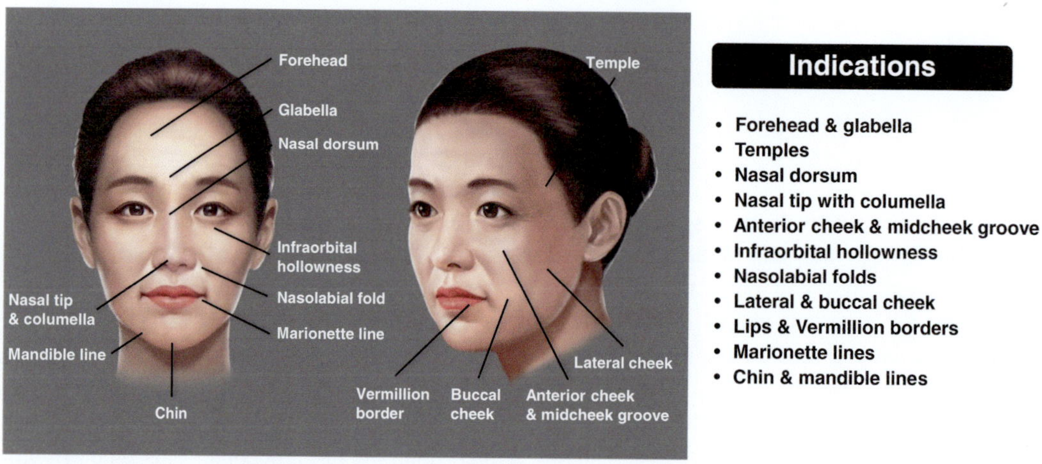

Fig. 11.8 Possible facial areas for combination treatment of volumizing threads with HA fillers

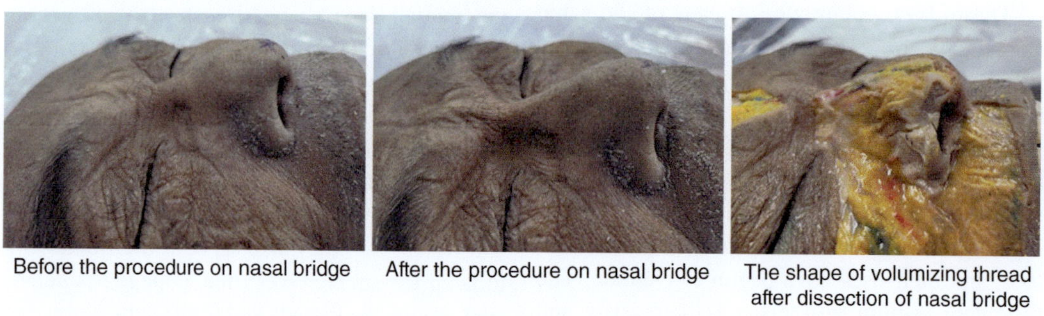

Fig. 11.9 Anatomical study for the effect of volumizing thread (i-THREAD Matrix Contour (HARD), HEALUX)

cedure with volumizing threads and fillers. In his book, *In Your Face*, David Perrett, who is a psychology professor in charge of the research center for social learning and cognitive evolution at the University of St. Andrews in Scotland, explains the criteria of human physical attraction by dividing them into absolute and relative. The absolute criteria are applied to anyone and include facial symmetry, similar to the standard proportion, emotions and facial expressions, skin conditions, and the severity of wrinkles. The relative ones include familiarity (people tend to like things that resemble someone familiar to them), differences in esthetic standards according to racial and cultural differences, and preference differences according to individual value systems. In other words, individual differences between an impression that someone is beautiful and another impression that someone is not beautiful depend on differences in the relative criteria of charm.

Of the absolute criteria for an attractive face, symmetry indicates normal genes and healthy conditions and offers visual stability to increase the degree of attractiveness. Biologically speaking, symmetry refers to a balanced state of overall facial features including the eyes, nose, mouth, head, eyebrows, and mustache with few differences. When a face is closer to such symmetry, it means better health and form that is visually favorable. This is why a symmetric face is considered more attractive than an asymmetric one.

There are two types of causes for an asymmetric face: congenital and acquired. Congenital causes can result in differences in size and imbalance between the right and left facial bones, differences in size and strength between the right and left facial muscles, and differences in length and volume between the right and left skin and soft tissues. Acquired causes include distorted or slanted postures in daily life (sitting with legs crossed, leaning to one side while standing, sleeping on one side of the body, etc.) and bad habits. Chewing food only on one side, smoking, and squatting can contribute to facial asymmetry. Other contributors include inflammation, tumors

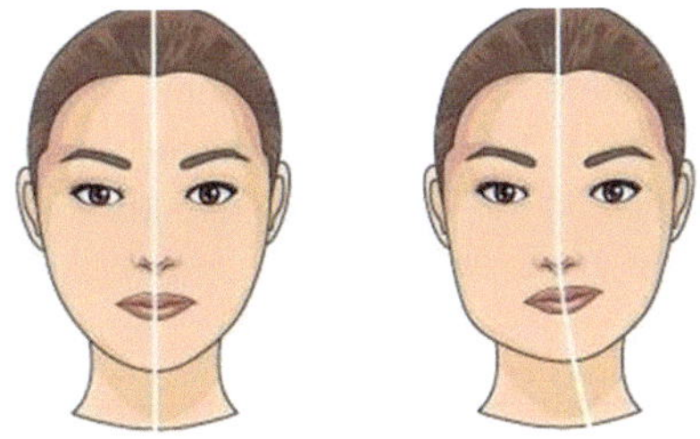

I. Congenital cause
(1) Inharmony & imbalance of facial bones
(2) Difference in size and strength of facial muscles
(3) Difference in tissue volume of left & right sides

II. Acquired cause
(1) environmental factors including bad habits
- eating, smoking, sitting, squatting, alcohol consumption, sleep position, dentures, etc
(2) Injury by accident
(3) Diseases - Bell's palsy, inflammation, tumors
(4) Psychological problems – stress, headaches

Fig. 11.10 Two main causes for an asymmetric face

in the facial nerves, and Bell's palsy, which is facial nerve paralysis due to psychological issues (Fig. 11.10).

Some studies reported that even faces with low innate asymmetry could increase in asymmetry over time due to aging and bad habits. In an experiment with enzygotic twins, the subjects had the same face when young. As they grew old, the twins with bad life habits and postures suffered more and more asymmetry.

Facial asymmetry due to acquired causes can be improved considerably by combining treatments with toxins, volumizing threads, and filler. This type of combination treatment enables a comprehensive approach to improve the entire face with a minimally invasive procedure. The goal can be achieving symmetry or maintaining the overall facial balance according to given situations.

Even patients who have received plastic surgery in the past can benefit from this option. It is even available to patients who have received plastic surgery for facial contour, including the nose, have complaints about their face shapes despite no particular side effects after the surgery, and wish to make their face shapes better. Such patients cannot easily choose to receive corrective procedures in many cases due to the burden of the removal of the current prosthesis and the need for another surgery. This option is helpful for such patients. It can improve the face shape to a certain degree with volumizing threads and fillers without inserting a new prosthesis or autogenous tissues after removing the current prosthesis.

11.5 Possible Target Areas and Applicable Methods for Each Area

11.5.1 Forehead and Glabella

Forehead wrinkles are usually corrected with toxins to simply paralyze the frontal muscles. Shallow wrinkles due to dermis atrophy can be easily corrected with toxins. There are cases of dents even in the subcutaneous layer and deep wrinkles like scars due to the enduring contraction of muscles. These cases can expect an improvement for the excessive movement of the forehead with toxins, but deep wrinkles cannot be restored to a flat state. When the entire expression muscles of the forehead, which move up and downward, are paralyzed with toxins, the patient may have an awkward expression like a frozen look and suffer from functional inconvenience such as difficulties with opening the eyes and swollen eyelids. If deep forehead wrinkles like scars are corrected with volumizing threads, they can improve deep wrinkles and tighten the forehead skin while minimizing discomfort.

Volumizing threads, which consist of many strands of thin threads that are overlapping and twisted, are effective for deep forehead wrinkles. When many mono-PDO threads in the thickness of 6-0 are inserted one by one, they can cause severe bruises due to hemorrhage. Volumizing threads can minimize the time and discomfort of a procedure by inserting many strands of threads at a time. Since they have thin threads entangled instead of thick ones, they give only a little foreign body sensation. Mono threads lack the strength to overpower the skin of the thick and hard forehead and glabella, but volumizing threads fill up space with many strands of threads that are inserted at a time. They can give volume effects by overpowering the hard skin and are better at maintaining form than a filler due to their lower movability. Once inserted, volumizing threads revive the dent through the volume of threads first. Then collagen is regenerated inside the spaces between the entangled threads, leading to the effects of tissue proliferation with connective tissues that are growing and filling the spaces. By inserting volumizing threads in the glabella with big wrinkles and dents due to the repetitive movement of the muscles, the doctor can improve the wrinkles and revive the dents.

In many cases, male patients with thick skin have wrinkle lines buried in the forehead and glabella. When threads are simply inserted under the wrinkle lines in such patients, they can be placed next to the target area. In this case, the doctor should make sure that the wrinkle lines are revealed by applying the pinching or holding technique to hold the skin around the wrinkle lines and pull it together to make the middle part bulge or the stretching technique to pull the skin next to the wrinkle lines outwards before accurately inserting threads under the wrinkle lines (Fig. 11.11).

The investigator prefers the cross technique, which inserts threads across the wrinkle line as explained in the previous chapter, to the linear technique which inserts threads along the wrinkle line for deep forehead or glabella wrinkles (Fig. 11.12). By inserting volumizing threads across the wrinkles askew like the fern leaf tech-

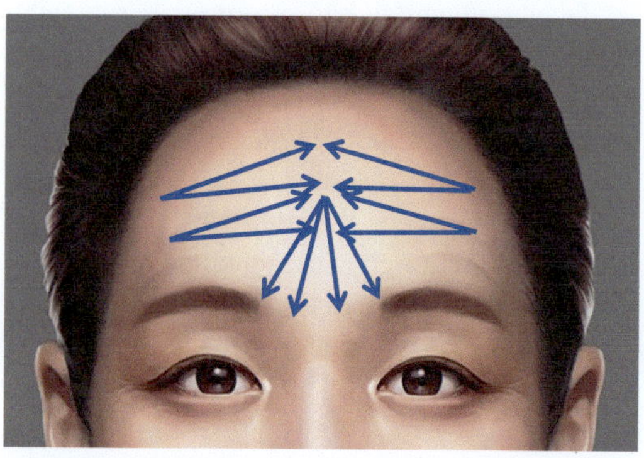

Fig. 11.11 Design of insertion and direction of linear technique for forehead and glabella (i-THREAD Matrix Soft & Hard, HEALUX)

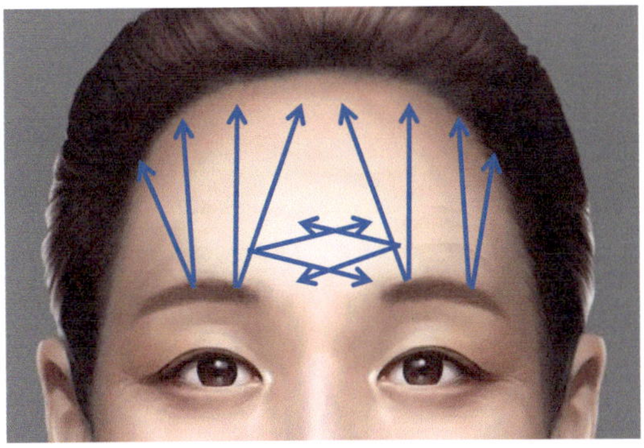

Fig. 11.12 Design of insertion and direction of cross technique for forehead and glabella (i-THREAD Matrix Soft & Hard, HEALUX)

nique used for a filler procedure, the doctor can spread the uneven and irregular forehead and glabella and revive the dented area. This way ensures that the area around the wrinkle line, which used to be buried and look sunken, becomes flat. Over time, the hollow part in the middle keeps its smooth state thanks to the tissue regeneration effects. There is another advantage to this volumizing thread procedure that builds a prop inside the hollow part. It can maximize the effects of fillers and toxins used along with the threads.

Volumizing threads have half of the threads inside a cannula as they are entangled or twisted in many layers. They need an entry point to get inserted in the skin. Setting an entry point might feel like a nuisance, but doctors can enjoy the benefits of minimized damage to many blood vessels in the forehead and glabella by using a cannula, unlike mono threads inside a needle. An entry for the cannula holding twisted threads can be made by marking an entry point to insert volumizing threads and making a needle puncture after local anesthesia. A cannula of 21G thickness is usually chosen for this procedure. If the patient is sensitive to pain, it would be a good idea to anesthetize the entry area for threads in advance as well. When making a needle puncture, the doctor needs to create an initial space for the cannula by inserting the needle only until the beveled needle eye and to be careful not to touch the muscles themselves by pricking the needle too deep.

When the insertion is shallow in the subcutaneous tissues, the shape of threads will be visible on the skin and give a foreign body sensation to the patient. The doctor should insert a cannula under the muscles and make sure that the tip of the cannula has reached the target area before pulling out only the cannula slowly by pushing its tip with a finger so that the threads exposed at the tip will not come out of the tissues. The entire length and depth of cannula entry should be adjusted to ensure that some of the threads will not come out through the entry point and that all the threads are buried right in the skin tissues. If some of the inserted threads come out and get pulled, even the threads inside will come out accordingly. In such a case, the doctor should cut the escaping threads and bury the remaining ones tight so that they will not come out again.

When the blood vessels in the glabella wrinkles suffer direct damage, it can cause heavy bleeding. This means that doctors should be extra careful when making a needle puncture for an entry point or inserting a cannula in the area. The branches of the supratrochlear artery pass in or above the muscle layer right under or next to the wrinkle line in the glabella. If threads are inserted in the subcutaneous layer in halves, there is a big concern with possible damage to the varied branches of blood vessels. It is thus important to pay attention to keep a certain depth so as not to cause damage to blood vessels during a procedure.

11.5.2 Temples

Temples refer to the concave parts under the superior temporal line (STL) where temporalis muscles or superior temporal septum (STS) begin. Korean people look even more sunken in the temple area due to the well-developed cheekbones and zygomatic arches as they are born with no volume or lose volume with aging. If a patient receives a procedure to make the area connected to the outside of the forehead above and the zygomatic arch below smooth by reviving the hollow temple area, the profile line in the upper part of the face will become smooth with an improve-

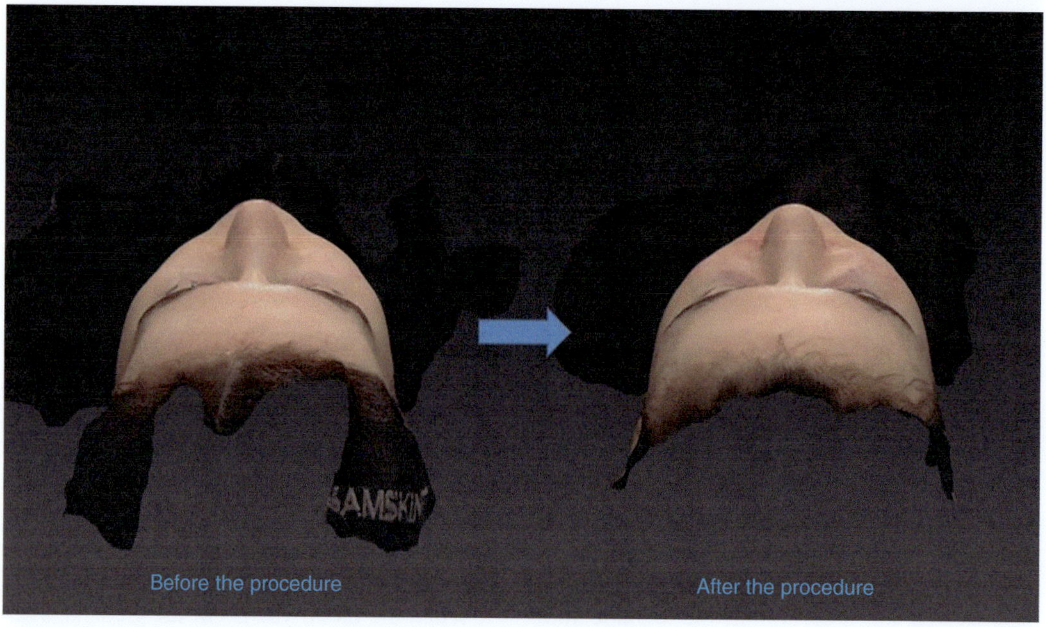

Fig. 11.13 Before and after the procedure on severely depressed temple area

ment to the uneven fierce-looking impression and the old-looking face (Fig. 11.13).

The doctor should know the anatomical layers first to improve the volume issue in the temple area successfully. The temporal bone area that makes the bottom of the temple is called the temporal fossa, above which there are temporalis muscles. There are superficial and deep layers in the temporalis muscles with the temporalis tendon between them. The deep temporal arteries and veins pass through the muscles.

Two fascial planes are wrapping the temporalis muscles above them. The upper fascial plane is called superficial temporal fascia (STF) or temporoparietal fascia (TPF). It wraps around superficial temporal arteries and veins and is connected to the frontalis muscles in the forehead, galea aponeurotica in the calvaria, and SMAS in the center of the face. The lower fascial plane is called deep temporal fascia (DTF), temporalis fascia, or temporalis muscle fascia. It starts at the superior temporal septum (STS) and gets divided into two layers, the superficial and deep layer, as it comes down. The two layers combine again in the upper part of the zygomatic arch or wrap around the arch separately. The deep layer ends as it attaches to the arch, and the superficial layer continues to go down. There can be individual differences.

There is space between the structures that make up the planes in the temple. There is the deep temporal fat pad (DTFP) as an extension of the buccal fat pad between the temporalis muscles and DTF. There is the superficial temporal fat pad (STFP or temporal fat pad) between DTF and the superficial and deep layer. It spreads in 3–4 cm or so along the upper boundary of the zygomatic arch. There is space comprised of fibrous tissues between STF and DTF, and it is like a compartment. It is divided into the upper and lower parts by the inferior temporal septum (ITS), and they are each called the upper and lower temporal compartments.

These days, it is generally believed that there is another fascia that is always separated regularly inside the compartment. Since it does not have an official name yet, it is called the innominate fascia, which means the anonymous fascia (Fig. 11.14). A cadaver study never fails to show the fascia that is always separated regularly like

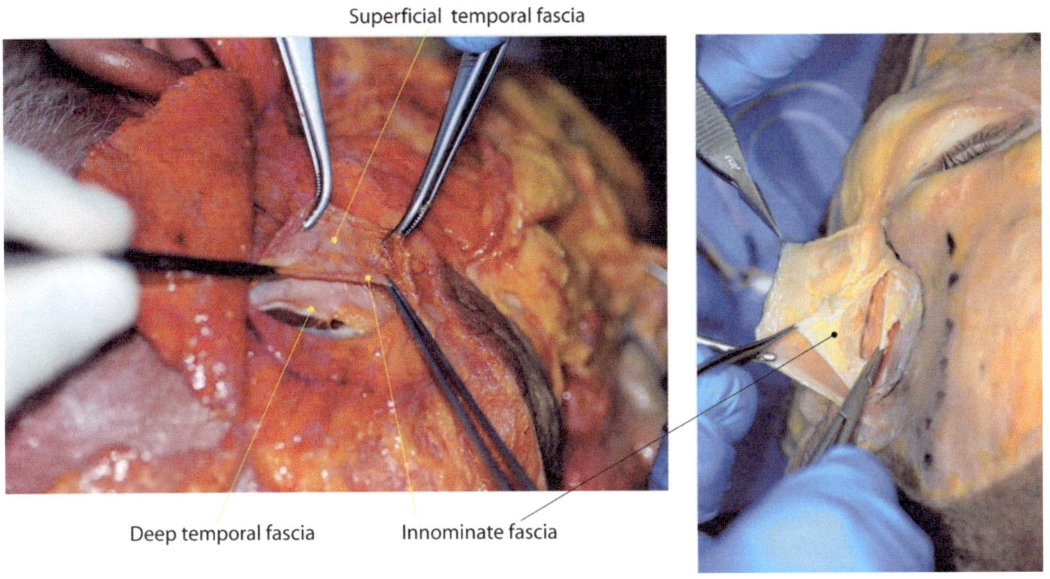

Fig. 11.14 Innominate fascia of temporal region

another layer. Some scholars argue that this fascia is connected even to the forehead and lateral cheek anatomically.

Like other parts of the face, the fascial plane is covered with a subcutaneous layer and skin above. There are many blood vessels and nerves that run across the target area in the temporal section, and a doctor should be careful with them during a procedure. They include the anterior branch of the superficial temporal artery (STA), the zygomatico-orbital artery, the middle temporal vein and sentinel vein, the temporal branch of the motor facial nerve, and the sensory zygomatico-temporal nerve. The following sections examine correlations between these anatomical structures and the upper and lower temporal compartments in the temporal area.

The upper temporal compartment is in a closed structure, being surrounded by STS and ITS which are the extensions of the temporal ligament adhesion, which is a hard structure that is connected from the interior supraorbital ligamentous adhesion. It is comprised of only soft tissues without any important blood vessels and nerves, and doctors can feel safe to do a procedure around it. Anchoring happens here during a cogged thread lift.

The lower temporal compartment is a triangular-shaped area under the ITS. Unlike the upper temporal compartment that has few fat tissues, it has increasingly many fat tissues toward the arch. Its upper part is blocked by the ITS, but its bottom facing the zygomatic arch is not blocked and has important blood vessels and nerves passing by. There are the temporal branch of the facial nerve, the medial and lateral branches of the zygomatico-temporal nerve (ZTN), and the sentinel veins around it. The temporal branch of the facial nerve is, in particular, known to run almost in parallel to the ITS boundary, but the cadaver studies show that there are individual differences (Fig. 11.15).

As for the superficial temporal artery (STA) and deep temporal artery (DTA) that provide blood to the temples, STA branches out from the external carotid artery (ECA) right away and ensures blood circulation in the temples, forehead, and calvaria. DTA branches out from the maxillary artery that is a branch of ECA and ensures blood circulation in the temporalis muscles around the temples (Fig. 11.16).

STA runs almost perpendicular to the preauricular crease before the tragus of the ear, diverges back and forth near the horizon of the superior

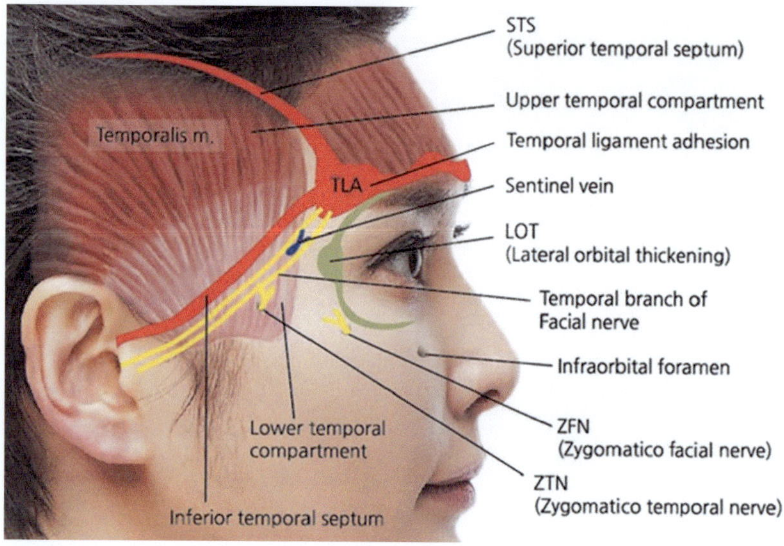

Fig. 11.15 Comparison of upper and lower compartments of temporal region

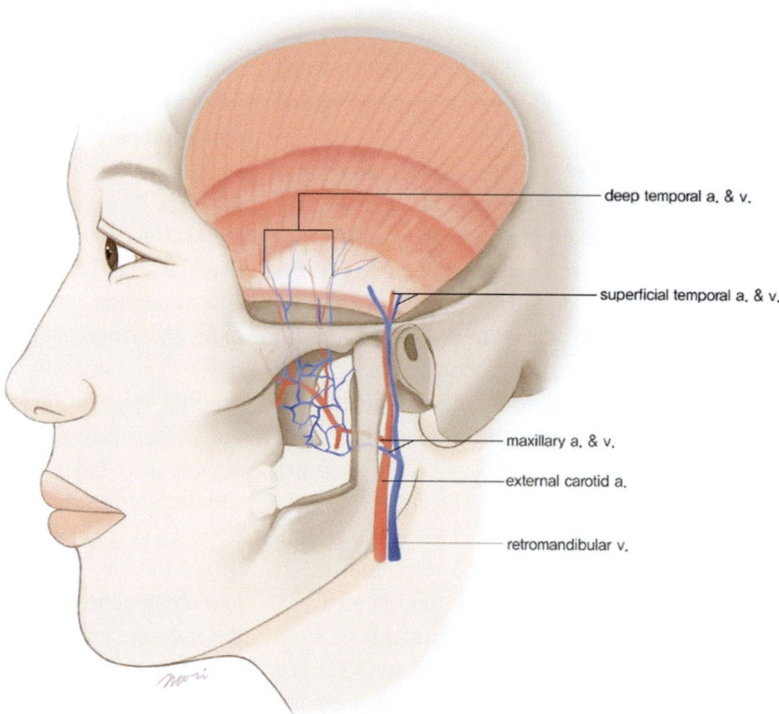

Fig. 11.16 Origin of superficial and deep temporal artery and vein

orbital rim, and leads to the anterior and posterior branches The anterior branch leans forward at an angle of 60° on average and runs in a superomedial direction, being surrounded by STF before returning to the lateral margin of the frontal muscles connected to STF. It is surrounded by the frontal muscles outside the vertical line from the lateral canthus. As it passes the vertical line, it gradually rises to the surface and forms a branch of STA in the subcutaneous tissues (Fig. 11.17).

There is another blood vessel that runs from the outside of the temporal area toward the fore-

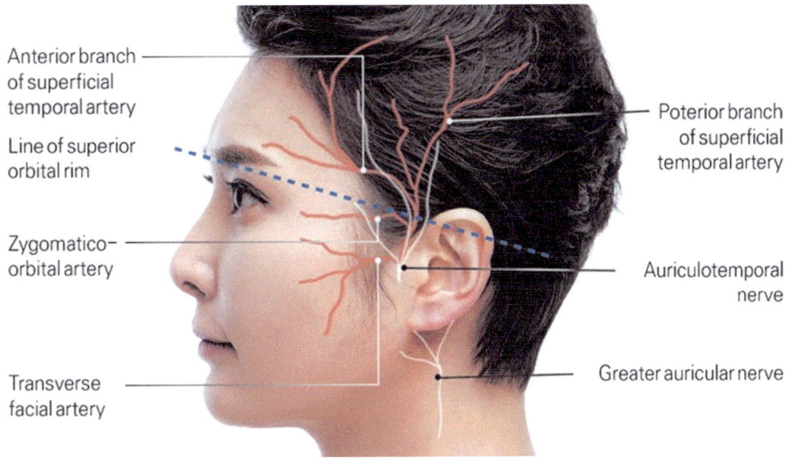

Fig. 11.17 Pathway of superficial temporal artery

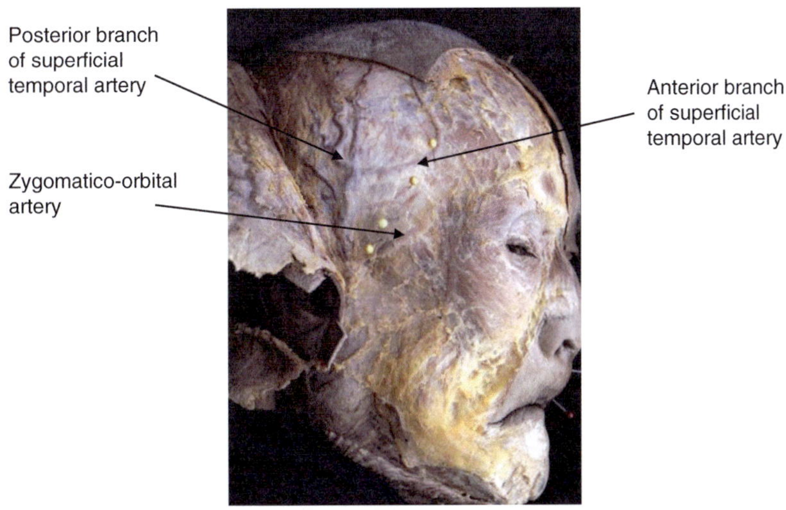

Fig. 11.18 Location of zygomatico-orbital artery

head. It is called the zygomatico-orbital artery. It is also called orbital artery in short. It branches out from the main branch before the superficial temporal artery is divided into the anterior and posterior branches. It is reported that approximately 80% of all Korean people have it. It usually comes out near the upper margin of the zygomatic arch and runs askew toward the lateral canthus over the arch before gradually rising and passing above the outer tip of the eyebrow (Fig. 11.18).

The volume of the temporalis muscles or STFP decreases for a congenital reason, due to weight loss, or according to aging. As people grow old, the volume of the buccal fat pad, which is a buccal extension of DTFP supporting the temples from the bottom, decreases along with the elasticity of the skin and soft tissues. As a result, the cheek areas around the mouth become hollow and depressed, leading to a reduced volume of DTFP. These developments raise a further need to restore the volume around the temples. The old approach is to revive the volume with fillers or fat transplantation only. This approach requires an excessive amount of filler or fat. The area will become hollow again over time, requiring the repetition of the procedure that uses an excessive amount of filler or fat. There is another approach using volumizing threads for contouring. The doctor can lift the skin and soft tissues of the sunken area by building support in the temporal area with the threads before a filler or fat transplantation to generate enough effects with a small amount of filler or fat. As for a space in which volumizing threads are inserted, the temporal space has some subcutaneous layers but few subcutaneous fat layers. When volumizing threads for contouring in a certain form are inserted in the space, there is a big chance that the area will look uneven after the procedure. This is why the space is not recommended. The compartment between the two fascial planes, STF and DTF, is a good space to insert volumizing threads.

Generally, volumizing threads for contouring in a cylindrical form are inserted. The elasticity of volumizing threads depends on the degree of hollowness and the thickness of the skin in the temple. The doctor marks an entry point to insert a cannula of volumizing threads and then makes a needle puncture after local anesthesia to make an entrance for the cannula containing twisted threads. The doctor can make an entry point above the zygomatic arch by drawing an imaginary circle with a diameter of 1 cm or so at the intersecting point of the upper margin of the zygomatic arch and the lateral margin of the lateral orbital rim and making an entry point in the circle (Fig. 11.19). By designing an entry point within the circle, the doctor can insert volumizing threads without any concerns about possible damage to the superficial and deep temporal artery, the branch of the facial nerve, the zygomatico-temporal nerve, the sentinel vein, and the middle temporal vein (Fig. 11.20).

Once reaching DTF that gives further resistance after STF gives the first round of resistance after the insertion of the cannula, the doctor should go in no further. By moving the cannula smoothly along the space between the fasciae, the doctor should insert volumizing threads in the upper and lower temporal compartments between STF and DTF around the hollow area. The risk of touching the important nerves and blood vessels below ITS can be reduced by moving the cannula in parallel to the location of ITS and making sure that it will not go down ITS at the entrance (Fig. 11.21). After lifting the hollow skin and soft tissues with volumizing threads to a certain degree, the doctor can complete the procedure by

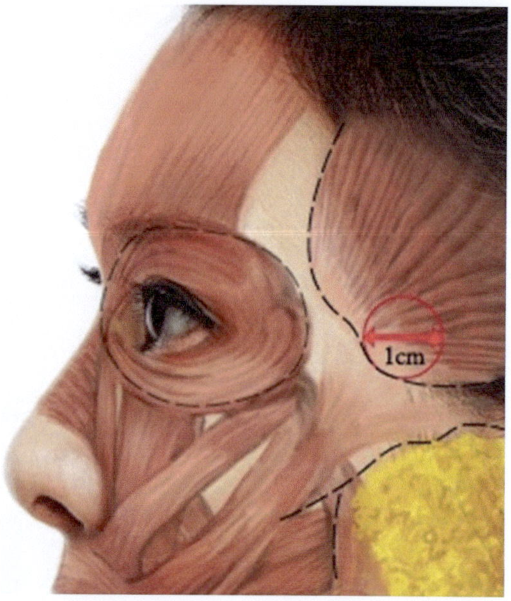

Fig. 11.19 Safe boundary of insertion point for temporal contouring

inserting a filler with the cannula in the same layer as the volumizing threads to fill the insufficient volume or make the boundary or surface smooth.

11.5.3 Nose

Rhinoplasty using a minimally invasive procedure is one of the most popular cosmetic procedures for Asians. These days there are many Western people who receive cosmetic procedures for the nose. In the past, doctors have usually used a filler. These days, they are using volumizing threads along with a filler to improve the nasal dorsum and tip with more certainty. In such cases, volumizing threads can also serve as a prop to elongate the nose in the skin and soft tissues in addition to increasing their volume. When only PDO volumizing threads are used, their hardness will disappear over time due to hydrolysis. By using a filler with PDO volumizing threads from the beginning, the doctor can postpone the hydrolysis and absorption of the threads

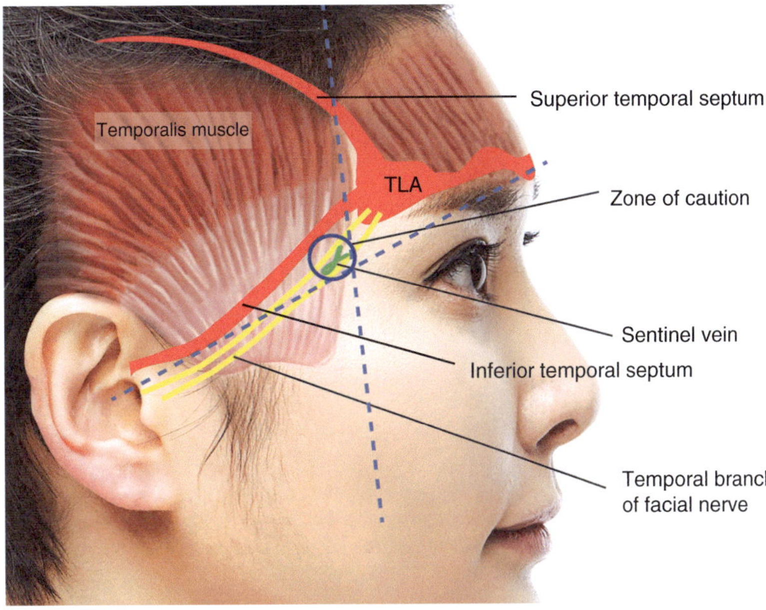

Fig. 11.20 Zone of caution for the sentinel vein and the temporal branch of facial nerve

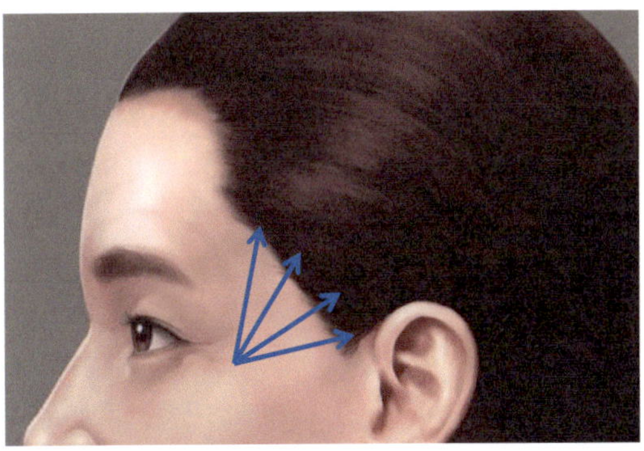

Fig. 11.21 Design of insertion and direction of volumizing threads for temporal contouring (i-THREAD Matrix Contour (HARD), HEALUX)

and prolong the duration of the procedure's effects.

This section will examine the anatomical layers of the nose for a procedure regarding the nose with volumizing threads. The soft tissues of the nose, including the skin, consist of five layers: the skin, the subcutaneous fat layer, the fibromuscular layer including the nasalis muscles connected to SMAS, the fat layer under the muscles, and the periosteum and perichondrium. As the proximal part of the nose has dynamic properties, there is space for the upper and lower layers to move smoothly around the fibromuscular layer. In the distal part, including the nasal tip at the bottom around the scroll area as the boundary between the lateral nasal cartilage and alar cartilage, the subcutaneous fat layer is replaced with dense collagen fibers and fat cells. The fibromuscular layer at the bottom is tightly connected to the dermis covering the upper part of the fat layer, and they cannot be separated. This makes the nasal tip look thicker along with the thick skin of the nasal tip.

Structurally speaking, a triangle appears where there is no cartilage at the intersection of the lateral crus of alar cartilage and the lower border of lateral nasal cartilage in the supratip area. This is called the weak triangle. It is covered only with the weak fibroareolar tissues under the skin and has no structures to strongly support it inside, thus being hollower than other parts and looking indented. Doctors should be aware that it is difficult to revive it fully anatomically only with a filler or fat transplantation (Fig. 11.22).

In most cases, the blood vessels in the nose run at the same depth as the fibromuscular layer or along the bottom plane right beneath. Their running depth becomes shallow as they rise toward the nasalis muscles. It would be a safe approach to insert threads in the deep fat layer under the fibromuscular layer to make enough

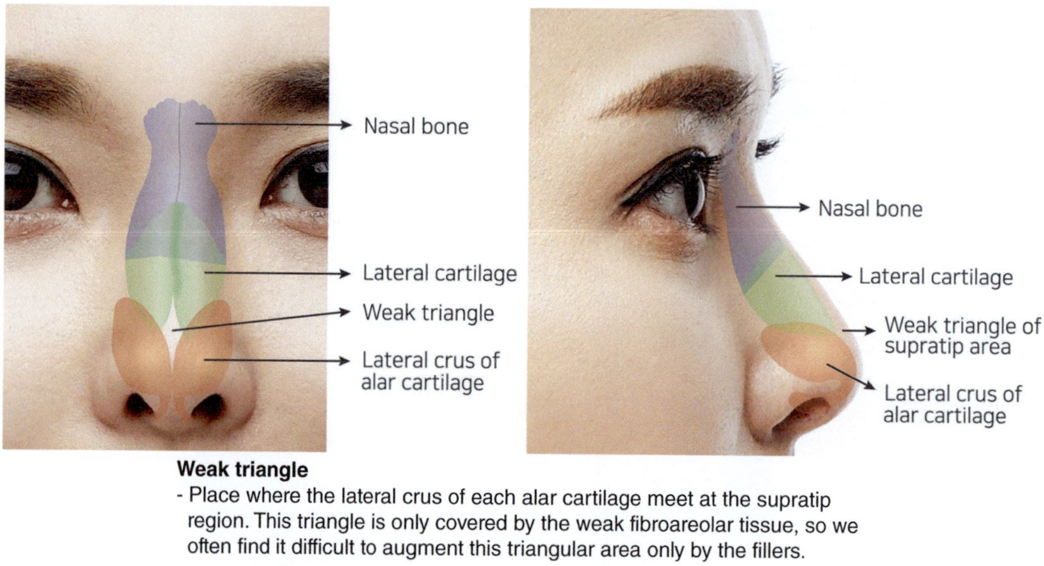

Fig. 11.22 Weak triangle on supratip region

Fig. 11.23 Vascular network of nose

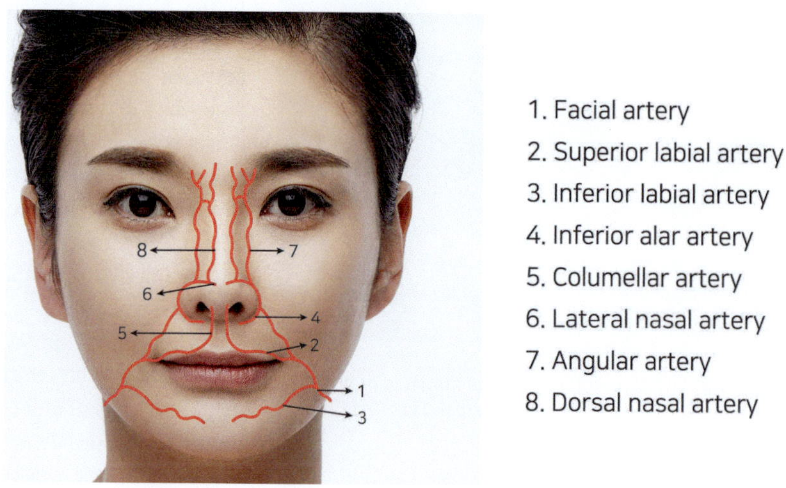

form while causing no damage to the blood vessels in the nose. The main arteries in the nose are the lateral nasal artery that branches out from the facial artery and the dorsal nasal artery that comes out from the ophthalmic artery. The columellar artery, which comes out from the superior labial artery which is a branch of the facial artery, passes through the nasal columella. The branches of the lateral nasal artery are usually responsible for the nasal tip, and the branches of the dorsal nasal artery and angular artery are responsible for the nasal dorsum (Fig. 11.23).

In the lateral nasalis muscle area, the possibility of hurting the main branches of the angular artery moving upward along the anatomical boundary between the nose and the medial cheek with a needle increases as the needle is closer to the medial angle. Doctors are thus advised to avoid as much as possible a procedure by the side of the nose. The branches of the lateral nasal artery that stretch to the nasal tip can be connected on the right and left across the central area, and doctors should be careful not to damage the blood vessels in any procedures at the center of the nasal tip. Unlike them, the two branches of the dorsal nasal artery in the nasal dorsum run slightly inclined to the margin rather than right in the middle. By keeping the procedure area right in the middle, doctors can reduce the risk of damage to the blood vessels. Some Asian people, however, have branches of the dorsal nasal artery crossing the middle area and reaching the other side. Doctors should keep in mind that they do not guarantee unconditional safety.

In a procedure around the nasalis muscles, doctors should be aware of the intercanthal veins running over the procerus muscles between the medial angles. They run between the medial angles in about 63%, move above the glabella in about 30%, and run a little below the medial angle in 7% or so. The intercanthal veins connect the angular veins on both sides like a bridge. In a procedure in the nasal root area, doctors can make sure that no intercanthal veins are hurt by holding the skin, including the procerus muscles below the subcutaneous layer, lifting it, and inserting threads deep under the muscles (Fig. 11.24).

The doctor should first check the upper limit of the nasal root area where volumizing threads will be inserted. It is important not to insert the threads upwards and make a so-called Beast or Avatar nose. The upper limit depends on the patient's taste, but it is generally a good idea to set the horizontal line connecting the highest point of the eyelash or double eyelid as the upper limit and do the procedure below it.

The doctor should mark the upper point of the nose before making an entry point for a cannula. The starting point at the bottom should be made at the infratip lobule between the nasal columella and nasal tip. In a procedure from this point to the nasal root area, the cannula moving upwards will pass a part (generally where a hooked nose appears) that protrudes a little bit and goes down again at the boundary of the nasal bone and lateral nasal cartilage. Once the cannula sets an upward direction, it may not be able to move down again. As the cannula cannot keep its insertion layer deep and moves superficially, there is a chance that it might damage the blood vessels. The doctor may have a difficult time controlling a cannula that is too long and will move up to the nasal root area, which means that an additional entry point would be a good idea right above the hooked nose and around it to lift the nasal root area. On the contrary, it would be a good idea to make an additional entry point near the nasal root or between the eyebrows in a procedure that moves in a top-bottom direction in the nasal root area (Fig. 11.25).

The doctor can insert a cannula through the entry point by lifting the bridge with the hand not holding the cannula. Here, the doctor should always keep in mind that the vertical central line should be maintained when inserting volumizing threads to avoid the possibility of damage to the dorsal nasal artery moving in the right and left of dead center and preventing the threads from going in asymmetrically.

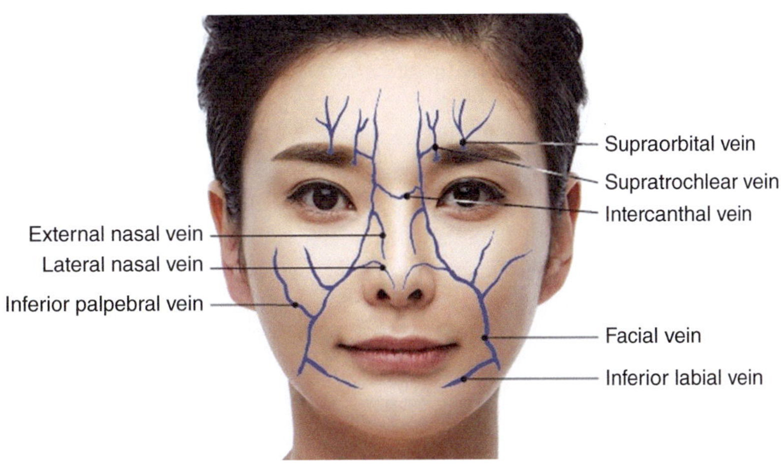

Fig. 11.24 Relationship of intercanthal vein with other veins

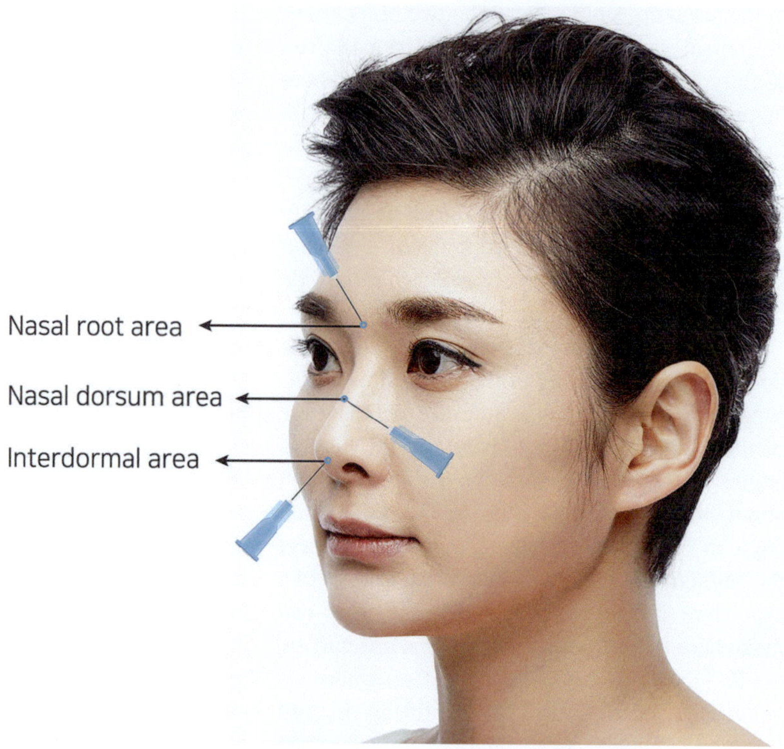

Fig. 11.25 Possible sites of cannula insertion for nasal shaping using the volumizing threads (i-THREAD Matrix Contour (HARD), HEALUX)

In the nasal tip, the fibromuscular layer is tightly attached to the skin above, which means that there is enough space for a cannula only in the deep fat layer under the fibromuscular layer. As a cannula is inserted in this layer, it could hurt the blood vessels that spread like a cobweb right under the fibromuscular layer. Thus, it is critical to always move the cannula smoothly (Fig. 11.26).

When threads are inserted too shallow in the subcutaneous tissues, their form might be visible on the surface and cause a foreign body sensation. When inserting a cannula under the muscles, the doctor should make sure the tip of the cannula has reached the target point completely and then pull out the cannula slowly while pressing its tip with a finger so that the threads exposed at its tip will stay in the tissues and not come out. The overall length and depth of a cannula insertion should be adjusted to prevent some of the threads from escaping through the entry point and make sure that all the threads are buried right in the skin tissues. If some of the inserted threads escape and are pulled out, even the ones inside will escape, too. The doctor should cut only the escaping ones and bury the remaining ones right inside the skin so that they will not come out. Doctors are advised to deeply insert threads inside for enough distance from the actual thread point so that no threads will be left at the insertion point.

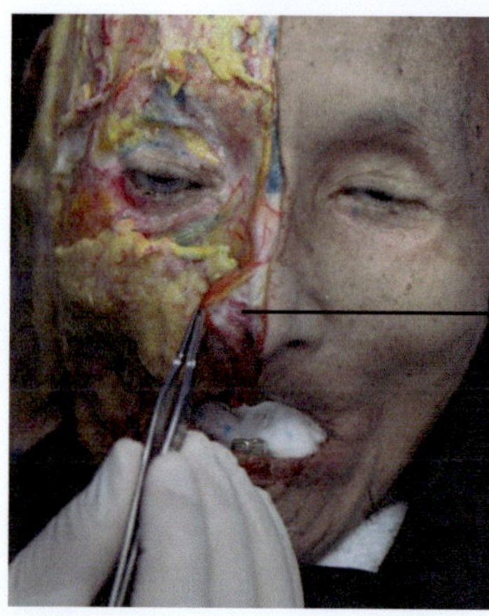

Fig. 11.26 Tight fibrous tissue on nasal tip region

After inserting the cannula again at the second entry point (near the hooked nose or nasal root), the doctor should insert volumizing threads through the same entry layer from the marked point in the nasal root area to the point that is not protruding above the hooked nose so that the area looks connected overall without any empty parts.

In recent years, there have been many volumizing thread procedures done for the nasal columella to lift the sagging nasal tip and increase the columella-labial angle that looks relatively pressed and hollow between the nasal columella and the upper lip in addition to filler procedures for the nasal tip to revive the volume of the flat nasal tip.

Like a filler, this procedure revives the volume of the nasal columella and, at the same time, makes the nasal alar narrow, thus improving the shape of the nasal columella. Like in a procedure at the nasal tip, doctors should always be careful about the movement of a cannula to reduce damage to the blood vessels that scatter around in the fat layer like a cobweb.

Similar to a procedure to revive the nasal dorsum and tip, this procedure makes an entry point at the infratip lobule point. A cannula should be erected perpendicular to the facial plane in the insertion area. Volumizing threads should be inserted from the anterior nasal spine between the footplates below the medial crus of alar cartilage to the top junction between the nasal columella and the nasal tip. When inserting the threads, the doctor should get as close to the medial crus deeper than the subcutaneous fat layer as possible not to cause damage to the branches of the columellar artery (Fig. 11.27).

When there is a need for a filler procedure after the insertion of volumizing threads to make the surface smoother, the doctor can insert a filler in the subdermal layer or subcutaneous layer through the same puncture site. When there is an uneven part after inserting a proper amount of a filler in the subcutaneous layer, the doctor can insert the filler superficially in the subdermal layer to make the surface smooth.

11.5.4 Infraorbital Hollowness and Midcheek Groove

As people get older, their expression wrinkles gradually become deeper around and under the eyes due to the movement of muscles around the eyes and cheeks. Even when they make no facial expressions, their wrinkles are visible. In the worst cases, they are left like a scar. In addition, the areas around the eyes will have grooves like a deep crack or wide hollowness due to changes in other anatomical structures, including the skin and soft tissues. In such cases, the muscles that make expression wrinkles around and under the eyes are weakened with the botulinum toxin, and the hollowness around the eyes is filled with a filler or fat transplantation.

When excessive amounts of toxins and fillers are used for wrinkles around and under the eyes,

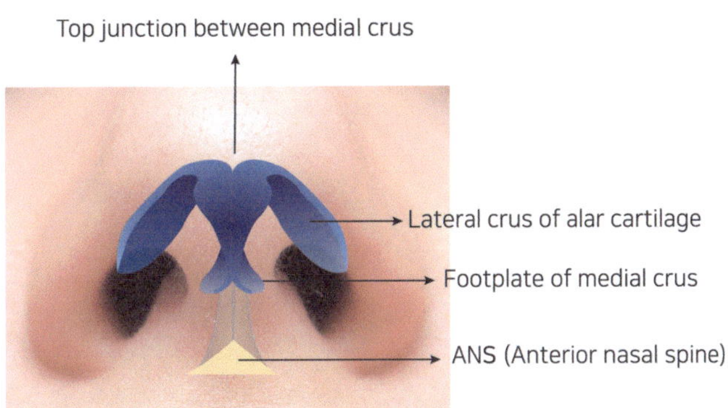

Volumizing thread insertion for the columella
: From ANS(between the footplates of medial crura of the alar cartilages) to top junction of the columella to increase the columello-labial angle in depressed & drooping nasal tip

Fig. 11.27 Anatomical structures of columellar region

they can make rather awkward facial expressions. After such a procedure, a bulging band might appear around and under the eyes. As the patients smile or make a facial expression, the band will be more prominent. Noncogged threads will be a better option than excessive amounts of a filler or toxin. As the threads that give elasticity are laid out in the crack area caused by wrinkles, they make the skin smoothed out and firm in the crack area and reduce the skin folding phenomenon during a smile. Volumizing threads are also a better option than a filler or fat transplantation for a hollow part. As volumizing threads are laid out in such a part, collagen regeneration will make the skin tissues tight. When they are combined with a filler or fat transplantation, the procedure will give maximum effect (Fig. 11.28).

This section examines the infraorbital symptoms and their related anatomical structures for a volumizing thread procedure that is effective and causes no side effects. Generally visible features can be used to distinguish an infraorbital groove and infraorbital hollowness. An infraorbital groove is a thick crack-like dent along the lower boundary of the orbital bone or around it. Infraorbital hollowness is a wide hollow area under the eye including the boundary. Infraorbital grooves and hollowness may appear separately according to individual differences in the infraorbital structures. As people grow old, these two symptoms can emerge together (Fig. 11.29).

Anatomists use the term, infraorbital groove, to refer to a groove in a bone rather than a ridge or wrinkle line in the infraorbital skin, but what shape such a groove takes in the skin is more important to clinicians. Whatever the causes might be, such a ridge in the infraorbital skin is called a tear trough in that it is a groove in which tears go down.

A nasojugal groove appears a little below a tear trough along the rim of the orbital bone. This wrinkle line is also called a nasolabial fold under the eye, stretching from the outer side of the nose to the front cheekbone. A nasojugal groove usually extends from the inner side of the midcheek groove toward the medial canthus. It becomes clearly visible when the levator labii superioris alaeque nasi (LLSAN) muscles attached to the lower boundary of the ocular muscle band contract due to the protruding and enlarged medial and inferior borders of orbicularis oculi muscles in the band. It is a little lighter than a tear trough that looks like a clear hollow crack. Its inner starting point is similar to that of a tear trough, but it looks more inclined downwards toward the outer part (Fig. 11.30).

Anatomically speaking, a tear trough is formed between the palpebral portion and the orbital portion of the orbicularis oculi muscles while a nasojugal groove is formed between the inner orbital portion of the orbicularis oculi muscles and the origin of the LLSAN muscle. The

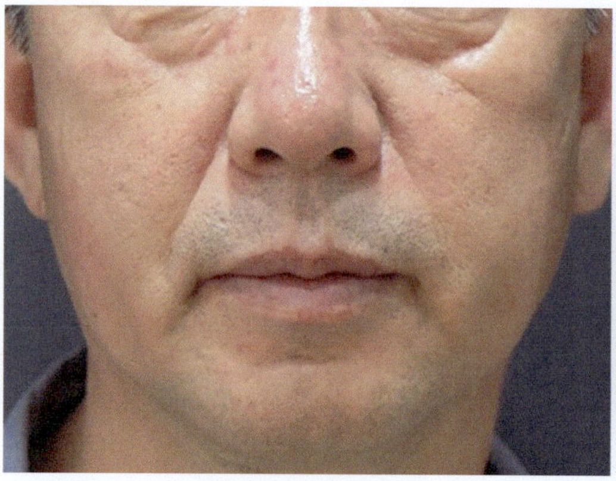

Before the procedure

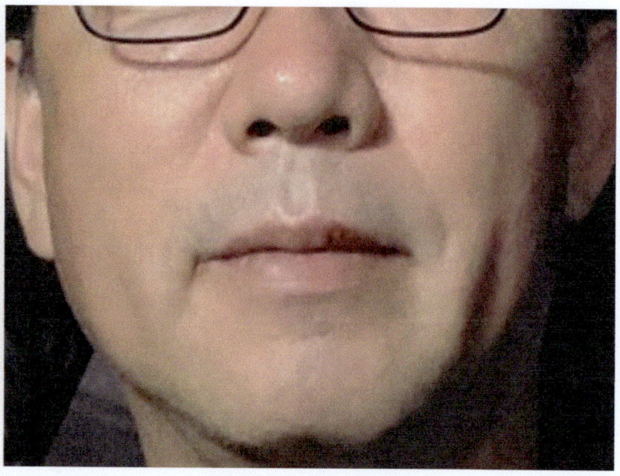

After the procedure

Fig. 11.28 Improvement of deep static groove and wrinkles of infraorbital region

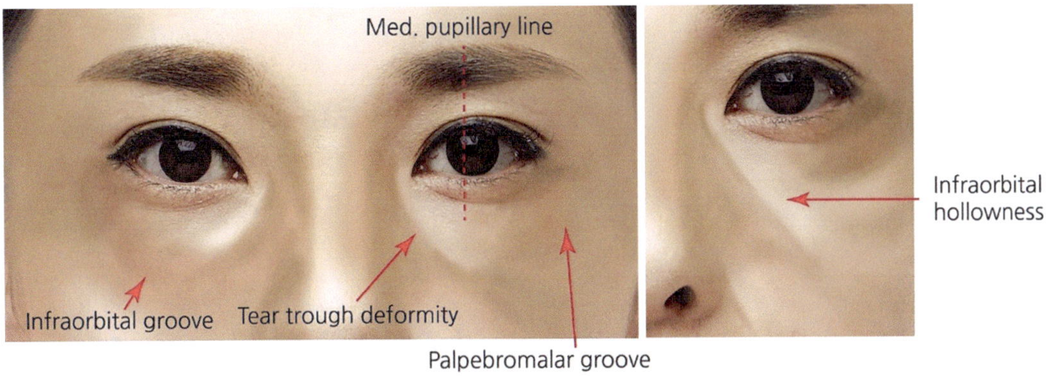

Fig. 11.29 Infraorbital groove (tear trough deformity and palpebromalar groove) and hollowness

Fig. 11.30 Tear trough deformity and nasojugal groove

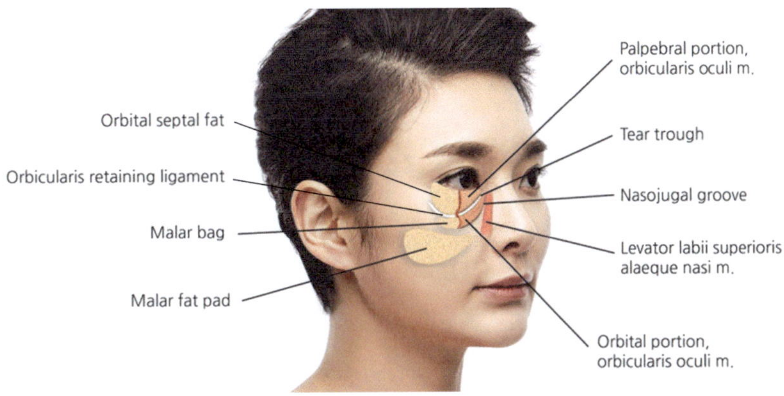

inner orbital portion of orbicularis oculi muscles becomes increasingly narrower toward the inside and gets attached to the medial canthal tendon by forming a band. A tear trough and a nasojugal groove that are each located above and below the inner orbital portion that is flat and narrow tend to get close to each other at the medial canthus as if they were attached to each other (Fig. 11.31).

As a nasojugal groove grows worse, it is connected like a single line to a midcheek groove, which is clinically called an Indian band. It has a crack-like hollow crease in the middle of the front cheekbone. The connection patterns may vary among people. In some people, they may appear to be connected to each other in a single line that is not cut off from the inside. In others, their connection may look cut off as the line bends a little in the middle. When patients have no nasojugal groove or a weak one, they may show a midcheek groove and tear trough deformity connected together. Even in such cases, a closer look will reveal a part where the connection is cut off. Anatomically, there is the zygomatico-cutaneous ligament that starts at such a part where the connection is cut off and continues long outwards. No matter what differences there are anatomically, doctors do not distinguish these cases clinically and call the entire line that looks connected and long a midcheek groove.

As seen in the figure, an entry point to insert a cannula is made outside the nasolabial folds. For the direction of volumizing threads, doctors employ the cross technique to cross the Indian band and the infraorbital groove from the bottom to the top. Inserting threads askew through the front cheek, the doctor is advised to have the threads go through the hard ligament tissues in the zygomatico-cutaneous ligament and around the eye rather than randomly deciding the depth and location of a thread. This approach gives the effects of volumizing threads pressing and

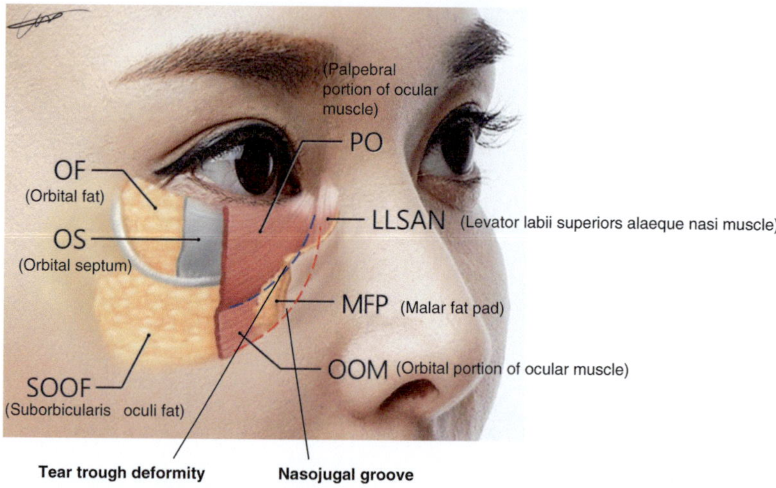

Fig. 11.31 Location of the tear trough deformity and nasojugal groove

smoothing out loose tissues inside the hard tissues. Several threads are inserted askew along the lower side of the orbicularis oculi muscles in a radial form according to the designed thread direction. The volumizing threads get caught inside the tissues after passing the ligament tissues in the front cheek and around the eye completely, reducing the concern with thread traveling even when the area around the eye moves. As the vector of the force working on the threads inclines toward the hard tissues, the front cheek area smooths out with the skin around the eye tightening. In terms of tissue regeneration, there is collagen regeneration from the front cheek area that the threads pass to the area around the eye. It pulls the skin upwards, making it tight (Fig. 11.32).

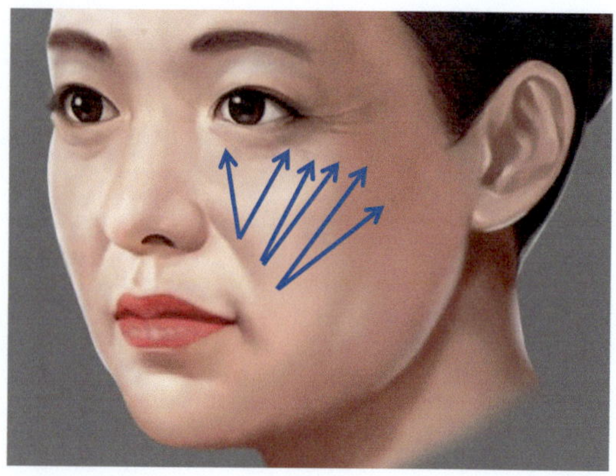

Fig. 11.32 Design of insertion and direction of cross technique using the volumizing threads for infraorbital hollowness and midcheek groove (i-THREAD Matrix Soft & Hard, HEALUX)

Some parts of the face have the skin folded repeatedly due to expression wrinkles. Even when the skin smooths out, the wrinkled parts still have the line marks. These wrinkles around the eyes that have established lines like a scar can be improved by inserting volumizing threads along the wrinkle line. In a procedure targeting periorbital lines, doctors need to make two entry points. As seen in the figure, the doctor makes one in the orbital rim margin outside the lines after checking the area prone to wrinkles as the patient has folds around the eye during a smile. The other entry point is made a little below the previous one. As the threads are inserted superficially under the dermis through the entry points from outside to inside, there is no problem even when threads are inserted in shallow skin inside the orbital rim. If an entry point is made too close to the eyelashes, threads may cause discomfort inside the skin. An entry point through which to insert threads had better be at least 5 mm from the lateral canthus and the lower eyelash margin. After the procedure, the patient will enjoy the effects of fainter lines as the skin around the eye with crack-like lines becomes tight with the skin surface folded along the lines smoothing out (Fig. 11.33).

When a patient has a part that looks a little hollow, a distinct boundary between the area with volumizing threads inside and the one with no

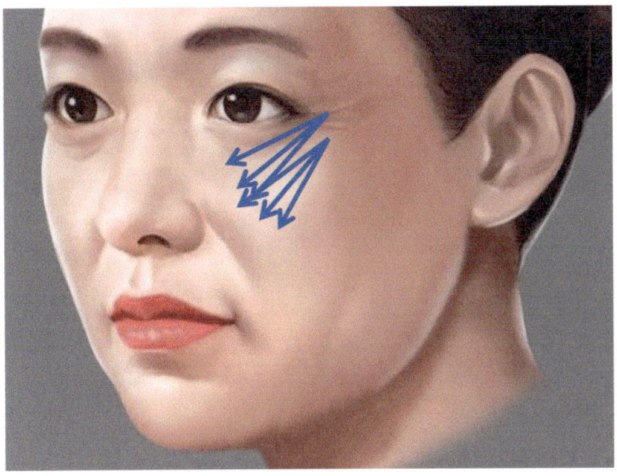

Fig. 11.33 Entry point and direction of volumizing threads for periorbital lines (i-THREAD Matrix Soft, HEALUX)

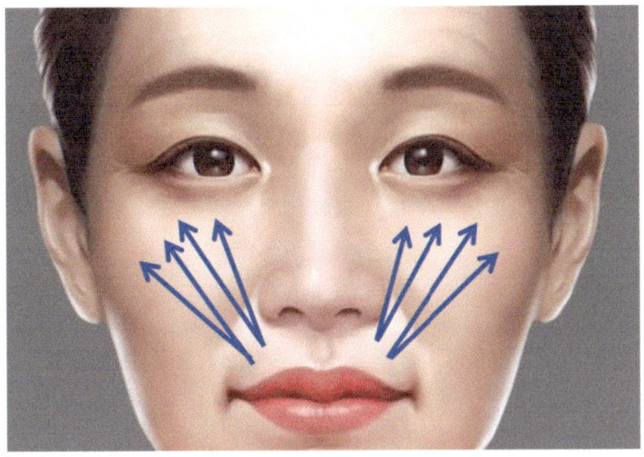

Fig. 11.34 Design of insertion and direction of cross technique using the volumizing threads for nasolabial folds (i-THREAD Matrix Soft & Hard, HEALUX)

threads inside, or an uneven surface after a procedure with volumizing threads, the doctor can make the entire skin surface smooth and fuller by inserting a filler in the subcutaneous or subdermal layer.

11.5.5 Nasolabial Folds

As explained in the previous chapter, it is important to consider that there are thickness and hardness differences between the upper and lower tissues of the wrinkle line next to the nose and around the mouth when trying to improve nasolabial folds with volumizing threads.

In the past, the popular choice of technique was to fill wrinkles by inserting fillers or non-cogged mono threads along the present wrinkle lines. As explained above, the investigator uses the cross technique with volumizing threads to make the folds fainter at the boundary between the hard tissues below the wrinkle line and the loose ones above it, such as nasolabial folds and marionette lines to smooth out the boundary.

The cross technique with volumizing threads makes an entry point a little above a wrinkle line next to the nose and the oral commissure. The distance between an entry point and the line depends on the length of a volumizing thread to be inserted. After making a needle puncture and inserting threads through the thick subcutaneous tissues tightly attached to the skin above the orbicularis oris muscles, the doctor should push the threads upwards perpendicular to the wrinkle line and across it as seen in the figure (Fig. 11.34). The tip of the cannula should be made to hold the retinacula cutis in the subdermal layer under the skin tissues and above the loose wrinkle line as it passes it. The area of volumizing threads that are inserted in the thick tissues below the wrinkle line works as support and ensures that the part above the threads presses and pushes the loose skin tissues above the line.

The volumizing threads that are inserted across the wrinkle line in this way make the loose tissues above the line flat by pushing and pressing them, thus improving the height differences of skin layers due to hardness differences between the upper and lower tissues of the line. If several volumizing threads are laid down perpendicular to the wrinkle line, collagen will be made and fill the space along the direction of the threads. As the loose skin tissues above the line become tight, the degree of the skin being pressed and folded next to the nose and around the oral commissure by expression muscles will be reduced (Fig. 11.35).

Volumizing threads can also be inserted along a wrinkle line to revive an area that simply develops a crack and looks hollow rather than pressing and smoothing out sagging tissues by using volumizing threads inserted in hard tissues as support similar to the technique explained above. This procedure does not only revive the hollow skin along the wrinkle line, but it also mitigates the

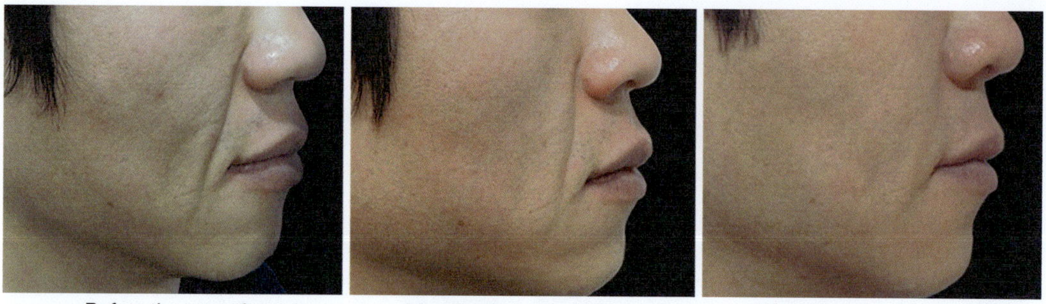

Fig. 11.35 Stretching and pressing effect of volumizing threads for nasolabial folds

degree of line folding during a smile or facial expression. Collagen regeneration occurs after the procedure, making the skin tighter. The crack-like lines, which used to be visible even when no facial expressions were made, become faint. Volumizing threads promote richer collagen regeneration in the skin than simple PDO mono threads, giving excellent effects to make the skin clear and tight.

11.5.6 Lateral Cheek Hollow

When the area below the zygomatic arch called the rear or lateral cheek is hollow, the protruding cheekbone looks prominent, and the face looks uneven. This requires a correction.

In many cases, if the hollowness is great, the masseteric cutaneous ligament and platysma auricular fascia develop from the inferior border of the zygomatic arch to the zygomatic ligament and the parotid-masseteric fascia attaches to the skin. When these ligament tissues develop, the skin is severely attached to the lower side of the zygomatic arch. Even a filler injection would not be enough to revive the hollow area. When a filler injection is forced, the filler will spread beside the hollow area and make the lateral part look bulgy and uneven. There is a good approach for such cases. The doctor should first weaken the strength of ligament tissues pulling the skin through tunneling with a cannula to create space. Then the doctor can build support by inserting volumizing threads below the pressed skin and injecting a filler to revive even a severely hollow area to smooth it out (Fig. 11.36).

This section will examine the blood vessels and nerves which are important structures that require careful attention in a procedure for areas with a lateral cheek hollow close to the SMAS layer.

There is the frontal branch of the superficial temporal artery and the zygomatico-orbital artery in the temporal areas above the zygomatic arch. The transverse facial artery runs parallel to the margin below the arch in the lateral cheek. There is the antegonial notch a little down the way. Doctors should be aware of the facial artery that is askew toward nasolabial folds and its branches. The following section will focus its explanations on the blood vessels that doctors should be cautious of in a procedure across the lateral cheek and buccal cheek below the zygomatic arch.

The superficial temporal artery from the external carotid artery moves up vertically before the ear and branches out into the transverse facial artery before the zygomatic arch. The transverse facial artery runs in the same depth as the facial nerve, being buried in the parotid gland in the lateral side of the face. As it moves to the anterior side of the face, it runs gradually shallow and produces branches moving to the malar region. In the lateral face, it runs deeper than the deep fascia, which means that there will be a reduced risk of damage during the procedure in the depth of the SMAS level (Fig. 11.37). It runs between the inferior margin of the zygomatic arch and the parotid duct. It is known to produce the perfora-

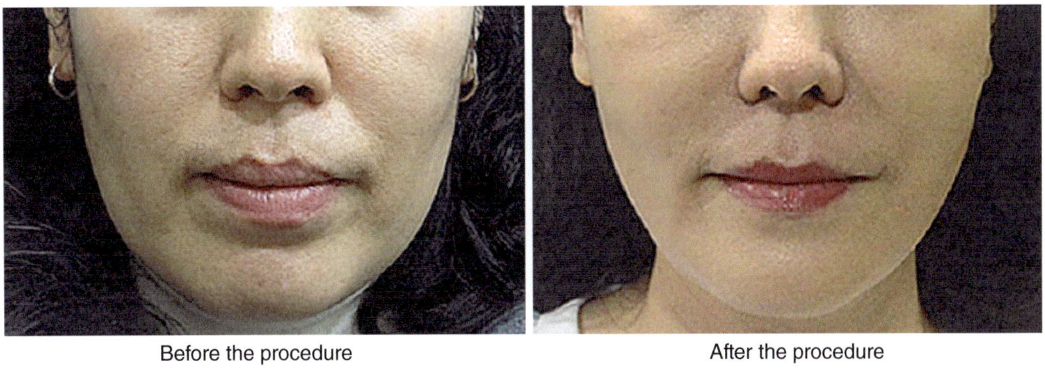

Fig. 11.36 Improvement of depressed lateral cheek hollow using the combination treatment of volumizing threads and HA fillers

Fig. 11.37 Origin of the transverse facial artery

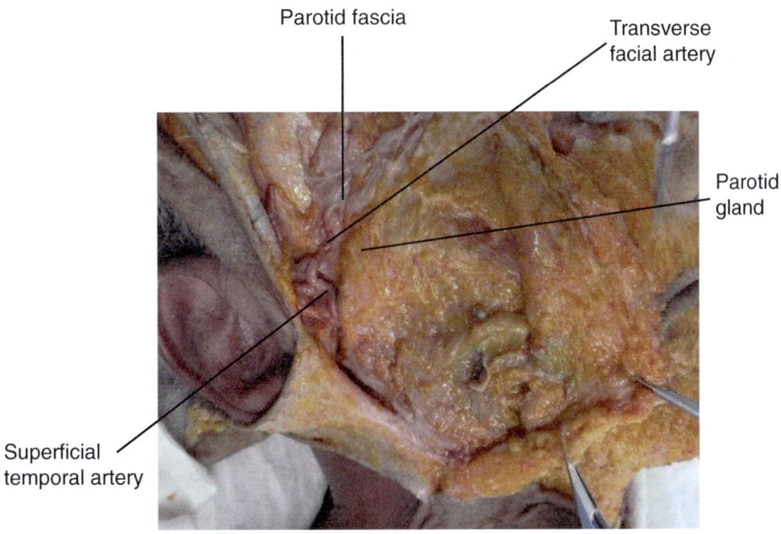

tor to move around the malar eminence after running parallel to the arch at a distance of 10 mm or so from it. The risk of damage will be reduced by setting a procedure direction in the cheek area below the malar region (Fig. 11.38).

The facial nerve responsible for the movement of the face comes from the stylomastoid foramen and diverges into the upper and lower division in the parotid gland. As it comes out of the parotid gland, it produces five branches. It is generally known that the face is divided into the later face, which is relatively fixed along the virtual vertical line made of five ligament tissues, and the anterior face, which is mobile and gets involved in facial expressions. Out of the parotid gland, the facial nerve is located safe in the deep layer below the deep fascia that is deeper than SMAS in the later face. As it passes the border of the anterior face with no deep fascia, it moves up to the bottom of the SMAS layer. Then, it gradually moves up to the surface layer, reaching expression muscles after the bottom of SMAS. In a procedure to target an area before the transition point from a deep layer to a shallow one, there is a possibility of hurting the facial nerve. In the lateral fat compartment around the transition point in the lateral face, however, the facial nerve is located deep below the parotid gland and parotid-masseteric fascia. If a doctor moves a cannula smoothly to insert volumizing threads around the SMAS layer, there will be no need to worry about hurting the facial nerve (Fig. 11.39).

The parotid duct (Stensen's duct) from the parotid gland passes 1/3 above the middle of the line between the tragus and the oral commissure by drawing a bridge-shaped arch. Like the buccal branch of the facial nerve, it is located below the parotid-masseteric fascia, which is a deep fascia, in the preparotid and premasseteric space. As it moves forward further, it runs deeper. It opens inside the mouth after the buccal fat pad. If a doctor properly keeps a procedure layer for a cannula, there will be no concern about hurting it (Fig. 11.40).

It is a good idea to make a puncture point for a cannula to go in at a point where a vertical line from the lateral margin of the lateral orbital rim meets a horizontal line from the oral commissure. After untangling the area that is entangled by ligament tissues to a certain degree by using a cannula before the insertion of volumizing threads, the doctor can insert volumizing threads upwards around the SMAS layer and lift the hollow area as seen in the figure. The threads should be made to support the skin and soft tissues so that the area will not get hollow again. Then a filler can be injected additionally in an uneven part or where the boundary is visible like other areas so that the entire surface will smooth out (Fig. 11.41).

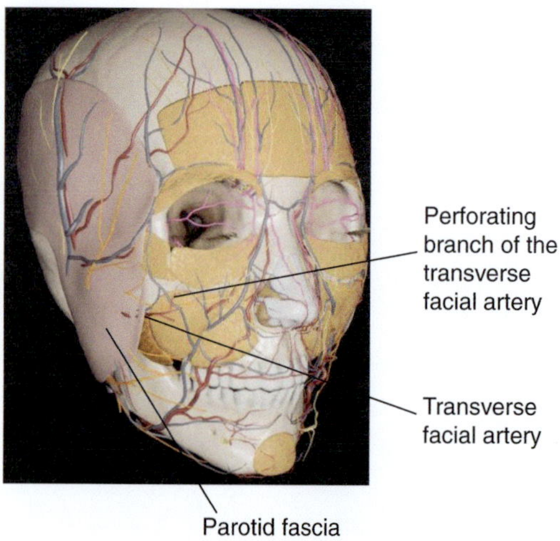

Fig. 11.38 Pathway of the transverse facial artery

11.5.7 Lips

There is the intermediate zone that is uplifted a little in a thin line form between the red mucous membrane of the lips and the skin. The boundary between the zone and the skin is called the vermilion-cutaneous border. The mucous membrane is further divided into the dry mucosa

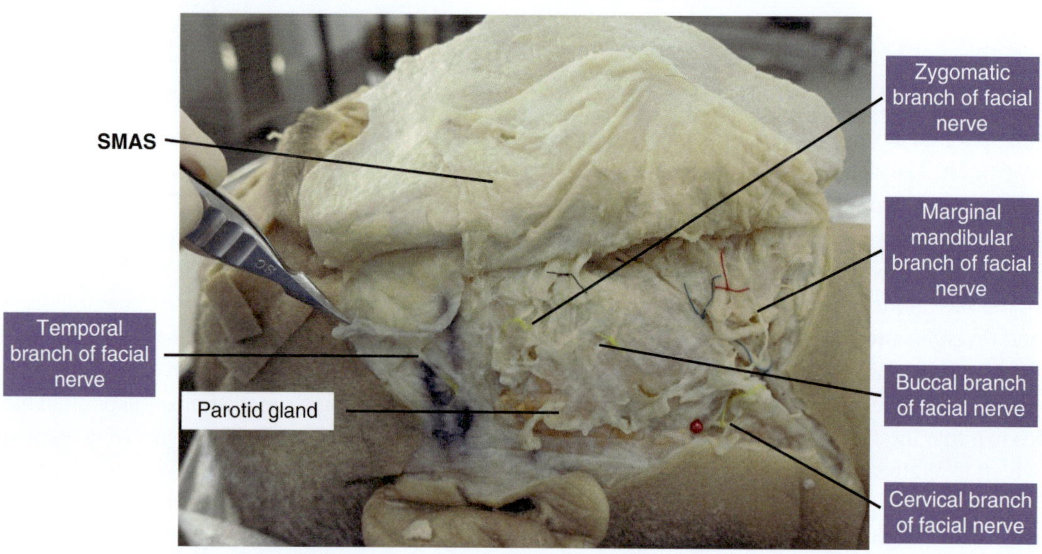

Fig. 11.39 Five branches of the facial nerve

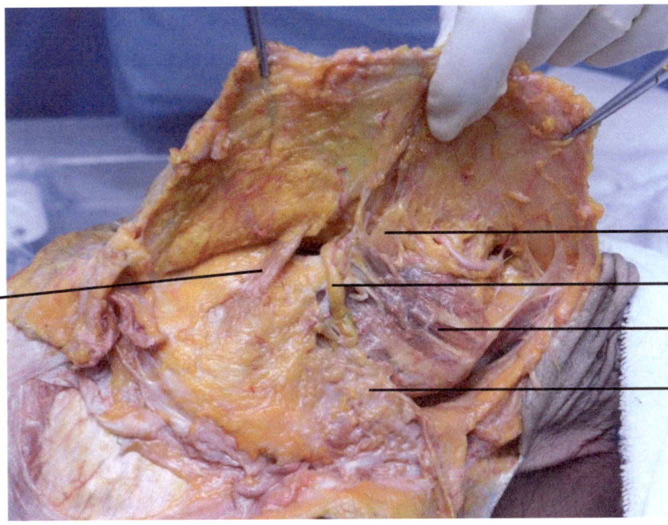

Fig. 11.40 Location and depth of the parotid duct (Stensen's duct)

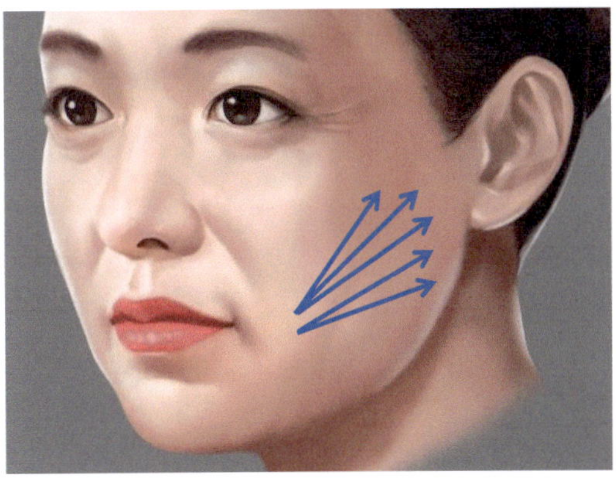

Fig. 11.41 Design of insertion and direction of the volumizing threads for lateral cheek hollow (i-THREAD Matrix Soft & Hard, HEALUX)

exposed to the outside and the inner wet mucosa (Fig. 11.42).

The lips consist of different layers. When seen from the outer lips, the skin along the red lip border and dry mucosa is in the outermost. The superficial fat spreads superficially below them. On the inside, there are the orbicularis oris muscles and the deep fat under the muscles. The wet mucosa is in the innermost part (Fig. 11.43).

There are cultural differences in the perceptions of what beautiful lips are according to race and region, but in most cases, beautiful lips are considered to be firm, have volume, and are distinct along the border. When lips are thin, have lost elasticity, look drawn inwards, and have a blurry border, they are considered far from beautiful; they are considered old. As for the reasons to inject a filler in the lips, the popular procedures in the past only revived the volume of the lips themselves. These days, a common goal is to enhance the overall face image by improving the shapes and forms of the lips. As people get older, in particular, there are changes to the shapes and volume of the lips. The lips, which used to face outwards, become thin and are drawn inwards. As a result, pouting reduces the red lip border, the lips become longer and flatter in the right and left, and the upper white lips become longer. The border between the lips and the skin becomes blurry, and the lip contour becomes less distinct. In addition, the oral commissure droops down and is drawn inwards, making the oral commissure sag and the upper lip look like it is covering the lower lip (Fig. 11.44).

When young patients start to suffer these changes to the lips, they need improvement to these changed forms as well as the volume of the lips to achieve satisfying results. These days, a procedure for the lips should enlarge the lips, improve the lip contour, and lift the lateral parts

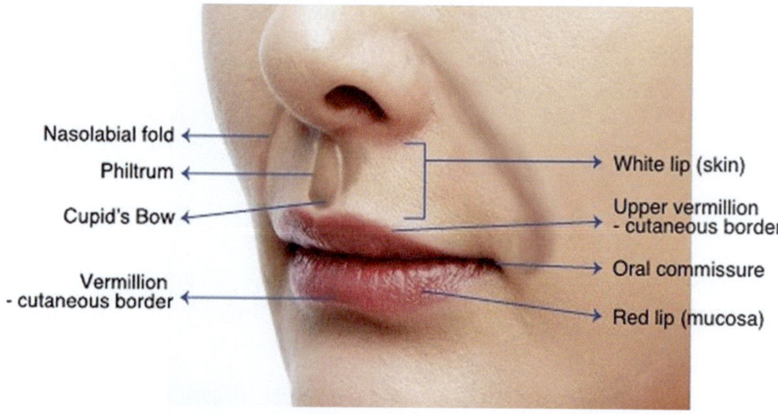

Fig. 11.42 The structures of lips

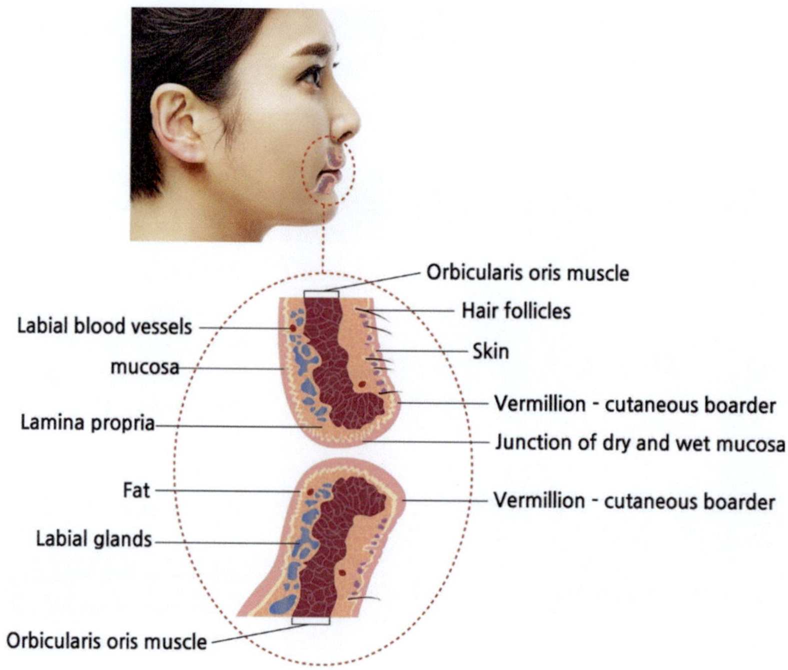

Fig. 11.43 Anatomical layers of lips

and oral commissures at the same time. Such procedures are not simple, and it is critical to choose the most appropriate method for the goal.

A recent study reported that although it was a natural phenomenon for the lips to decrease in volume according to aging, there was no clear information about which parts would decrease and how much. Some argue that the overall volume of the lips is maintained as the superficial fat tissues of the lips increase while the volume of muscles decreases along with the border between the skin and the mucous membrane. When the lips age, the mucosa of the vermillion reduces definitely rather than the reduction of the entire lip volume. The intermediate zone disappears, and the lips become flat. Like the fat layers of other parts of the face, the superficial fat increases its volume according to aging with the deep fat layer reduced. The study reported that the doctor should revive the volume of the lips whose volume seems to decrease due to aging by targeting the deep fat layer between the wet mucosa of vermillion and the muscles called suborbicularis oris fat layer.

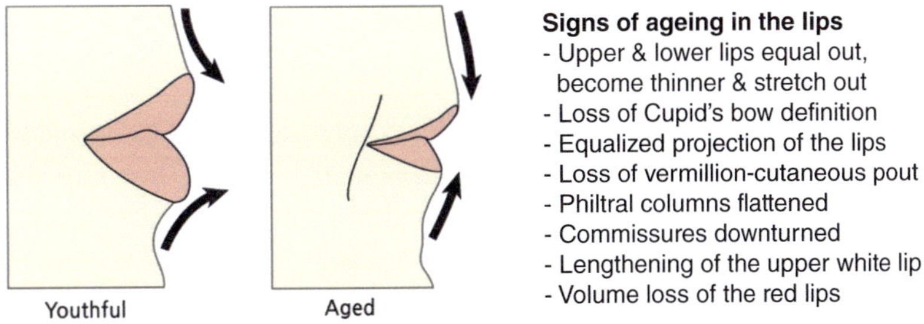

Fig. 11.44 Aging changes of lip and philtrum

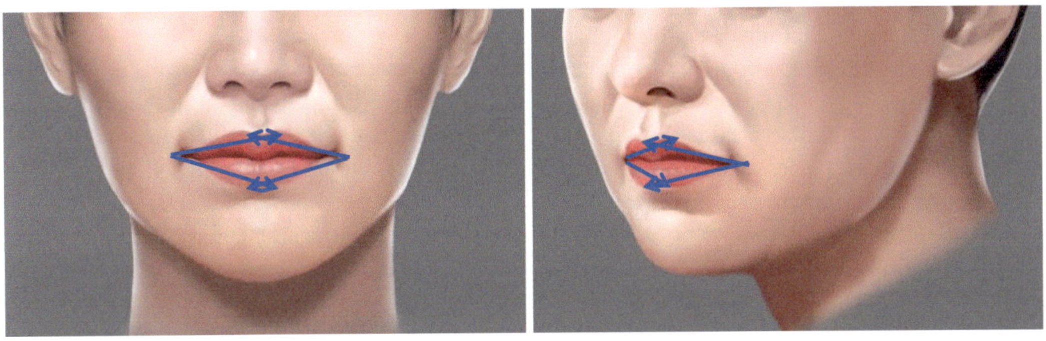

Fig. 11.45 Design of insertion and direction of the volumizing threads for lips (i-THREAD Matrix Contour (HARD), HEALUX)

The investigator now feels that a procedure should revive the volume of the orbicularis oris muscles or the layer below them through the border of the dry-wet mucosa to create further eversion effects for lips that are thin, have a blurry contour, and are drawn inwards while reviving their volume fully.

A simple filler is not enough to generate full effects to improve the contour, volume, and shape of the lips simultaneously. Volumizing threads should be inserted to fully endure the external force and maintain the shape of the lips in addition to the sufficient eversion of the lip tissues that are drawn inwards. The lip area should continue to move as people make facial expressions, speak, and eat in daily life. When choosing volumizing threads for the shape and volume of the lips, it is especially important to consider flexibility, which refers to the ability to stretch and contract smoothly without any discomfort when the patient opens and closes the mouth. An entry point for the insertion of volumizing threads should be made a few millimeters from the oral commissure to reduce damage to the superior and inferior labial arteries from the facial artery by a needle puncture. Volumizing threads should go in below the mucous membrane at the dry-wet mucosa border along the orbicularis oris muscles via a cannula. The depth should not be too shallow. They will revive the volume of the lips that are thin and look drawn inwards, making the entire lips more everted and fuller (Fig. 11.45).

After witnessing the lips become inflated and everted overall after the insertion of volumizing threads, the patient might wish to make the border of Cupid's bow distinct in the middle of the lips along with the red lip border. The doctor can fulfill the patient's additional wish by injecting a filler in the subdermal layer including the dermis. The injection depth should not be too shallow in the dermis to prevent any lumps, but an injection that is deep under the muscles in the skin or under the mucous membrane inside can cause damage to the branches of the superior and inferior labial arteries and lead to many side effects due to severe hemorrhage. Doctors should always be careful.

11.5.8 Marionette Lines and Prejowl Sulcus

A marionette line appears as the line extends from the oral commissure. As the fat down and inside a line reduces with the deposition of the fat (jowl fat) up and outside the line, a border emerges. The mandibular ligaments at the bottom of a marionette line pull the tissues inside the line and prevent them from moving, making the border distinct. In such a case, volume asymmetry can be corrected by fat absorption or transplantation and a filler. Volumizing threads can also be used. By inserting them perpendicular to the line, a doctor can make the border between the two fat layers less distinct.

For the cross technique with volumizing threads, a doctor needs to make an entry point inside a marionette line as seen in the figure. Its location depends on the length of volumizing threads (Fig. 11.46).

After volumizing threads are inserted upwards at the entry point across the line, the area of the threads serves as a support in the thick tissues below the line. The upper part of volumizing threads presses and pushes the loose skin tissues above the line. After volumizing threads are inserted perpendicular to the line, collagen will be produced along the direction of the threads with the loose skin tissues above the line tightening. These improvements can reduce the degree of the skin being pressed and folded around the oral commissures due to the expression of muscles when the mouth area moves.

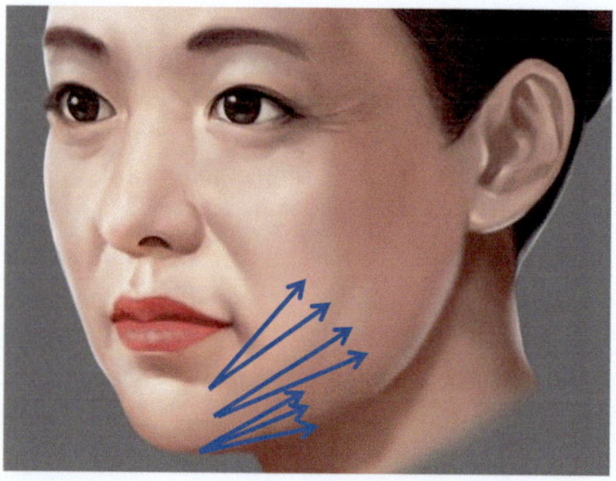

Fig. 11.46 Design of insertion and direction of cross technique using the volumizing threads for marionette line and prejowl sulcus (i-THREAD Matrix Soft & Hard, HEALUX)

When inserting volumizing threads inside a marionette line, doctors should be careful not to hurt the mental artery and nerve from the mental foramen below the oral commissure. The mental foramen is often located around the middle point of a vertical line from the oral commissure to the borderline of the mandible.

In old patients, a marionette line is accompanied by prejowl sulcus due to the sagging of the skin and soft tissues in the lower face. The jawline area below the line is pressed and does not look smooth, making the area above the line look more bulgy. The mental lateral part has a thinner fat layer and skin than the mentum, and the mandibular ligament along the jawline is attached to the skin and pulls it tight. When these ligament tissues severely press prejowl sulcus, a filler is not enough to revive the area and smooth it out fully. When a filler is combined with volumizing threads, it can generate even better effects (Fig. 11.47). In such a combined treatment, the doctor should create enough space for volumizing threads and fillers through tunneling between the hard ligament tissues before moving a cannula smoothly forward to insert volumizing threads and fillers.

As for an entry point for a cannula, a doctor should make a needle puncture at the anterior border of the hollow and pressed area around the border between the mentum and mandible body. Then, the doctor should insert the cannula laterally and then the volumizing threads along the depressor anguli oris and platysma muscles or the fat layer under the muscle (Fig. 11.46). For an uneven area after the insertion of volumizing threads, the doctor can smooth it out by injecting a filler in the subdermal layer or subcutaneous layer through the same puncture site.

The overall shape of the oral commissure will improve after the doctor moves the sagging tissues outside a marionette line upwards and revives the hollow and pressed area before the line. When the patient wishes to make the folded

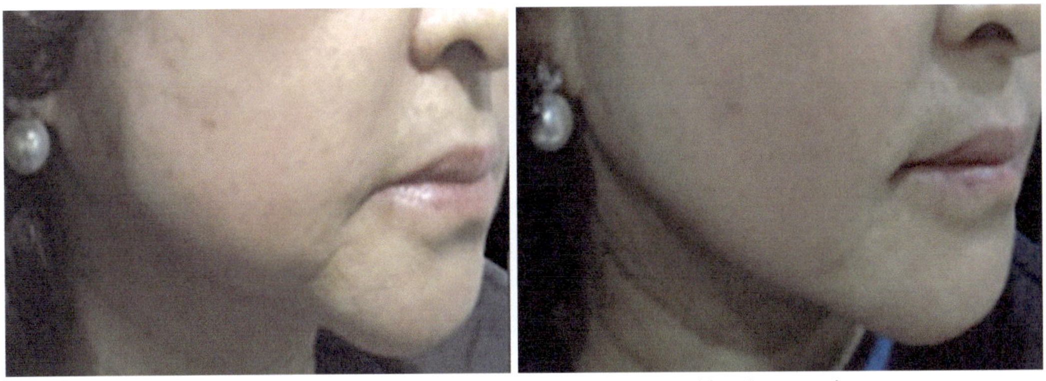

Fig. 11.47 Improvement of marionette line and depressed prejowl sulcus using the combination treatment of volumizing threads and HA fillers

border between the hard and loose tissues faint, the doctor can use softer volumizing or mono threads. By inserting threads parallel to the line and a little inside the line, the doctor can improve skin layer differences due to the hollow area. After volumizing or mono threads are laid out along the line, collagen will be produced in the direction of the threads. As skin tissues become tight, they will reduce the symptoms of the skin being pressed and folded before the line.

11.5.9 Chin and Jawline

Westerners usually have a narrower face and have fewer cases of weak mentum than Asians. They used to receive many procedures to make the mandibular angle and jawline distinct or to smooth out an uneven jawline for an improved facial contour rather than procedures to revive the mentum. Koreans have a shorter mandible than Westerners or a short chin and used to receive relatively more surgeries or procedures to revive the mental area. These days, however, Koreans have gradually changed in facial shape as well as body type. Orthodontics has become common during childhood. The cases of a very weak mentum and one drawn backward have decreased considerably compared to the past. In these cases, it is important to make the overall jawline form, including the mentum, distinct as in the cases of Westerners.

The combination of fillers and toxins is a good option for patients who have a blurry contour in the mentum and jawline, have a mentum that looks relatively weak due to the protruding area around the mouth, and have a mentum that looks pressed by the contraction of the mentalis muscles due to excessive force applied when the mouth is closed.

In general, an entry point for a cannula to insert threads is made at the border between the chin and mandible body. It is 2–3 cm from the middle of the mentum sidewards. The investigator makes a puncture with a 21G needle and pushes an empty 21G cannula into the area where the cutaneous insertion of the mentalis muscles in the mentum and the mandibular ligament pull the skin as well as where the mandibular septum is connected to the skin along the jawline so that volumizing threads can make a smooth entry. When the cannula does not move smoothly and feels blocked by some hard fibrous tissues, the doctor keeps pushing the cannula into these hard tissues by creating space between them.

As seen in the figure, a doctor inserts a cannula at the entry point medially and laterally and then volumizing threads along the muscle layer or the fat layer below the muscles (Fig. 11.48). After inserting volumizing threads, the doctor might need a filler injection to make the surface smoother. The same puncture site can be used to inject a filler in the subdermal layer or subcutaneous layer. When injecting a filler in the subcutaneous layer, the doctor should be careful not to have the filler flow down the jawline by injecting it a little above the inferior border of the jaw. When there is an uneven area after a proper amount of filler is injected in the subcutaneous layer, the doctor can smooth the surface out by injecting a filler superficially in the subdermal layer.

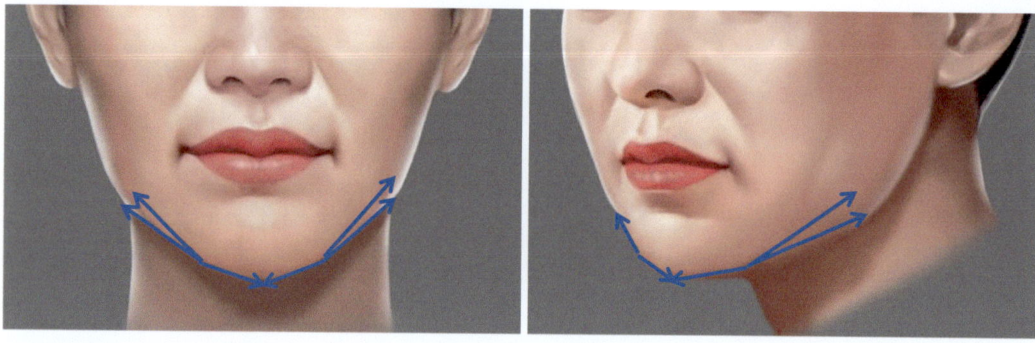

Fig. 11.48 Design of insertion and direction of the volumizing threads for chin and mandible line (i-THREAD Matrix Contour (HARD), HEALUX)

Evaluation of Procedural Outcome 12

Contents

12.1 Typical Method of Evaluating the Results of Thread Lifting

The effectiveness of thread lifting is generally evaluated using the GAIS score (Table 12.1).

The GAIS score consists of two main points. First, the lower the number, the better the effect is considered to be. Second, the GAIS score does not objectively evaluate the effectiveness of the procedure but rather speaks to the degree of subjective improvement. It would be beneficial if the effectiveness of thread lifting could also be measured through an objectively quantified evaluation tool. The evaluation method using Morpheus, which will be discussed later, was a device that, albeit modestly, helped in the objective evaluation of treatment results. Recently, with the advancement of technology, it has become possible to evaluate the degree of improvement objectively and quantitatively with the aid of devices that apply AI.

Table 12.1 Global Aesthetic Improvement Scale (GAIS) score

	Degree	Description
1	Exceptional improvement	Excellent corrective result
2	Very improved patient	Marked improvement of the appearance, but not completely optimal
3	Improved patient	Improvement of the appearance, better compared with the initial condition, but a touch-up is advised
4	Unaltered patient	The appearance substantially remains the same compared with the original condition
5	Worsened patient	The appearance has worsened compared with the original condition

S. M. Oh et al., *The Art and Science of Thread Lifting Based on Pinch Anatomy and Moving Plane*,
https://doi.org/10.1007/978-981-97-5516-5_12

12.2 Evaluation of the Outcomes Using the Morpheus

12.2.1 Simulation Using the Morpheus

12.2.1.1 Treatment Result Simulation

It is difficult to objectively evaluate the effects of thread lifting, but it is possible to demonstrate the extent of changes. In the case of Morpheus equipment, it is possible to simulate volume changes, as well as the direction and area of movement.

Figures 12.1 and 12.2 show a comparison between the simulated results of midface thread lifting, anterior cheek filler, and chin filler using Morpheus equipment and the actual treatment results. It is evident that there has been a significant change in the patient's appearance.

Recently, programs that can simulate before and after treatments based on artificial intelligence are being developed. Compared to before, simulations are faster and more convenient.

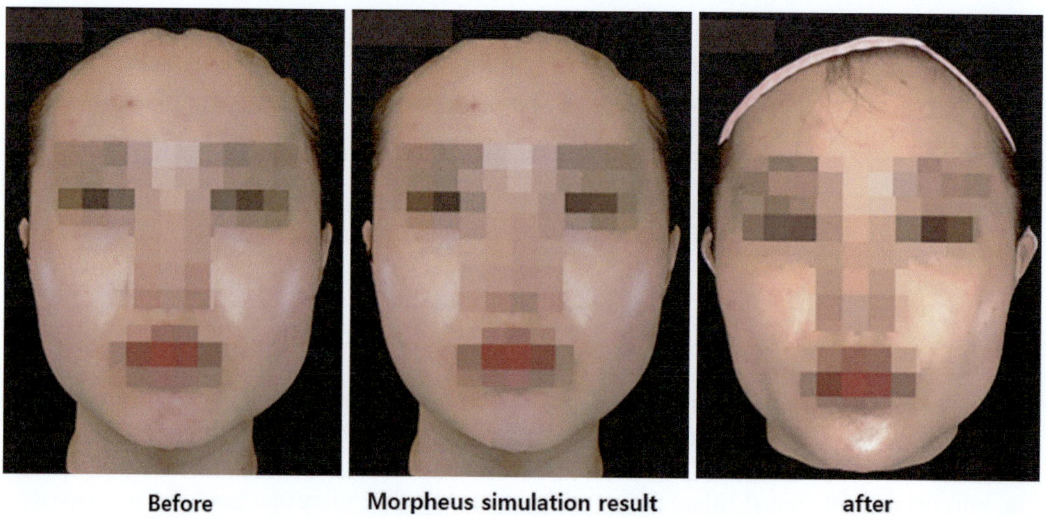

Fig. 12.1 Simulation vs. actual result—frontal view

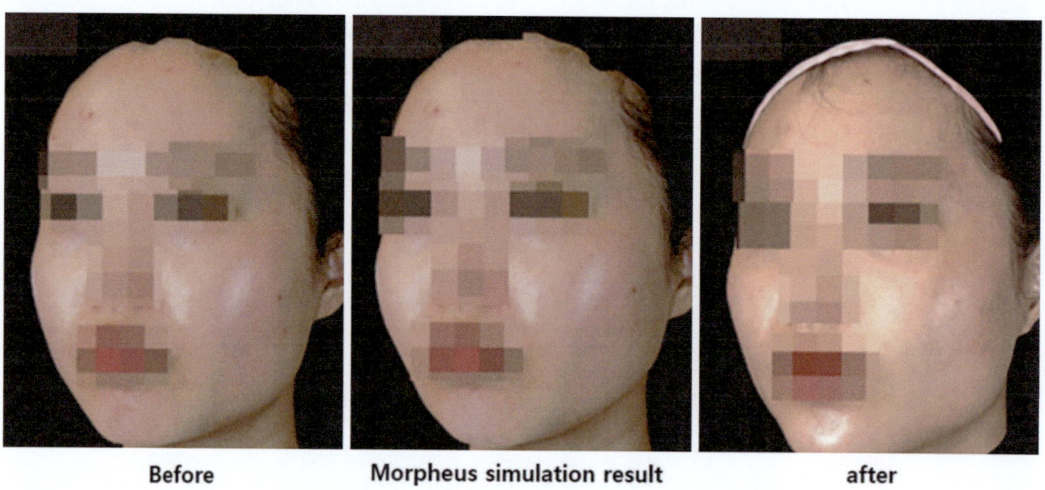

Fig. 12.2 Simulation vs. actual result—oblique view

12.2.1.2 Effectiveness Evaluation

Figure 12.3 shows a simulation of the volume changes after the thread lifting, anterior cheek filler, and chin filler mentioned above, using Morpheus. The image was captured using the Morpheus system, then the desired procedures were simulated, and based on this, a virtual post-treatment photo was created for comparison.

The areas marked in green indicate where volume changes are visible in the before and after photos, meaning that these are the areas where new volume has appeared. Analyzing the image, the volume changes in the anterior cheek and chin areas are the result of filler treatments. However, it is notably observable that there are volume changes in the temple area, which was not simulated to have filler injected. Despite this, an increase in volume is evident. The reason for this and the production process can be understood through a series of photos from Fig. 12.4a–f.

12.2.1.3 Interpretation of Results

It can be seen that thread lifting can be simulated through Morpheus. At the same time, it is also possible to evaluate the effect of thread lifting through the increase in volume in the temple area. Additionally, the Morpheus functionality allows for the quantitative assessment of the increased volume in the green areas. Although not perfect, it can be used to analyze the effects of thread lifting in a different way than the GAIS score.

12.2.2 Evaluation of Actual Pre- and Post-treatment Photos Using the Morpheus

Increased volume (green areas) after the actual treatment. Areas where volume increased after the actual treatment are marked in green. The green areas on the frontal hairline and the left side of the neck appear to be errors (Fig. 12.5).

Looking at the areas of increased volume (green sections) after the actual treatment, it includes the temple area. This is thought to be due to the lifting effect.

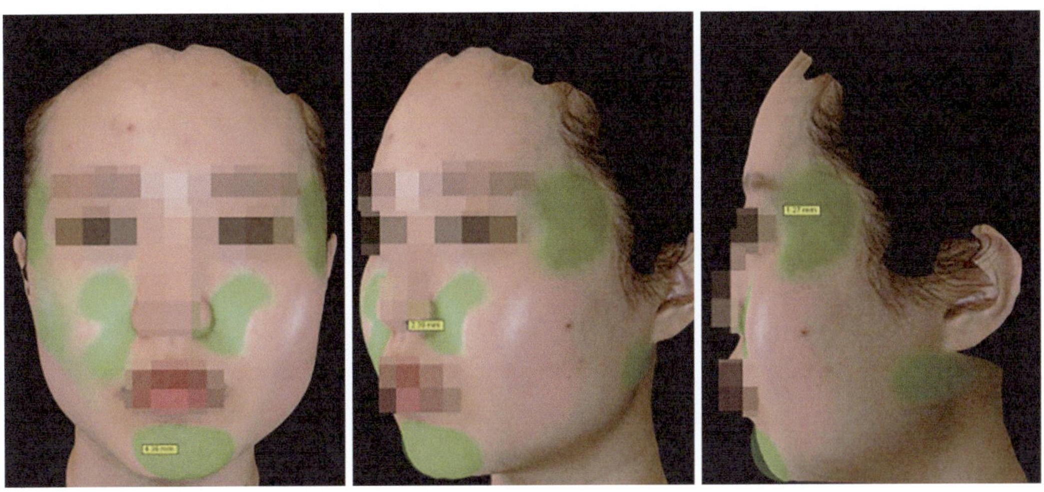

Fig. 12.3 Treatment result simulation using the Morpheus

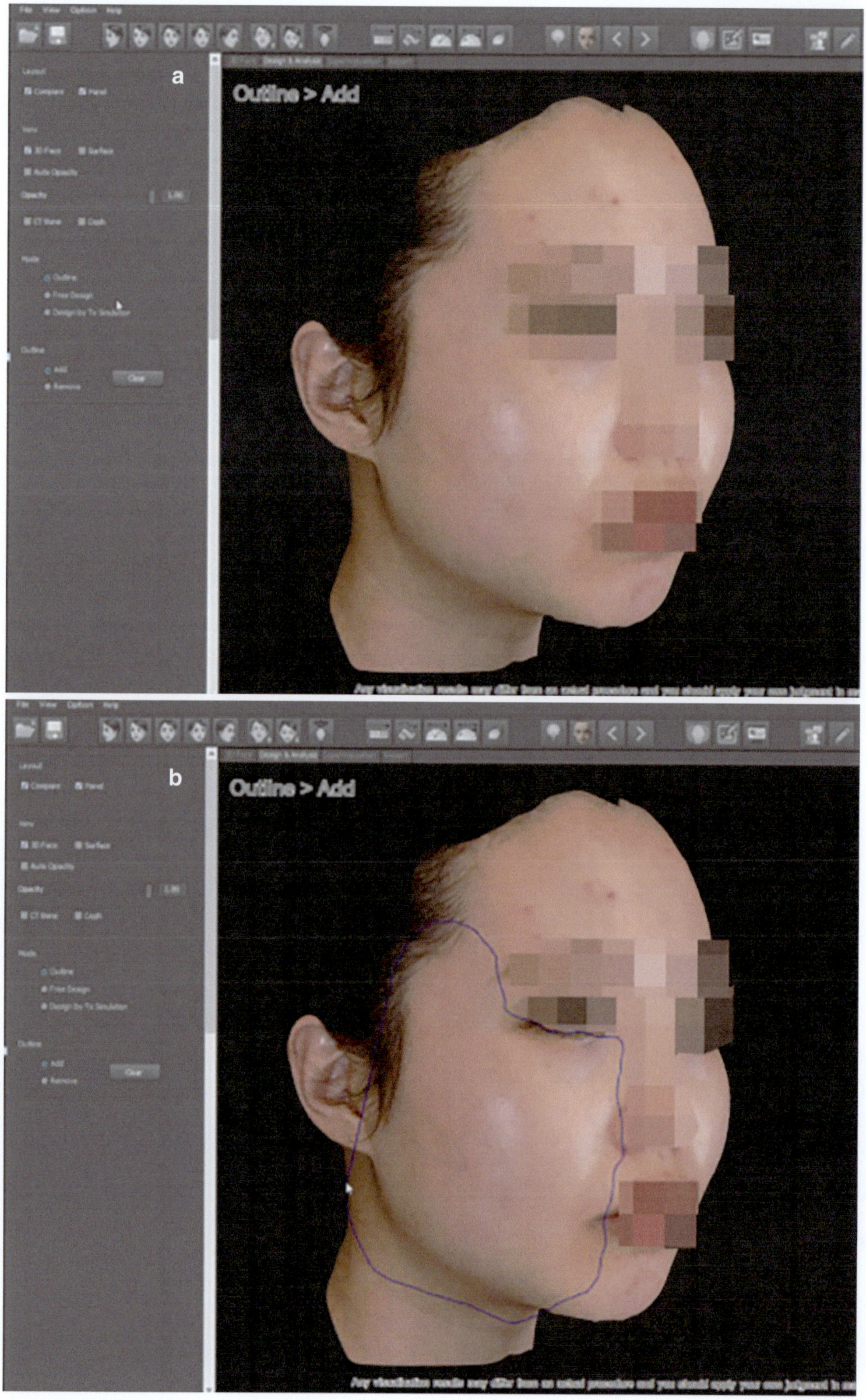

Fig. 12.4 (**a**–**f**) Simulation process using the Morpheus

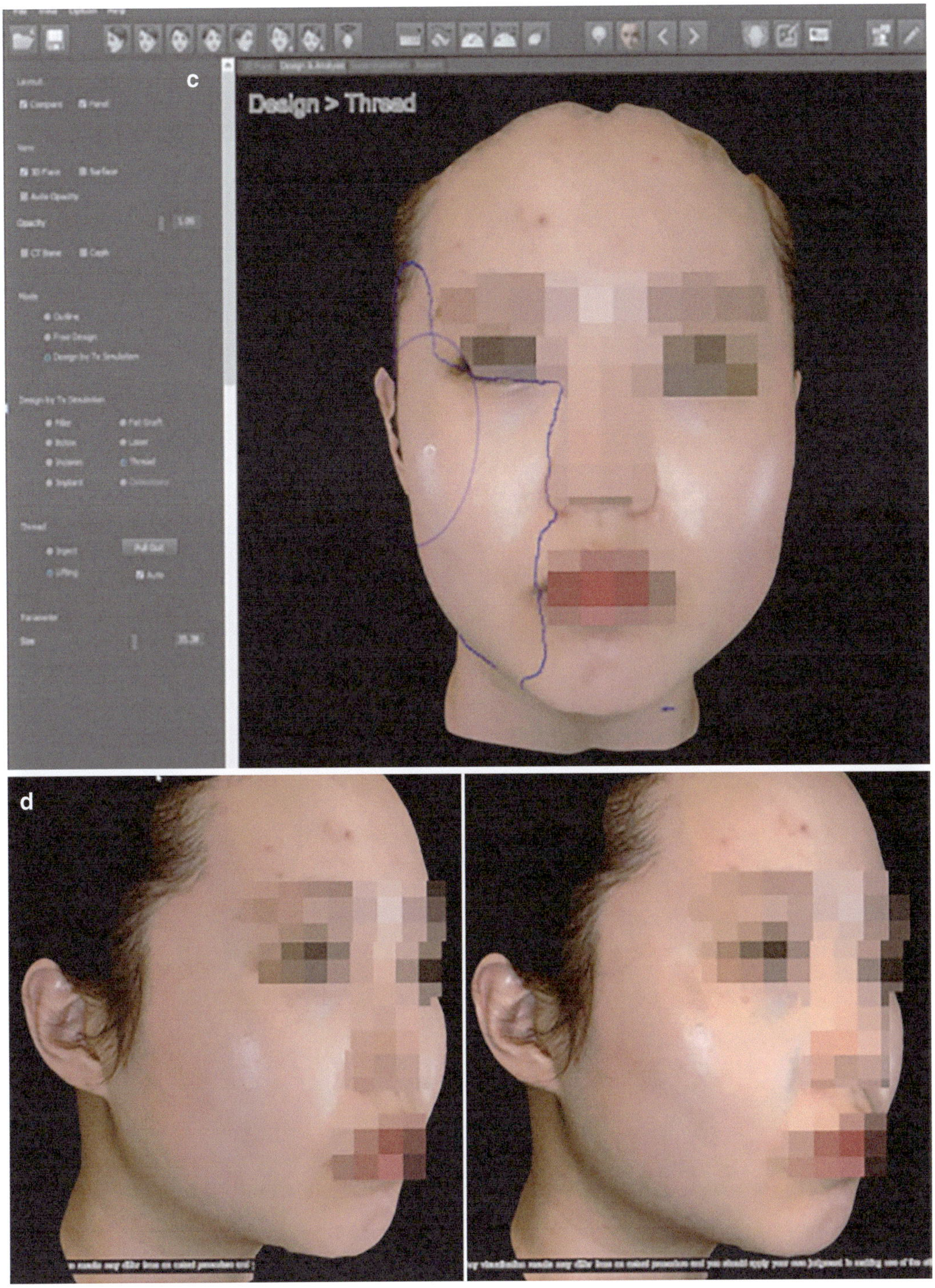

Fig. 12.4 (continued)

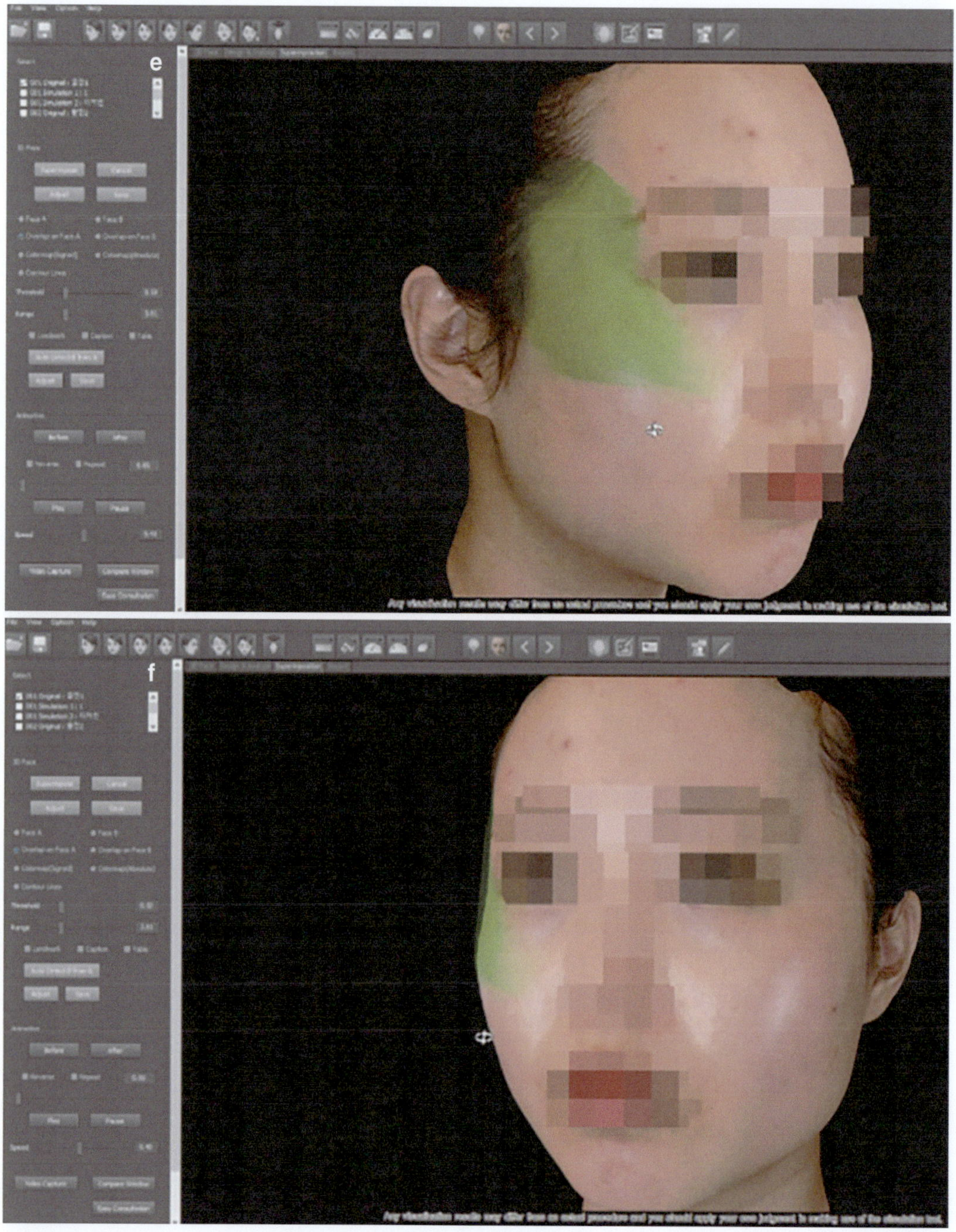

Fig. 12.4 (continued)

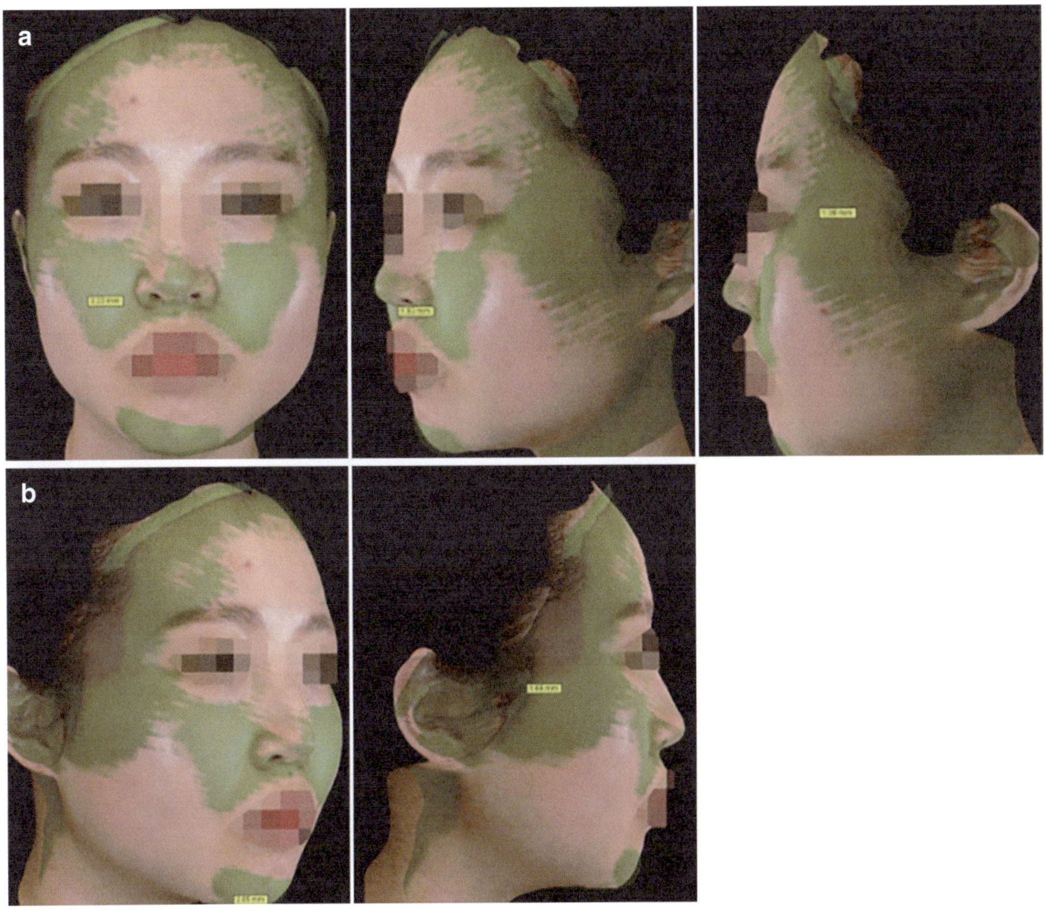

Fig. 12.5 (**a**) Evaluation of actual pre- and post-treatment using the Morpheus. (**b**) Evaluation of actual pre- and post-treatment using the Morpheus

12.3 The Potential and Future of Pre-treatment Prediction or Post-treatment Result Evaluation System

Currently, pre- and post-treatment prediction programs based on artificial intelligence are in use. For example, Crisalix company has developed the FACE App, a 3D virtual cosmetic surgery program dedicated to the face (Fig. 12.6). Currently, the service is provided with a feature that predicts the results before and after filler treatments, and it can generate before and after prediction photos in real time.

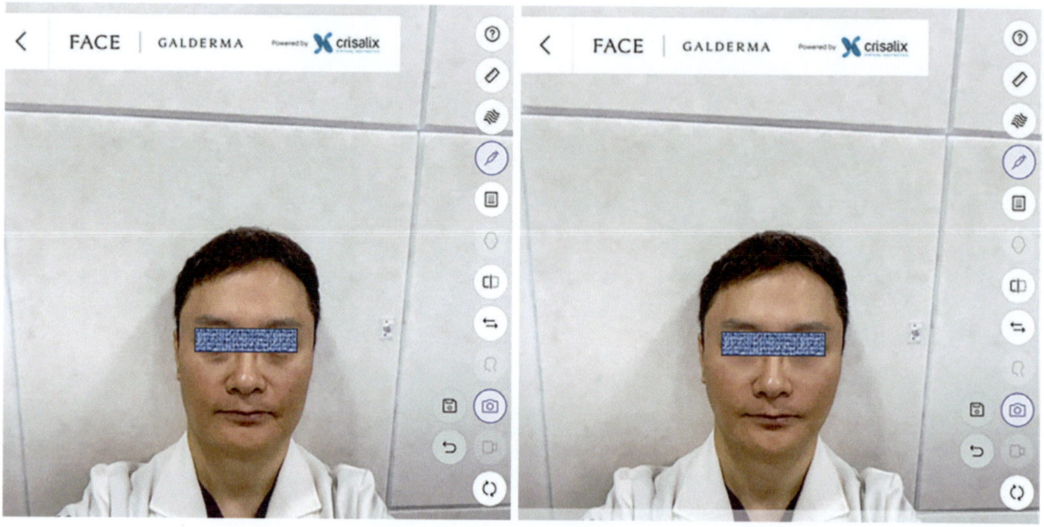

Fig. 12.6 FACE App, an AI-based pre- and post-treatment simulation tool

Overall Adverse Events of Thread Lifting and Its Management

13

Contents

13.1 Common Complications

13.1.1 Dissatisfaction

The most common complaint from patients after thread lifting might be dissatisfaction due to the effects not meeting expectations. This dissatisfaction often occurs, especially when threads without cogs are used, or even with cogs, if shorter threads are utilized for the procedure. However, patient satisfaction has been improving significantly due to the upgraded manufacturing methods of the threads and the advancement of techniques. Properly explaining the expectations based on the type and number of threads and the patient's facial condition can reduce dissatisfaction with the effects after the procedure. Aligning the patient's expectations with the post-treatment results can also increase satisfaction. The overall satisfaction with thread lifting procedures needs to increase for thread lifting to become more popular and evolve. The causes of dissatisfaction after thread lifting can be divided into four main factors. Although this is a subjective classification

S. M. Oh et al., *The Art and Science of Thread Lifting Based on Pinch Anatomy and Moving Plane*,
https://doi.org/10.1007/978-981-97-5516-5_13

by the authors, categorizing and approaching them can help in administering appropriate post-treatment. The causes of post-treatment dissatisfaction are as follows:

13.1.1.1 Excessively High Expectations of the Patient

As with all cosmetic treatments, it is important to be careful when advising treatments to patients with excessively high expectations. When the patient's expectations differ from those of the medical team, thorough discussions are needed to close the gap between them. The treatment should proceed only after this gap has been somewhat reduced.

13.1.1.2 Patients Who Are Difficult to Treat

The results of thread lifting can inevitably vary depending on the degree of facial aging and the characteristics of the face. Unlike surgical treatments, thread lifting does not involve the removal of tissue. Instead, it is a process of repositioning tissues by pulling and gathering them together. If the simulation of this pulling and gathering process does not anticipate good results, the actual treatment outcomes will likely be similar. For such patients, it may be more appropriate to recommend other treatment methods, including surgical options. Forcing a treatment on patients who are unlikely to see good results from the outset can only lead to dissatisfaction.

13.1.1.3 Structural Limitations of Thread Lifting Products

Various thread lifting products exist, each with its own principles. As explained in detail earlier, good results can be achieved by accurately understanding the histological changes induced by the threads inside the tissue, the subsequent changes in the face, and the mechanisms involved, and then performing the procedure. If the practitioner attempts to achieve outcomes that are difficult to expect based on the mechanism of the thread product being used, the desired results can never be achieved. It is crucial to clearly understand the principles of each product, compare the desired level of outcome with what the practitioner aims to achieve, and select the correct product accordingly.

13.1.1.4 Issues with the Practitioner's Technique

Upon clearly understanding the principles of thread lifting, it should be performed with a delicate, patient-customized design. If a uniform technique and design are applied identically to all patients, satisfaction is bound to decrease.

13.1.2 Stiffness and Pain

Pain is inevitable after a thread lifting procedure. At this time, it is important to carefully check the extent of the pain, its association with the treated area, whether there is accompanying heat sensation, whether the pain worsens when making facial expressions, and whether there is accompanying swelling.

13.1.2.1 Pain Due to Infection

Pain primarily occurs at the entry or exit points. Four symptoms—warmth, swelling, redness, and pain—all appear. If the patient's symptoms are related to an infection, it is advisable to start treatment as soon as possible. There can be a special form of infection associated with thread lifting where hair gets embedded at the entry point. If examination reveals hair has entered, it must be removed carefully. Care must be taken to ensure the hair does not break during the removal process. If the hair is completely embedded and not visible, it generally does not cause problems; however, if persistent inflammation occurs, it is essential to check whether the hair at the entry point is causing the inflammation.

In rare cases, there may not be clear signs of infection, but the entry or exit points continue to swell without accompanying warmth or pain, sometimes along with fluctuation symptoms. Even if the presence of an infection is unclear, if there is persistent swelling, it is recommended to attach an 18G needle to a syringe and perform aspiration. In cases where fluid or pus has accumulated, aspiration may be possible. Additional treatment is necessary in such cases.

If an infection is suspected, treatment with antibiotics is necessary. The choice of appropriate antibiotic depends on how much time has passed since the procedure. Especially if an infection is found within the scalp 2–4 weeks after the procedure, it is advisable to suspect a mixed infection and use levofloxacin. Generally, it is more effective than first- and second-generation cephalosporins. It is recommended to continue the medication for at least 3 days after the symptoms have subsided.

13.1.2.2 Pain Caused by Hematoma

If there was significant bleeding during the procedure and it was difficult to stop, a hematoma can develop later on. Upon examination, the swollen area may progressively spread and be accompanied by bruising. Severe swelling can occur, and the patient is likely to experience pain. Active compression should be used to minimize the swelling. Over time, it will naturally subside, so it is important to reassure the patient. This is because if pain caused by a hematoma is suspected, it can be resolved through observation and compression, assuming there is no infection.

13.1.2.3 Pain Caused by a Cog Catching on Skin Tissue

Dimpling can occur if the barbs of the cog engage too strongly in a specific area. This can happen if the procedure is not carried out at a uniform depth or if the cog catches strongly beneath the dermis at the exit point, leading to such symptoms. Pain may also accompany this. Dimpling caused by thread lifting is one of the well-known side effects and causes significant discomfort to the patient, so it is important to resolve it as quickly as possible. If pain is due to a cog catching in a specific area, massage or molding can be used to release the cog if within a few days to a month of the procedure. However, if it is more than a month later, a process to separate the entangled tissue by dissecting the cog from the dermis is necessary.

13.1.2.4 When the End of the Thread Irritates the Skin

If the end of the thread is not smooth and is finished sharply, it can irritate the skin at the end of the thread. In severe cases, it may even puncture the skin. Recently, to make the ends smoother, some threads are designed to bend at 180° at the excess length. This is to prevent the sharp ends of the threads from piercing through the skin. Since the development of this type of thread, the frequency of thread ends irritating the skin has decreased.

If the skin is irritated by the end of the thread, it typically appears as if the end of the thread is pushing through the skin. In such cases, the end of the thread should be removed without delay.

13.1.3 Swelling

Swelling is the most common complaint of patients with thread lifting with bruising. There are many reasons why the face swells after thread lifting may be different. First, the tissue actually swells and the second cause is that the tissue moves to one side. Minimizing local anesthesia before the procedure is also helpful to minimize the cause of swelling of the tissue, and it is important to perform it neatly at once. It is fine enough to do thin monofilament thread procedure with topical ointment anesthesia. But when you put a thick cogged threads, it is difficult to do without local anesthesia at all. Weak sedation can reduce the amount of local anesthesia, thereby reducing the postoperative swelling. Temporary swelling due to such procedure or anesthesia is somewhat reduced by 3–5 days.

The most irrigating type of swelling to the patients is the swelling of the cheek area rather than the entire swelling of face after the procedure. When using cogged threads, the mechanism of lifting the lower tissue upward is used. The movement of tissues is most intense when using the U- or V-shaped long cogged thread at the temporal region or I-shaped bidirectional cogged threads, rather than I-shaped multidirectional cogged threads. Therefore, it is better not to use the U- or V-shaped long cogged threads, even if the patient needs a lot of tissue lifting force. When the cheek shows signs of enlargement, it can last up to 2 weeks to 1 month. In patients who are worried about cheek protrusion even if we use I-shaped short or medium length cogged threads, it is recommended to plan the procedure in a way that fills the area below the zygomatic arch, not the zygomatic area. In addition, it may be better to use I-shaped multidirectional cogged thread that can minimize the cheek protrusion even if the lifting effect is slightly reduced, so it is most important to choose the most suitable thread according to the patient's facial condition and purpose of the procedure.

13.1.4 Bruising and Hematoma

Bruising or hematoma can occur during the procedure, and the causes include damage to the dermal plexus by the thread during needle use, vascular damage around the entry point, and vascular damage along the cannula's path. Additionally, the causes of bleeding vary depending on the type of thread used and the technique applied. It is important to be mindful of the anatomical structure of each area and to take care to prevent bleeding.

13.1.4.1 Damage to the Dermal Plexus Caused by Needle-Based Threads

When using threads with sharp-pointed needles for the procedure, bruising inevitably occurs. This happens due to damage to the dermal plexus, even if there is no major vascular injury (Fig. 13.1).

To prevent this type of bleeding, it is recommended to insert slightly deeper into the subcutaneous layer rather than within or just below the dermis, or to use a blunt-ended cannula.

13.1.4.2 Entry Point Bleeding

This usually occurs when creating an entry point with a needle, especially when designing around the hairline or temple area. It is important to create the entry point in a location where it does not intersect arteries or veins, by feeling for the pulse of the arteries (pulsation) and carefully observing the veins visually (inspection) (Fig. 13.2).

Attention should be paid to the superficial temporal artery and vein (STA, STV), and the sentinel vein (SV).

As a preventive measure, it is beneficial to habitualize precise visual and tactile examination while designing. In the supine position, the sentinel vein is more visible, and the STA is more palpable, so the design should ensure they are avoided (Fig. 13.3).

13.1.4.3 Bleeding Along the Path of the Cannula

Severe bleeding can occur during the insertion of a cannula. In such cases, the bleeding is due to damage not to the dermal plexus but to a major vessel or its branches, and it can lead to hematoma formation. This is especially more likely with sharp-ended cannulas. Even with a blunt-ended cannula, care should be taken as tissue damage and bleeding can occasionally occur in areas where the tissue is dense.

Generally, the tensile strength of vessels is higher compared to that of subcutaneous fat. Although not specifically using facial vessels and

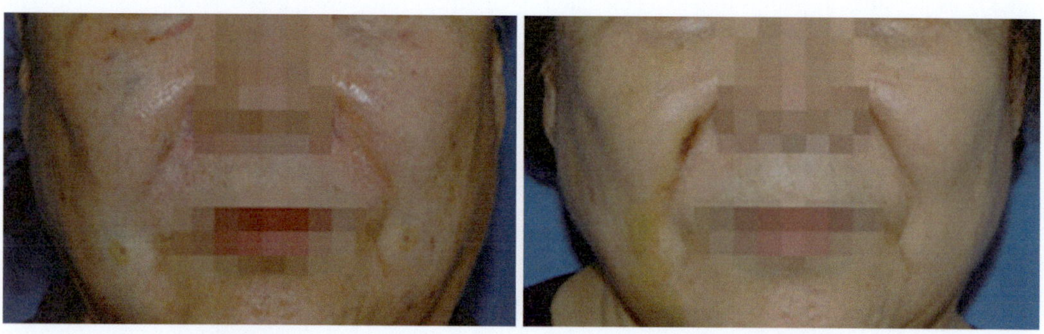

Fig. 13.1 Bruising due to bleeding after thread lifting—in cases where mono-PDO needle-based threads were inserted

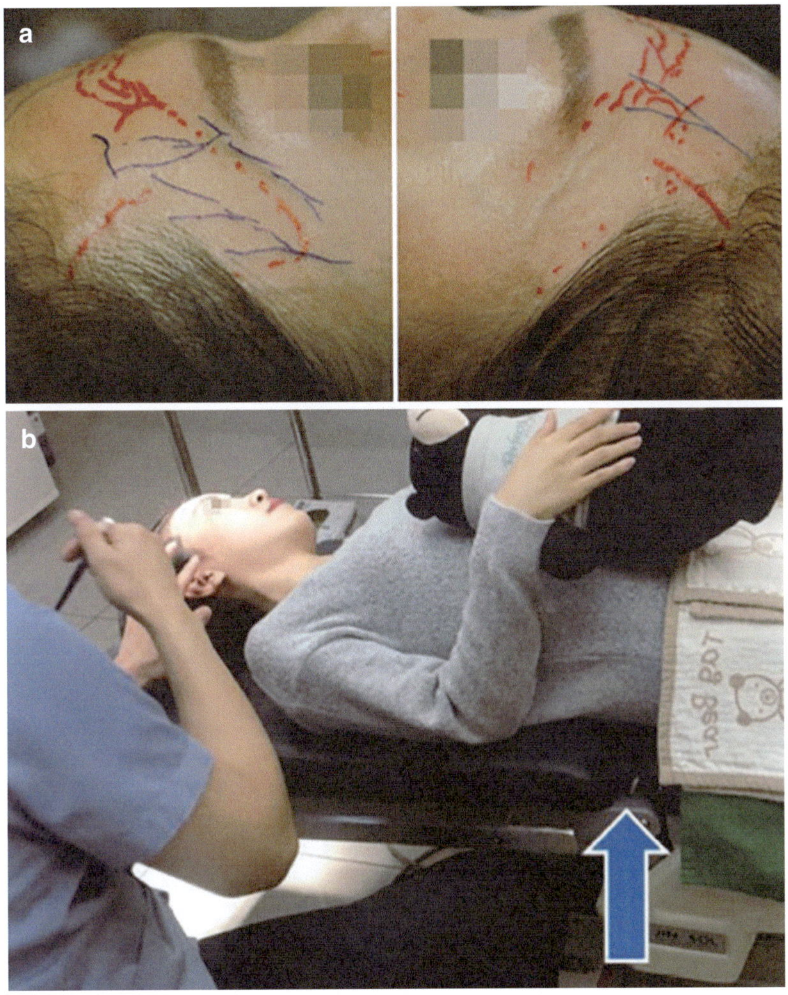

Fig. 13.2 Design for preventing bleeding at the entry point. (**a**) The left image is of the right side of the face, with the sentinel vein marked in blue. The right image is of the left side of the face, before marking the sentinel vein (visible to the naked eye). (**b**) If visual inspection and palpation of the vessel are difficult, placing the patient in a supine position or tilting the waist further down can make the vessels easier to observe and facilitate the design

fat in their research, there are studies from which we can infer. Tibor Balazs et al. collected tissue from the coronary vein of pigs to measure its tensile strength. Denise et al. collected human subcutaneous fat tissue to measure its tensile strength. Although the objectives of the studies were different, both measured the tensile strength of specific tissues. Combining the independent results of each study shows that the tensile strength of pig coronary veins is 990–2550 mN/mm^2, whereas that of human fat is 10.4–13.7 mN/mm^2, indicating a significant difference in magnitude.

This suggests that when using a blunt cannula to gently advance through the fat layer, there is a higher likelihood of smoothly passing through the fat layer around the vessels, even when encountering them. Therefore, by identifying the path of major vessels and carefully advancing the cannula, especially feeling for resistance at points where it meets major vessels, vascular damage can be minimized. Especially when vessels are stimulated, patients tend to report sharp pain. Therefore, by delicately monitoring the patient's pain and proceeding with caution, it is possible to minimize bleeding.

Occasionally, bruising accompanied by swelling can occur a few days after the procedure (Fig. 13.4). This is rare after treatments with cogged threads. Even if there was no bleeding at the time of the procedure, it is thought that the repeated irritation from the cogs can damage the vessels. Slight bruising with some swelling can appear around the eyes or temples without severe

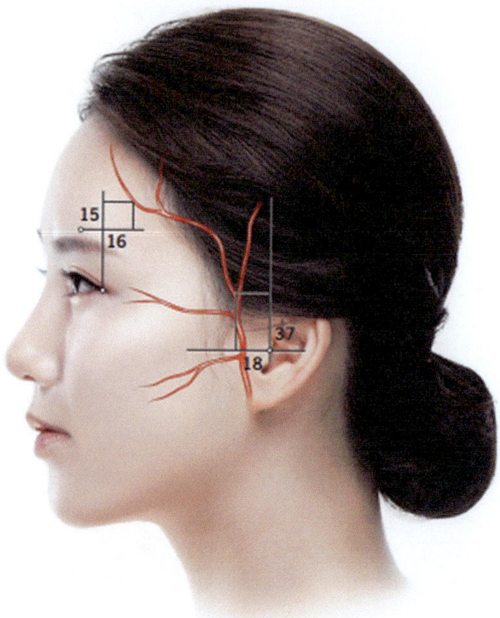

Fig. 13.3 Vessel associated with bleeding at the entry point—superficial temporal artery

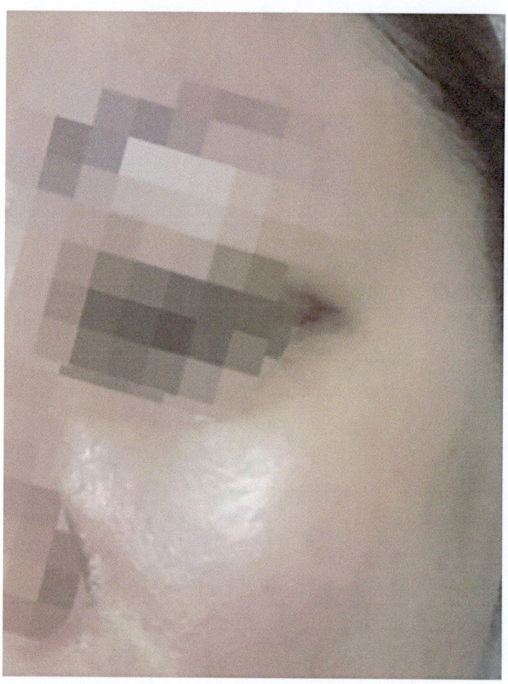

Fig. 13.4 Bruising and swelling that occur several days after the procedure

hematoma. No special treatment is needed, and improvement can be achieved with compression alone.

13.1.5 Dimpling

Dimpling is often mentioned as a side effect of thread lifting. It can occur immediately after the procedure or several days to weeks later, but it is rare for it to occur after a month. The dimpling may appear suddenly and disappear on its own, but patients may visit the clinic complaining of the cosmetic inconvenience. While it can be unsettling not knowing how to handle it the first time it occurs after thread lifting, molding with the fingers can easily improve the condition. Since the likelihood of occurrence varies depending on the type of thread used and where it is inserted, explaining the possibility of dimpling and how to manage it to patients in advance can also help in building rapport with clients.

13.1.5.1 The Principle Behind the Formation of Dimples

To understand the principle behind the formation of dimples after thread lifting, it is essential to first know the difference in the density of fibrous tissue within the fat tissue according to different facial areas (Fig. 13.5). The parts where the thread is inserted and the cogs catch well are areas where a certain amount of fibrous tissue is distributed within the fat tissue. This is necessary for the cogs to maintain their position without slipping after lifting, ensuring good effectiveness. However, if the fibrous tissue within the fat tissue is too abundant and dense, it can be difficult for the cannula or needle to pass through. Additionally, the cogs may become firmly anchored in positions other than their intended locations, making dimple formation more likely.

Facial fat tissue is divided into superficial and deep fat in some areas, while in others, it exists as a single layer of fat. The critical factor is the density of the fat tissue. Fat tissue that is soft like

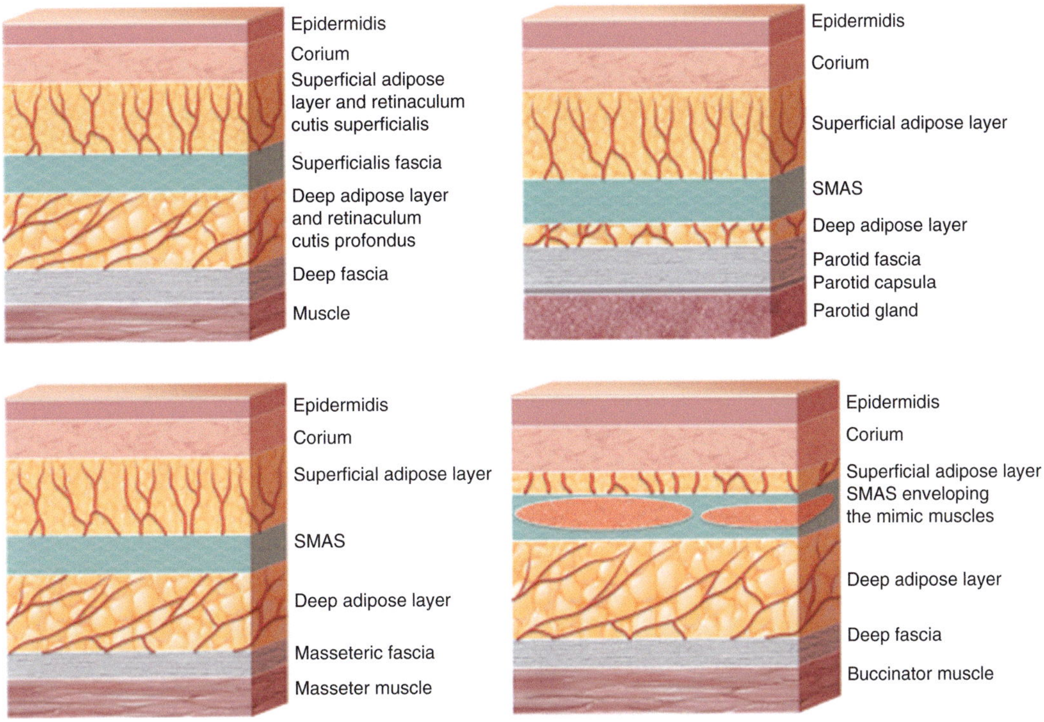

Fig. 13.5 Differences in the distribution of subcutaneous connective tissue by facial area

cheese allows the cannula/needle to pass through easily, but fat tissue that is dense with a lot of fibrous tissue is difficult to penetrate. Understanding which parts of the face have soft or dense fat tissue makes the procedure easier.

When the Insertion Depth of the Cog Is Not Uniform

If the insertion depth of the thread is not uniform, dimples can occur when some cogs catch on the firm subdermal layer, while others catch in the looser subcutaneous fat layer (Fig. 13.6a, b).

To avoid vascular damage and ensure uniform depth of thread insertion, various pinch techniques are used. However, if the force used to pinch is not properly regulated, it can instead induce skin dimpling. Even when the subcutaneous fat layer is lifted uniformly with a pinch and insertion seems even, dimples can unexpectedly form. Clinicians with experience in liposuction may have encountered similar issues with fat indentation due to the same principle. As shown in Fig. 13.6b, if the thread or needle is not inserted at the correct mid-level depth but is skewed to the side, rather than the middle of the pinch, dimpling can occur.

Indentation at the Cutting Site

When performing lifting by pulling the thread out through the opposite side (exit point) using a cannula, pinpoint indentations can occur at the exit point area. This happens when the cogs of the thread buried around the cutting site catch on the fibrous tissue of the firm dermal layer and subcutaneous fat layer (Fig. 13.7).

When Some Cogs Catch Unevenly in the Dermal Layer

In Fig. 13.8, the dotted red circle indicates the area where the cog catches on the dermal layer of the skin. When a thread with strong cogs unevenly catches on parts of the subdermal layer, the skin area where the cogs strongly catch can become indented.

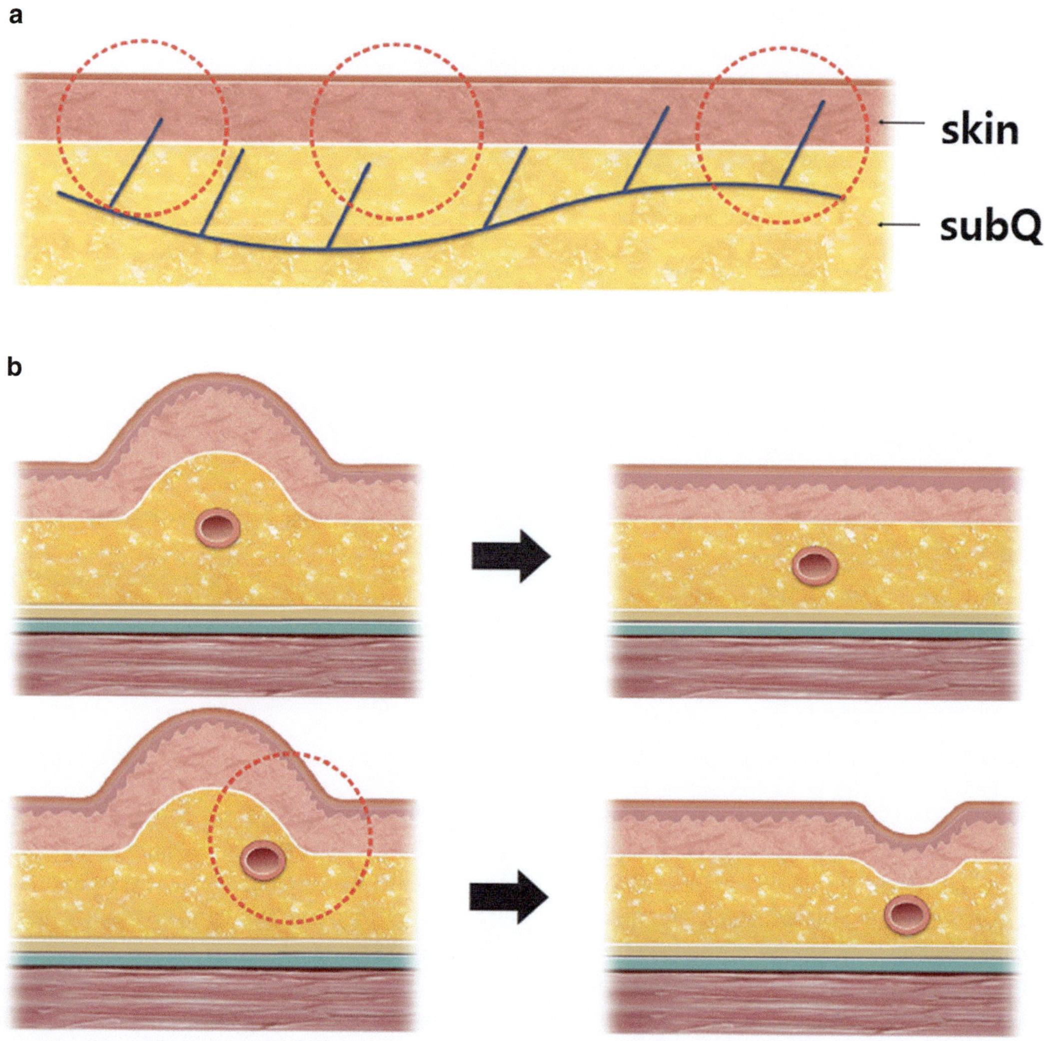

Fig. 13.6 Principle behind the formation of dimples—when the insertion depth is not uniform

13.1.5.2 Types of Dimples by Facial Area

Dimples Along the Thread Path

Dimples along the insertion path can be resolved as follows: Wear a glove on the left hand and place the index finger on the inside of the mouth at the dimple location, then snap the right hand's index finger below the dimple and pull in the direction of the thread's extension. At this moment, the dimple should release with a snapping feeling, and the cog will fix in its original position (Fig. 13.9).

Sometimes, a dimple does not appear immediately after the procedure but manifests suddenly after laughing heartily or eating with the mouth wide open. Such dimples are caused by facial expression changes (contraction of the zygomaticus muscle) during which the tissue where the thread is inserted moves along with the muscle, and suddenly, a dimple forms when the cog fixes in a different location (about 2–4 mm upper lateral) from its original position. Dimples caused by facial expression changes are likely to occur in areas within about 2FB distance from the corner of the mouth, where the subcutaneous tis-

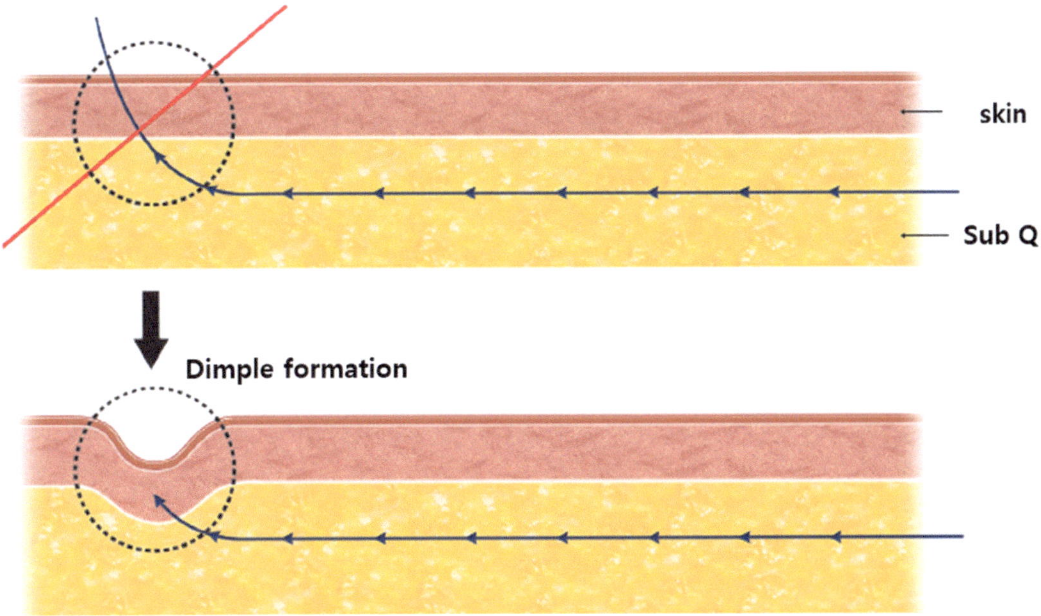

Fig. 13.7 Principle behind the formation of dimples—indentation at the cutting site. The end part of the thread must be sufficiently buried into the subcutaneous layer. If it catches in the subdermal layer, indentation occurs

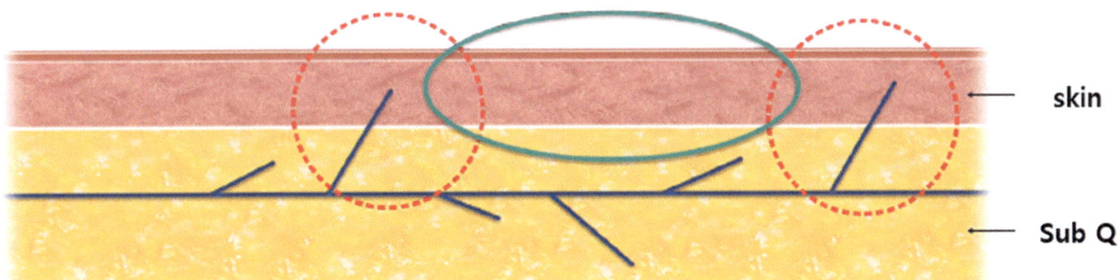

Fig. 13.8 Principle behind the formation of dimples

sue is very dense. In this case, wear a glove on the left hand, place the index finger inside the mouth at the dimple location, and with the right hand's index finger, snap below the dimple and pull in the lower medial direction. The dimple should release with a snapping feeling, and the cog will fix in its original position (Fig. 13.10).

Dimples most commonly occur between 1 and 2 weeks after the procedure rather than immediately post-treatment, and they rarely form after a month. Even after resolving with massage, there can be cases of recurrence. Therefore, it is beneficial to demonstrate how to resolve it using two fingers while showing the patient in the mirror, so they can self-manage if it recurs at home.

When inserting the thread into the inside of the face, the possibility of dimple increases if the thread is inserted close to the mouth corner. In Fig. 13.11, dimple by facial expression can be prevented by inserting only the blue line without thread (3) and (4) going to the orange oval area.

Exit Point Dimple: Temporal Tagging Method

This is the case that occurs immediately after cutting the thread of the exit point, which is the last step of the procedure (Fig. 13.12). However, if you push while giving a snap with your hand, it will be simply unfolded. Sometimes, dimples may occur around the exit point as shown in

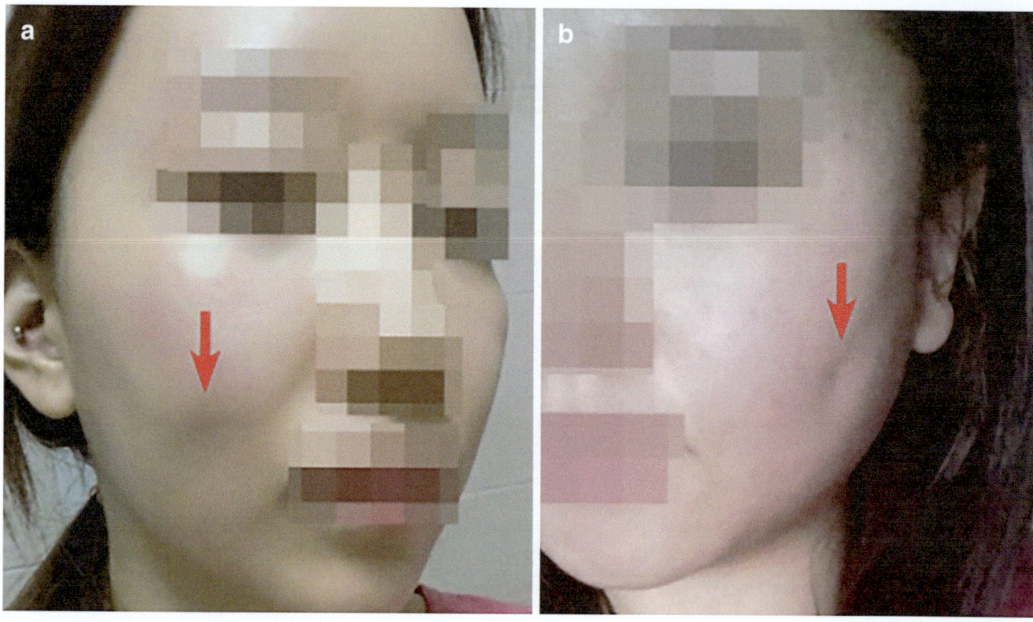

Fig. 13.9 Causes of dimples—dimples along the insertion path. (**a**) Insertion method without a separate exit point. (**b**) Exit point of temporal tagging method

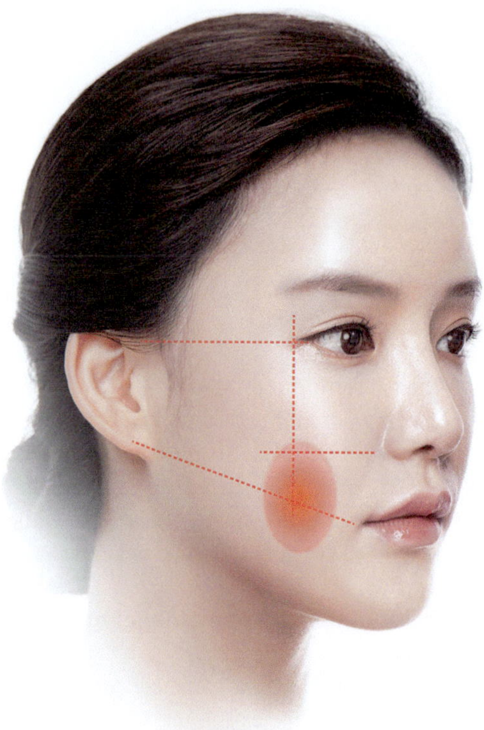

Fig. 13.10 Common sites for dimple occurrence—dimples tend to form in areas where the subcutaneous fat tissue is fibrous or there is significant movement due to facial expressions

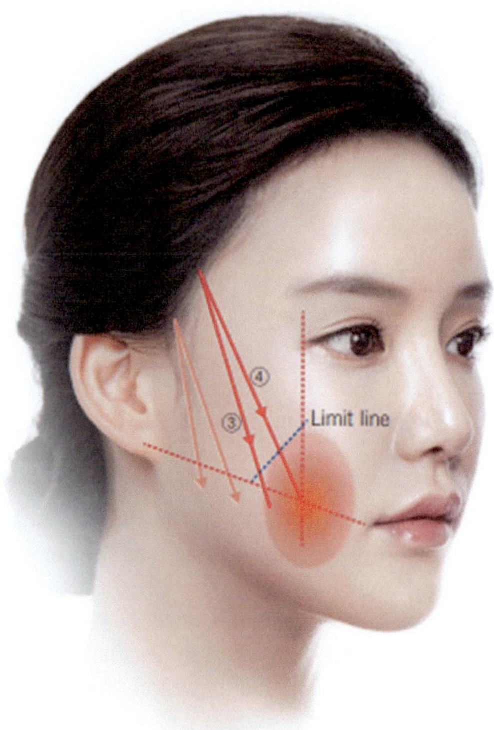

Fig. 13.11 Dimple prevention

Fig. 13.9 after several days after the procedure. In this case, it can be solved in the same way as the treatment of dimples along the insertion path.

13.1.5.3 Entry Point Dimple: Temporal Tagging Method

Principle of Entry Point Dimple

Since thread lifting essentially involves pulling sagging skin, some may think that proper lifting requires certain areas to be slightly folded or wrinkled. As the pulled skin does not disappear, if the lower part is pulled, the upper part may fold or wrinkle.

So, a dimple can form at the entry point. When a fixation point is formed inside the hairline, even if some skin is pulled, the dimple may not be easily visible because it is located inside the hair. However, it is recommended to avoid creating dimples in areas that are not easily visible whenever possible.

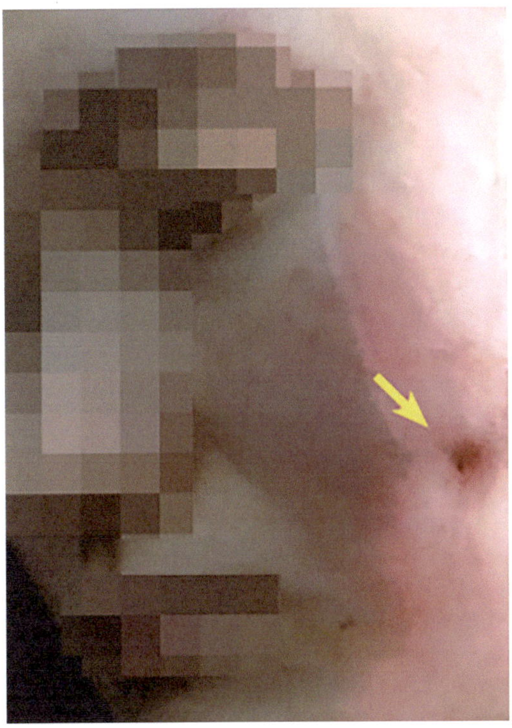

Fig. 13.12 Exit point dimple

Prevention of Entry Point Dimple

To prevent entry point dimpling, it is important to create adequately sized holes when making the entry point. Additionally, ensure that the passage for the thread, which passes through in a U-shape, is well established to facilitate easy passage. It is especially crucial to prevent the thread from catching on the dermal sublayer at the two points where the needle enters (Fig. 13.13).

Solutions

Using scissors, dissect the dermal tissue, separating the dermal tissue caught on the thread.

13.1.6 Skin Fold

Within about 3–4 days after a thread lifting procedure, some patients may visit the hospital complaining that "the threads are sticking out." In reality, the threads are not actually protruding, but the skin may appear swollen along the path where the threads have passed, resembling furrows or ridges in a field.

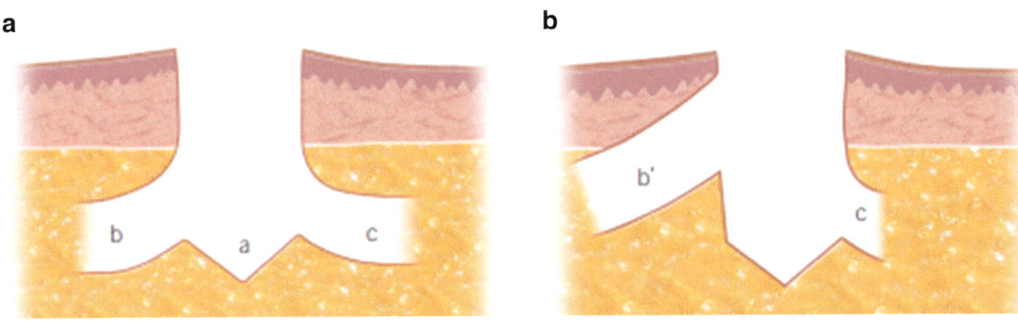

Fig. 13.13 Cause of entry point dimple and prevention. (**a**) good entry point (**b**) A wrong entry point

13.1.6.1 Check Point

Check whether the folds are visible even when at rest, or if they only appear when making facial expressions. Also, assess whether the skin feels uniformly smooth to the touch or if there is a sensation of threads being caught.

13.1.6.2 Causes and Solutions

If excessive forward and backward movements with a cannula or needle are performed for the insertion of a single thread, relatively large tissue damage occurs, and swelling develops along the path of the thread. In such cases, during examination, the thread may not be palpable, and spontaneous recovery occurs.

In cases where multiple threads are inserted, but only one is excessively pulled, skin fold symptoms can still occur. This can be treated by increasing the number of threads and evenly distributing the tension on the skin.

Skin fold symptoms can also occur when the depth of the thread insertion is shallow. In such cases, instead of immediately removing the cannula, retrying with a slightly deeper insertion of the thread into the subcutaneous tissue layer resolves the issue.

Additionally, skin fold symptoms can occur when the number of threads is insufficient compared to the amount of lax tissue that needs to be pulled. In this situation, increasing the number of threads can resolve the issue. This can be achieved by supplementing short threads in the middle portion of the existing threads.

13.1.7 Bulging of Entry Points

When inserting too many threads through a single entry point, it is easy for the ends of multiple threads to gather and protrude toward the entry point. During the final stages of the procedure when cutting the threads, it is important to sufficiently remove the ends of the threads to bury them completely within the skin. However, even with this precaution, threads may still protrude when making facial expressions, especially around the eyes or temples. If the path of the threads intersects with facial expression muscles, it is crucial to ensure that the ends of the threads are buried deep enough at the entry point. This is because if the threads move along with the facial muscles' movements, they may protrude back toward the entry point.

13.1.7.1 Frequent Area

When creating an entry point at the junction of the horizontal line of the lateral canthus and the hairline, there is a higher probability of dimpling in individuals with significant movement of the zygomaticus major muscle. The likelihood increases if the cutting is not done sufficiently during the procedure. Additionally, there is a higher probability of dimpling when inserting multiple thick threads into one hole (especially when inserting 3–4 or more threads of 2-0 thickness into one hole).

When inserting threads from the zygoma beneath the lateral canthus toward the temple to pull, it is important to ensure that the threads are sufficiently buried within the connective tissue (Fig. 13.14). If the ends of the threads are too close to the entry point, they may protrude back toward it due to smiling movements.

13.1.7.2 Solutions

In general, in areas near the hairline, dimpling usually disappears spontaneously and leaves no trace. However, if dimpling occurs in the zygomatic area and worsens due to facial expressions, it may not naturally disappear. To prevent this, some portion of the ends of the threads should be removed to increase the distance from the entry point. Due to the elasticity of the threads, it is advisable to avoid creating entry points on the curved areas of the face. Whenever threading, it is crucial to keep the path of the threads as straight as possible, and if it is unavoidable to traverse a curve, ensure that the threads travel sufficiently straight after passing the curve to minimize such side.

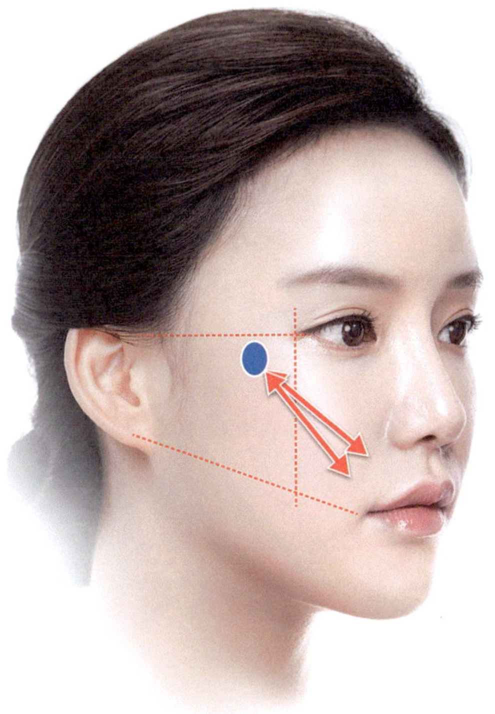

Fig. 13.14 Entry point area where bulging is prone to occur

13.1.7.3 Preventions

When designing the entry point, observe the movement of the skin according to the movement of the frontalis muscle. Proper cutting is essential, and the most important aspect is ensuring that the threads are buried deep inside the skin so that the ends of the threads are sufficiently distant from the entry point. Placing the entry point at eyebrow height or higher results in less visibility (Fig. 13.15).

13.1.8 Protrusion of Threads

After the procedure, patients may visit the hospital complaining of "protrusion of threads" several days or weeks later. Thread protrusion can be broadly categorized as follows: firstly, protrusion outside the skin (Figs. 13.16 and 13.17), intraoral protrusion (Fig. 13.18), and imminent protrusion.

13.1.8.1 Protrusion Outside the Skin

13.1.8.2 Protrusion in the Oral Cavity

13.1.8.3 Thread Near Protrusion (Fig. 13.19)

13.1.9 Migration of Threads

Thread migration typically occurs several weeks after the procedure, with the causes being as follows:

Threads without cogs move easily. When using unidirectional cogged threads, if a secure anchoring point is not created, the thread can easily migrate. Incorrect cutting of bidirectional cogged threads can also lead to migration (Figs. 13.20 and 13.21), as can poor storage conditions that weaken the thread, making migration more likely.

13.1.9.1 Thread Without Cogs

After the insertion of a thread without cogs, it may migrate and become visible just beneath the skin or appear in a state just before protrusion. This is particularly observed when inserted in areas with frequent facial expressions, such as just below the lips, and may become visible beneath the thin skin along the jawline.

13.1.9.2 Incorrect Cutting of Bidirectional Cogged Threads

13.1.9.3 Damage to the Thread Due to Prolonged Storage

PDO, the primary material used in thread lifting, becomes brittle and loses its strength when exposed to moisture in the air. Among cogged threads, bidirectional cogged threads are prevented from migrating due to the cogs facing opposite directions. However, even these can easily break and migrate after insertion if not stored properly.

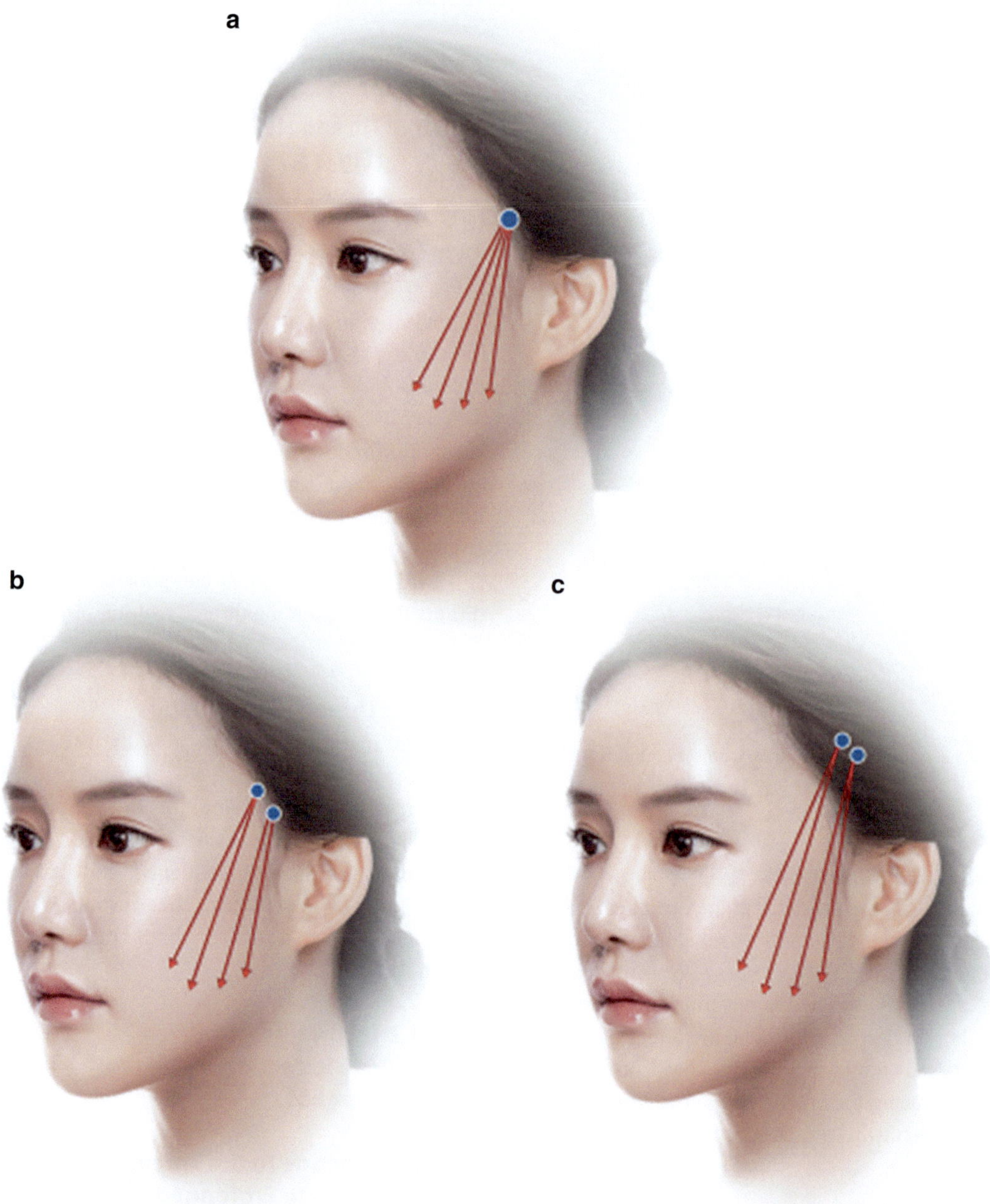

Fig. 13.15 Occurrence of bulging depending on entry point location and number of threads. (**a**) If there is one entry point and four threads are inserted, there is a high probability that entry point bulging will occur. (**b**) By setting two entry points and inserting two threads at each, entry point bulging can be prevented. (**c**) It is a good preventive measure to place the entry point higher than the hairline so that it is not exposed

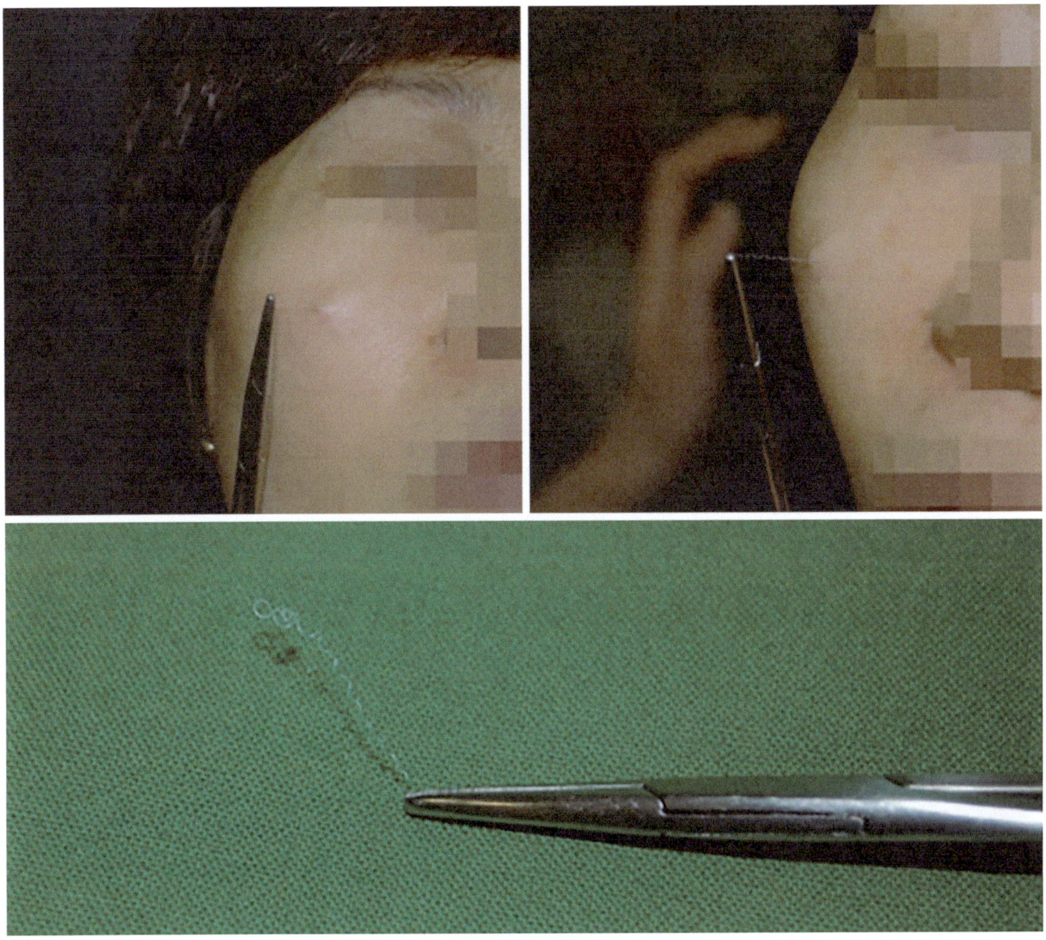

Fig. 13.16 Thread protrusion and removed thread—this patient visited the hospital with thread protrusion a few days after surgery with a twist-type PDO thread inserted into the lateral cheek. Pull the end of the protruding thread with the needle holder and remove it

13.1.10 Relapse

The major disadvantage of thread lifting is its insignificant effect, or the tissues may get drooped too soon. Thread lifting is often described to be effective for 1–2 year. However, even with a thread that lasts for 2 years, it is difficult for the effect to last for 2 years. The effect of cogged threads is most significant in the first 6 months with cogs firmly holding the tissues. However, as the cogs get absorbed and have decreased lifting effect, it is natural that the tissues return to its original position. Therefore, before cogged thread lifting procedure, the limitations of product should be recognized and inform the patient that the effect is not permanent. As with tightening procedures using lasers, such as Ulthera or Shrink, the thread lifting procedure should also be performed periodically.

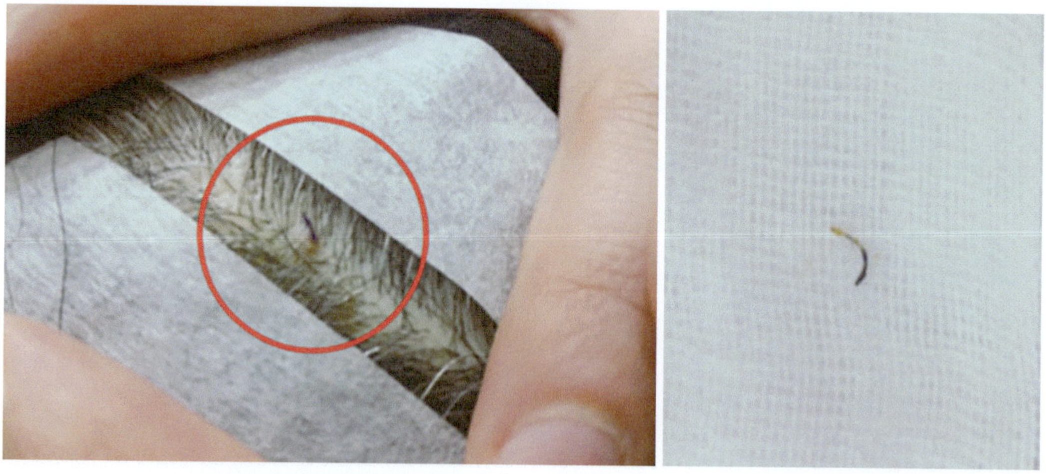

Protruded thread **Removed thread**

Fig. 13.17 Thread protrusion and thread removal—bidirectional cog type PDO thread inserted into the temporal region. A few days after the procedure, the patient visited the hospital due to thread protrusion at the entry point. The end of the protruding thread was pulled and removed using the needle holder

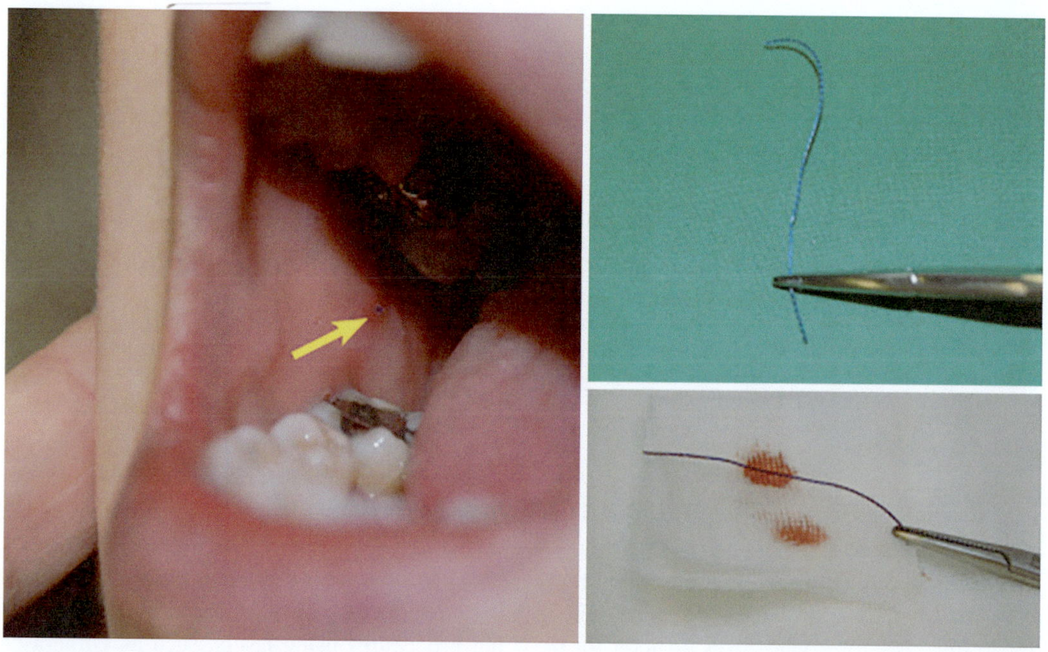

Fig. 13.18 Thread protrusion and removal—a bidirectional cogged PDO thread inserted into the cheek. The patient came in several days after the procedure due to pain and the thread protruding into the mouth (the patient felt the thread "snap" while laughing loudly during a meal with friends). The protruding end of the thread was grasped with a needle holder and removed

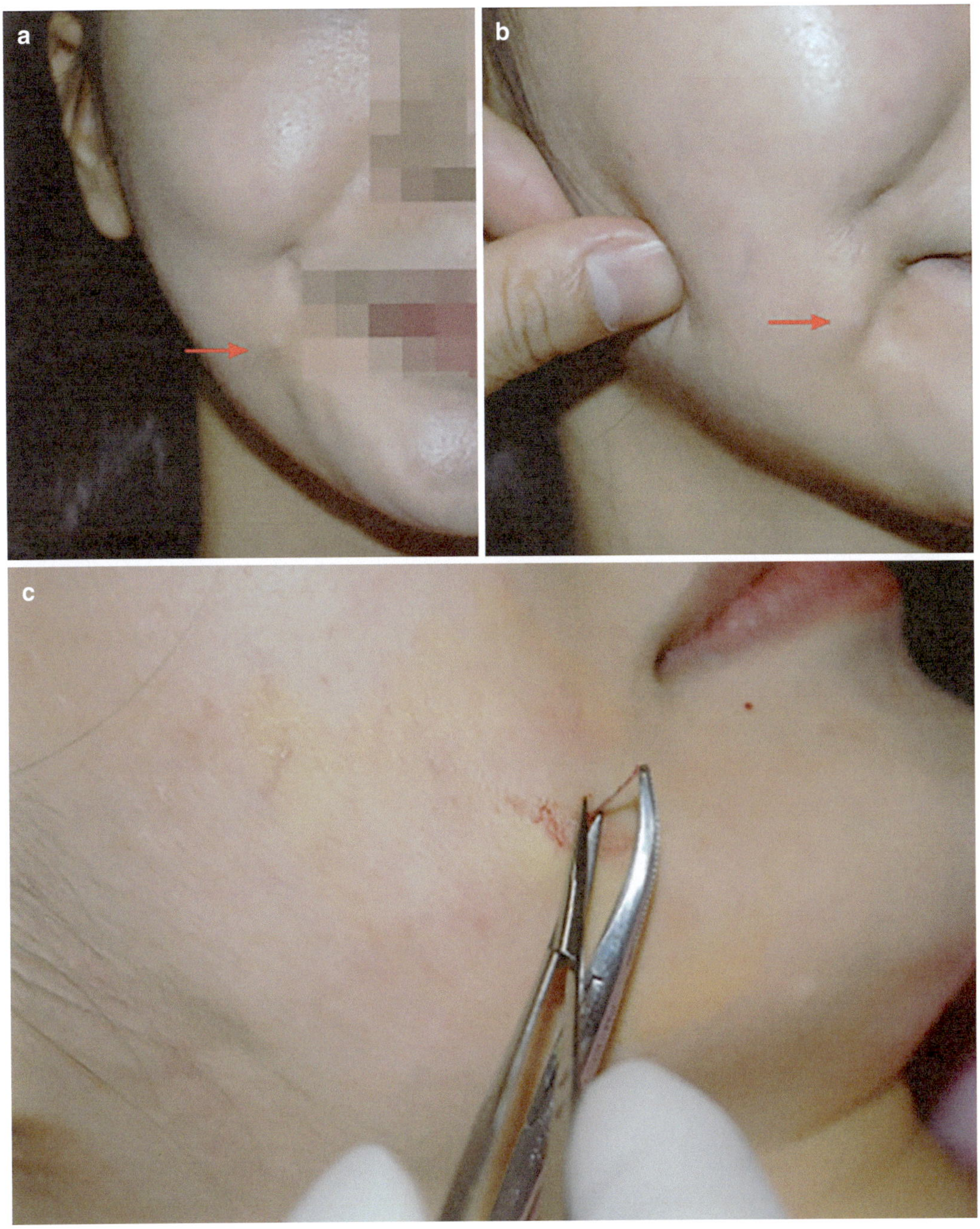

Fig. 13.19 Thread protrusion and removal. (**a**) More visible when making facial expressions. (**b**) Push with the opposite hand before making an incision to make it more visible. (**c**) Grasp with mosquito forceps and cut a portion with scissors

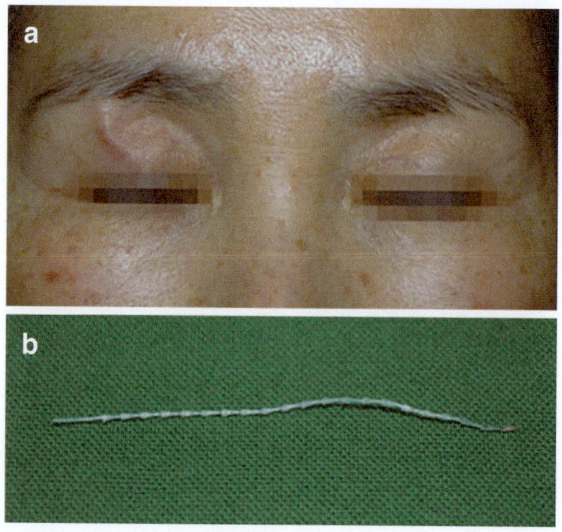

Fig. 13.20 Thread migration (after eyebrow lifting) and removed thread. (**a**) A bidirectional cogged PDO thread was inserted for eyebrow lifting (forehead lifting), and the patient came in 8 weeks post-treatment feeling "like the thread was coming out through the eyelid." After a stab incision, the entire thread was removed. For eyebrow to hairline lifting, cogs need to be inserted sufficiently in both directions, but in this case, they were not fully inserted, and the middle part of the bidirectional cogs was cut. Consequently, only the cogs in one direction remained, and the thread slowly migrated downward, appearing as shown in the figure (refer to Fig. 13.21). (**b**) A closer look at the removed thread, 8 weeks post-treatment, shows that while the characteristic blue color of PDO has disappeared, the shape of the cogs is still maintained, which is noteworthy

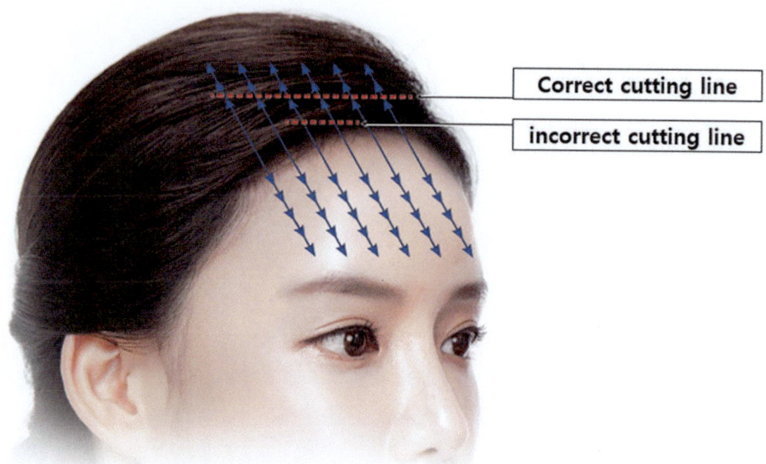

Fig. 13.21 Cause of migration in bidirectional cogged threads—incorrect cutting. Since the reverse-direction cogs serve to create anchoring points, if all reverse-direction cogs are removed then the thread is likely to migrate in the direction of the cogs. It is essential to leave some reverse-direction cogs intact

13.2 Unusual Complications

13.2.1 Temporary Paralysis of Facial Nerve

After thread lifting, there are instances where facial expressions become asymmetrical, surprising both the patient and the practitioner. This is particularly noticeable when patients try to open their eyes wide and look in the mirror but find that their eyebrows do not lift properly, or when they speak and discover asymmetry in their facial expressions. This can occur unilaterally or bilaterally.

13.2.1.1 Etiology

When local anesthesia is used for pain control, it can anesthetize not only the sensory nerves but also the motor nerves. During a thread lifting procedure using a cannula, the likelihood of completely severing an entire branch of the facial nerve with the cannula is very low. Therefore, in most cases, the effect is due to the anesthesia of the motor nerves caused by the spread of lidocaine.

13.2.1.2 Clinical Presentation

Difficulty closing the eyes occurs when the orbicularis oculi muscle is paralyzed, which can happen when excessive anesthesia is applied to the zygomatic area, leading to paralysis of the facial nerve's zygomatic branch. Difficulty opening the eyes occurs when excessive anesthesia in the temple area paralyzes the facial nerve's temporal branch. Asymmetry of the mouth occurs when the zygomaticus major/minor and risorius muscles are paralyzed, typically due to excessive anesthesia of the lateral cheek causing paralysis of the facial nerve's buccal branch.

This can be noticed immediately after the procedure while looking in the mirror, but sometimes, patients may only contact the clinic after returning home (about 3 h post-procedure). In these cases, the issue was not evident immediately after the treatment but became apparent once the patient was at home.

13.2.1.3 Solution

Typically, natural recovery occurs within a few hours or a day.

13.2.2 Permanent Facial Nerve Injury

Facial nerves are generally firmer than the surrounding fat or fibrous tissues, so the likelihood of damage is low when the procedure is performed carefully or when using a cannula.

Although very rare, if the facial nerve's temporal branch near the zygomatic arch is damaged, a side effect can occur where one eyebrow drops due to paralysis of the frontalis muscle.

At this time, the facial nerve's temporal branch near the zygomatic arch runs deeper than the superficial temporal fascia. Therefore, when crossing over the zygomatic arch, lifting the SubQ layer through PINCH manipulation and inserting the cannula through the loosened SubQ layer can reduce the possibility of nerve damage (Fig. 13.22).

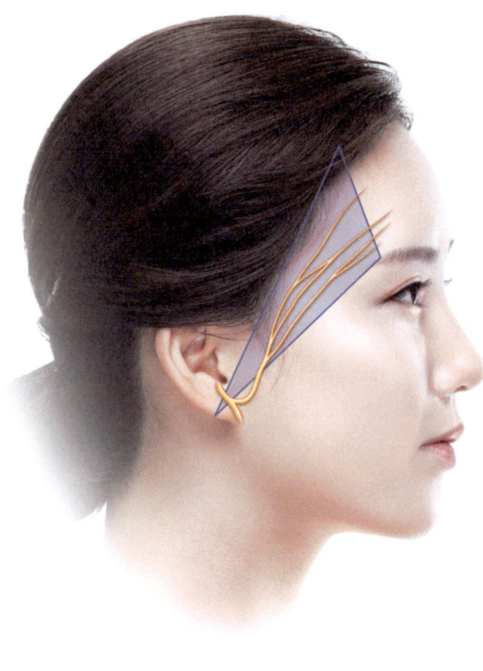

Fig. 13.22 Facial nerve temporal branch pathway

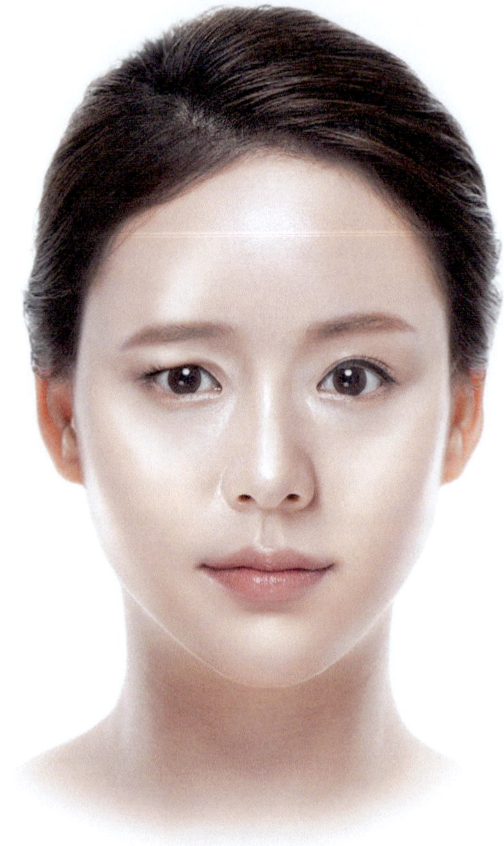

Fig. 13.23 Symptom of facial nerve temporal branch damage

Even if symptoms of a drooping eyebrow occur, most cases are due to temporary paralysis caused by the anesthetic solution, and improvement is usually seen within 24 h. However, if the condition persists for more than 24 h, immediate contact with a facility capable of micro-neurosurgery is necessary to assess nerve damage and, if necessary, perform a repair surgery. Nonetheless, such cases are rare (Fig. 13.23).

13.2.3 Sensory Nerve Injury: Greater Auricular Nerve Injury

Continuous pain can occur if a great auricular nerve injury happens while performing lifting in the neck area. This can occur when tagging the thread in the deep area below the mastoid process or when traversing deeply in the lateral neck area (Fig. 13.24).

When inserting threads behind the mandibular angle and below the ear, they should be gently maneuvered to prevent nerve damage.

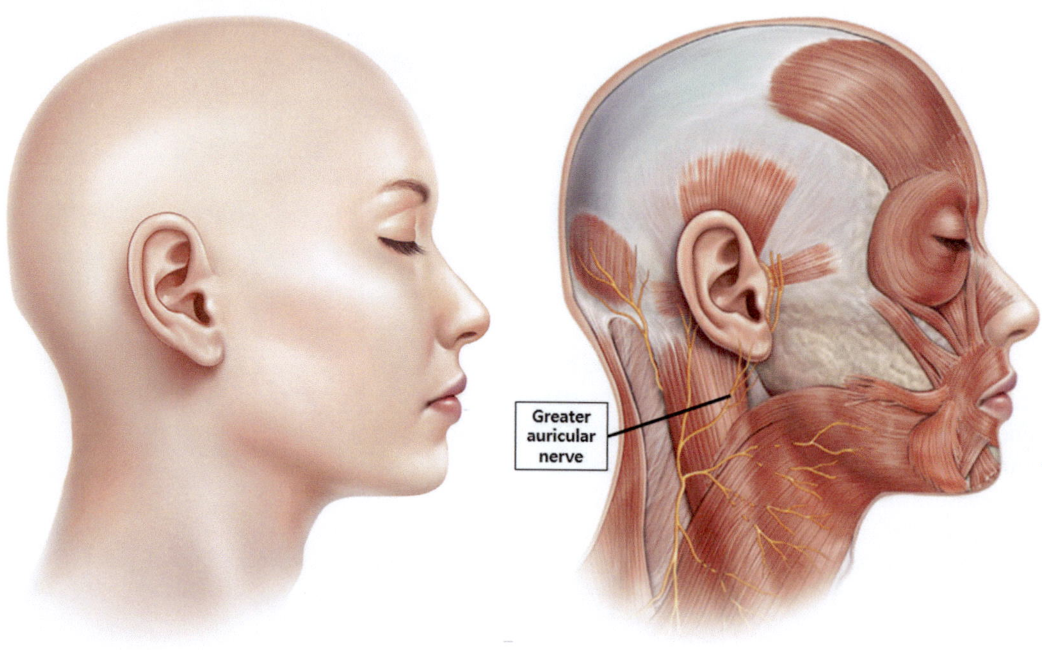

Fig. 13.24 Great auricular nerve pathway

13.2.4 Elevation of Lateral Canthus

Complaints of lifted eye corners after thread lifting occur only when an excellent lifting technique has been used. Typically, this occurs with the temporal tagging technique (U-technique).

13.2.4.1 Etiology

In Fig. 13.25, the occurrence may happen when the distance between the fourth thread and the lateral canthus is less than two fingerbreadths (FB).

13.2.4.2 Solutions

Design the entry point and trajectory to ensure a distance of at least two fingerbreadths between the fourth thread and the lateral canthus. After designing, simulate the lifting process and carefully check how much the lateral canthus moves. Be mindful not to pull the fourth thread too forcefully during traction.

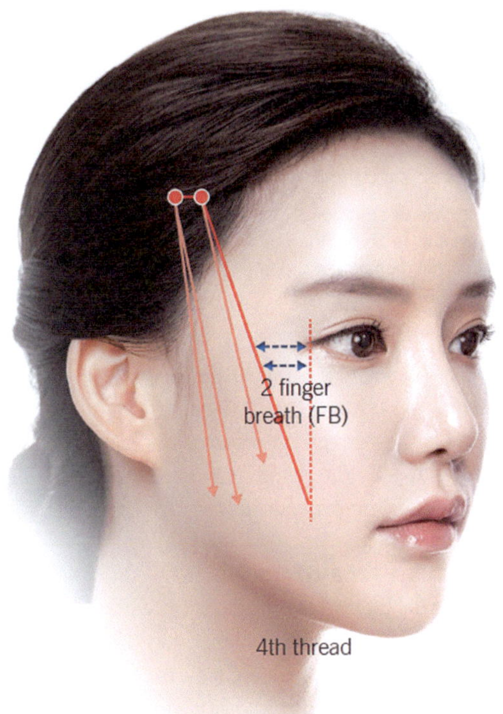

Fig. 13.25 Cause and prevention of the upward lifting of the lateral canthus

13.2.4.3 Prevention

Before the procedure, it is crucial to explain the possibility of the lateral canthus rising. While slight elevation of the lateral canthus may occur immediately after the procedure, it typically returns to normal within 2–3 days as swelling subsides. However, some patients may be particularly sensitive to any changes in the position of the lateral canthus, so caution is necessary.

On the other hand, occasionally, younger patients may prefer the lateral canthus to be elevated. By showing the patient a detailed design process before the procedure, satisfaction may actually be enhanced.

For middle-aged patients who are concerned about sagging around the eyes or eyebrows, slightly lifting the lateral canthus can also increase satisfaction.

13.2.5 Sunken Cheek

There is a slight depression in the side of the face called sunken cheek in English, which is considered attractive in Western cultures. However, Korean women tend to dislike this feature. While some people may not have this feature when they are young, it becomes more pronounced as they age, and eventually, almost everyone develops it (Fig. 13.26). Some patients who originally had cheek depressions may complain that their cheeks appear even more sunken after lifting procedures. They may also complain of asymmetry. These are issues that can arise if not addressed with the patient before the procedure. Understanding the causes and clinical significance of cheek depressions is essential for avoiding problematic situations between the practitioner and the patient (Fig. 13.27).

13.2.5.1 Anatomical Structure

This is a structure formed by the zygomatic ligament and the masseteric cutaneous ligament. There are individual variations in the location on the cheek and the angle of the sag.

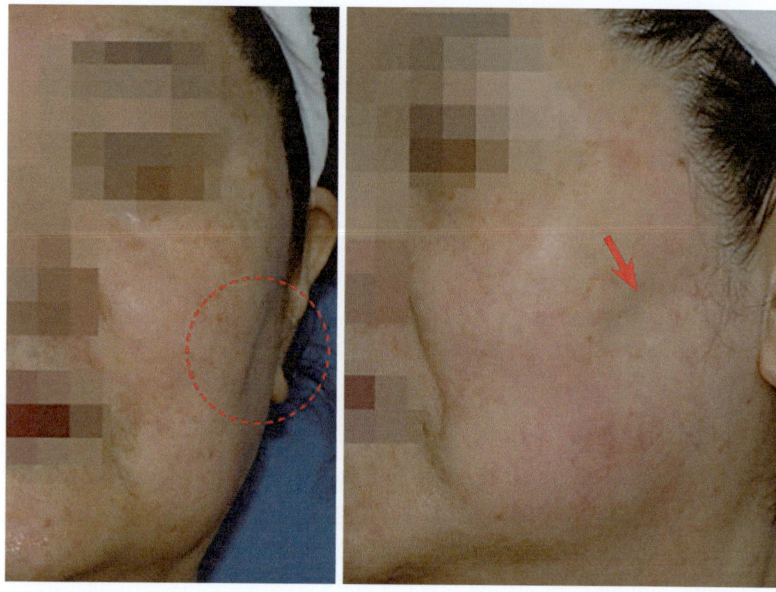

Fig. 13.26 Lateral cheek hollowing—it occurs in everyone as they age. Because it is an area with tight skin adhesion, caution is required during thread lifting procedures

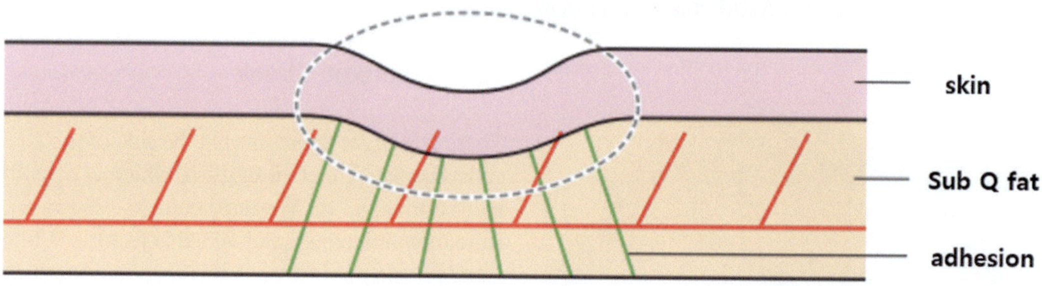

Fig. 13.27 Cause of indentations—when a cog catches on tightly adhered areas. (1) The green line represents existing adhesion → the skin originally sinks. (2) In the red cog thread, the cog length remains consistent. However, in some cases, cogs catch in the subcutaneous layer and in the epidermal layer of some sunken areas, exacerbating existing indentations

13.2.5.2 Clinical Significance

When pushing the skin infero-laterally with your hand, you can observe a peculiar phenomenon. While the skin in other facial areas moves up or down along the direction of the finger when pushed up or down, in this area, pushing the skin supero-medially results in it moving in the same direction, but pushing it infero-laterally causes the skin to retract inward (i.e., an inner vector is at play). Unlike other facial areas where the skin moves along an upward/downward vector with the finger, in this area, it operates on an upward/inner vector. This area is composed of minimal fat and consists mainly of ligaments and fibrotic tissue, making it difficult to penetrate during procedures. Moreover, once the cog is engaged here, it tends to stay fixed and may contribute to further ptosis after the procedure (Fig. 13.28).

13.2.5.3 Precautions

Before the procedure, we confirm with the patient if there is any sunken in the cheeks. Simultaneously, we also check for any asymmetry between the right and left sides. We explain that even though the cheeks may lift well, this particular area may not be adequately addressed.

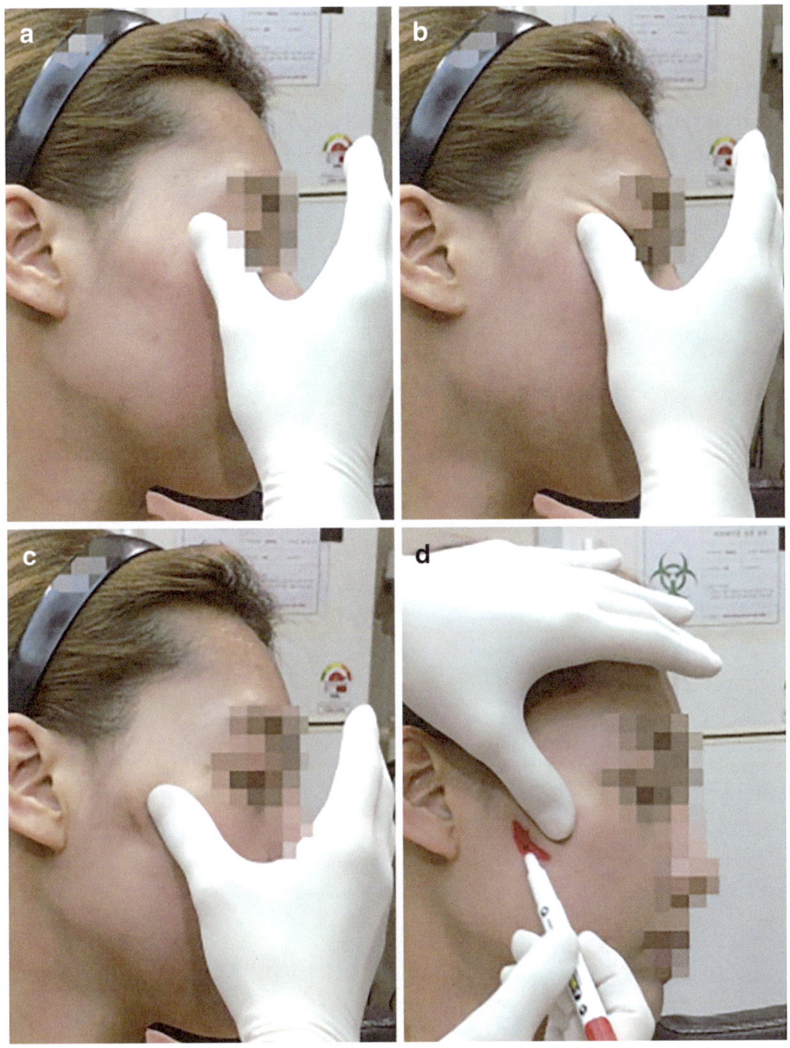

Fig. 13.28 Sunken cheek area marking: (**a**) In the static state, (**b**) When lifting the skin of the zygomatic arch upward, it rises well (upward vector). (**c**) When pulling down the skin of the zygomatic arch, it does not descend well and tends inward (inward vector). (**d**) Use a pen to mark the sunken cheek area with a triangle or diamond shape

13.2.6 Penetrating Salivary Gland

The most serious complication of thread lifting is the penetration of salivary glands. The salivary glands that clinician should take extra care on are the parotid gland in the periauricular region and, when performing the double chin thread lifting, the submandibular gland (Fig. 13.29).

Of course, both of these salivary glands are wrapped around the deep fascia of the face and neck, making them difficult to access. However, thread lifting with a sharp-ended needle (two-way needle with a needle attached to a thread) may cause the clinicians to penetrate the salivary glands if patients move during the procedure, such as tightening the masticatory muscle due to pain (Fig. 13.30).

If the thread completely penetrates the center of the salivary gland, the symptoms will be more severe and the extent of the symptoms may not be so great if only the gland is slightly rubbed or invaded partially.

Symptoms are usually found on the 2–7 days after the procedure as the salivary glands swell unilaterally, and may be accompanied by a feeling of warmth and some pain. Of course, it may be confused with the inflammatory reaction, but the inflammatory reaction is accompanied with more red skin and more sense of warmth, when compared to the salivary gland injury. The important differential diagnosis point is that when the salivary glands are damaged, the protruding symptoms get worse before and after the meal.

In order to make an accurate diagnosis, it is necessary to check whether the saliva is leaking using the sialogram, but it would be difficult to be examined for diagnosis in all cases if there are only mild symptoms. Therefore, it is a good idea to initiate treatment if clinical signs of salivary gland injury are found, assuming the gland is damaged in actual.

The most important treatment is to press the site, which is best done through a facial band like Jobst, and if you are sure the mouth is salivated a lot, you should also consider setting up a drainage through the skin. In addition, antibiotics such as amoxicillin and steroids such as dexamethasone should be administered together with anticholinergic drugs such as scopolamine or atropine to reduce salivation. And if the damage to salivary gland is clearly suspected, it is helpful to reduce the overall salivary gland function by injecting botulinum toxin into overall salivary glands.

If there is a response to these treatments or if the extent of the damage is small, the symptoms usually get relieved to normal range in about 2 weeks. However, close observation is required because if the symptoms get worse, the inserted thread may need to be removed.

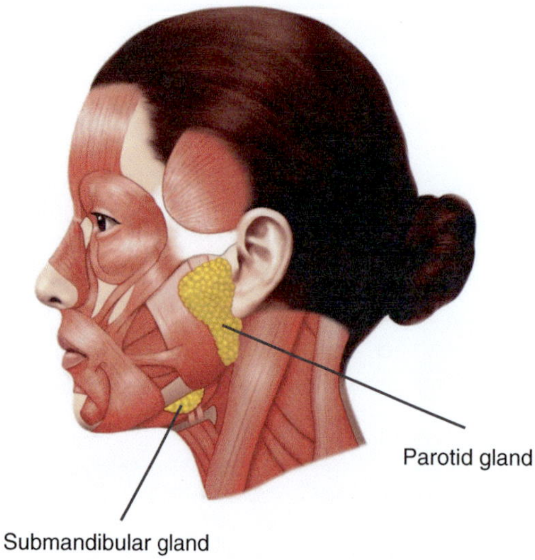

Fig. 13.29 Parotid and submandibular glands

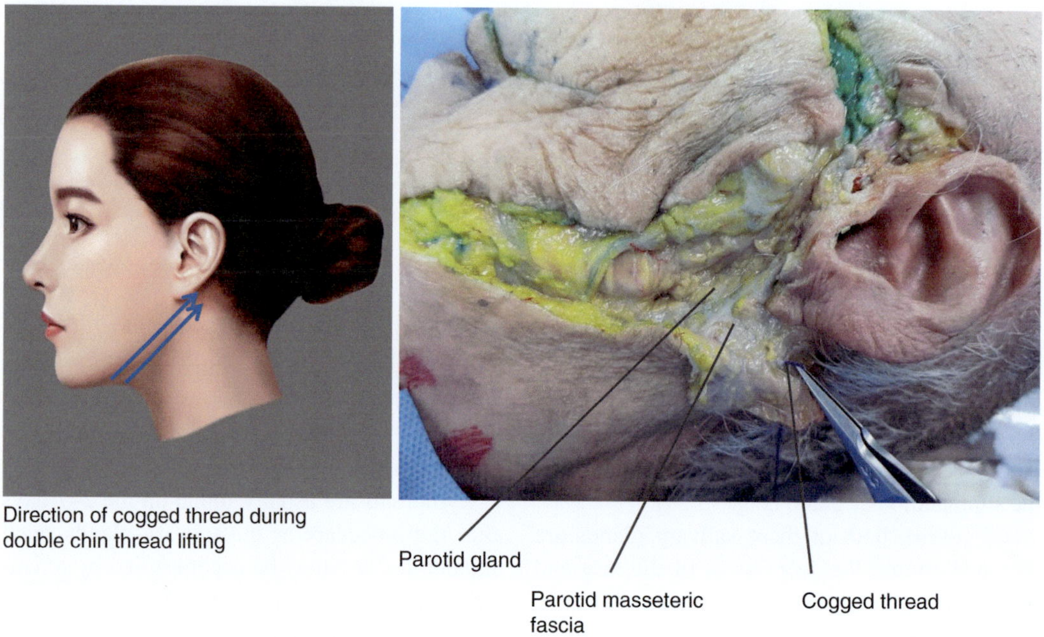

Fig. 13.30 Cogged thread inserted into parotid gland through parotid-masseteric fascia during double chin thread lifting

13.2.7 Infection

13.2.7.1 Thread Lifting and Infection

According to Park et al., during the era when non-absorbable thread lifting was predominantly performed, cases of chronic inflammation such as foreign body granulomas, in addition to infections, were rare but occurred. Wu et al. mentioned the possibility of infection or formation of granulomas with cog thread lifting. Fortunately, most complications, including infections, were not severe and were easily treatable. However, Benny Yau et al. reported a case of mycobacterium abscess infection following facial thread lifting, highlighting the possibility of rare but severe infections. Infections after absorbable thread lifting procedures are considered to be less frequent than those after non-absorbable thread lifting procedures. With thorough adherence to surgical hygiene in the operating room, infections in the thread insertion site or surrounding tissues are unlikely to occur. Moreover, PDO (polydioxanone), which is commonly used in absorbable thread lifting, has a smooth surface and can be processed into a monofilament form, making it relatively resistant to infections.

However, cases of mycobacterium infection have been reported in South Korea after thread lifting procedures using PDO. Shin Jung Jin, et al. reported a case of a 47-year-old woman who presented with erythematous plaques on both sides 2 weeks after receiving PDO thread lifting performed by a non-medical practitioner. The patient initially sought treatment at a local hospital and, with no response to 1 week of antibiotic therapy, was referred to a comprehensive hospital, where she was ultimately diagnosed with Mycobacterium massiliense infection. Recently, meta-analysis studies on various side effects following such thread lifting procedures have been published. In particular, infection cases comprised a significant portion, and cases requiring surgical intervention due to unsuccessful non-surgical methods have also been reported. Therefore, as medical professionals preparing for such procedures, it is crucial to always consider the possibility of infection and strive to maintain a sterile environment before and after the procedure.

13.2.7.2 Prevention of Infection

To prevent infection, thorough disinfection around the entry point should be ensured, and caution should be exercised to avoid infection during the procedure manipulation.

While the use of betadine for facial areas is cautious due to the risk of discoloration, betadine should be used for disinfection in the entry point area, even if it covers a minimal range. It is essential to disinfect the entire skin within the cannula manipulation range, and it is crucial to tidy and disinfect any hair along the trajectory. During the procedure, attention should be paid to prevent hair from getting tangled at the entry point, and thorough education on disinfection of the entry and exit points should be provided after the procedure.

13.2.7.3 Treatment at Infection Case

Infections occurring after thread lifting are generally easily treated with antibiotic therapy. However, in extremely rare cases, as seen in the aforementioned case involving mycobacterium infection, a prolonged course of treatment involving drainage and susceptibility-guided antibiotic therapy is necessary. In cases where infections do not respond well to antibiotics, consideration should be given to surgical intervention, and aggressive treatment is required. In the mycobacterium infection case mentioned in the previous paper, long-term treatment with clarithromycin and amikacin was administered after drainage.

Antibiotics used may vary depending on the timing of infection. Immediately after the procedure, antibiotics for skin infection prevention, such as first-generation cephalosporins, are typically used. However, in cases of infection detected 2 weeks after the procedure, broad-spectrum antibiotics should be considered due to the possibility of mixed infections. Particularly in cases of infections occurring after 2 weeks of fixation thread lifting involving the superficial musculoaponeurotic system (SMAS), it is recommended to use broad-spectrum antibiotics such as levofloxacin, which can cover Gram-negative bacteria.

Further Reading

Abhinitha P, et al. Unusual termination of facial artery associated with the presence of premasseteric branch-a case report. J Surg Acad. 2014;4(2):62–4.

Abraham RF, et al. Thread-lift for facial rejuvenation: assessment of long-term results. Arch Facial Plast Surg. 2009;11:178–83.

Agarwal CA, Mendenhall SD, Foreman KB, Owsley JQ. The course of the frontal branch of the facial nerve in relation to fascial planes: an anatomic study. Plast Reconstr Surg. 2010;125:532–7.

Alghoul M, et al. Retaining ligaments of the face: review of anatomy and clinical applications. Aesthet Surg J. 2013;33:769–82.

Balazs T, et al. Mechanical properties of coronary vein-in vitro evaluation of longitudinal and transversal samples. Biomech Hungarica. 2010;3:3.

Bartlett SP, et al. Age-related changes of the craniofacial skeleton: an anthropometric and histologic analysis. Plast Reconstr Surg. 1992;90:592–600.

Beer GM, et al. The causes of the nasolabial crease: a histomorphological study. Clin Anat. 2013;26:196–203.

Boenisch M, et al. Influence of polydioxanone foil on growing septal cartilage after surgery in animal model. Arch Facial Plast Surg. 2003;5:316–9.

Brandt MG, et al. Biomechanical properties of the facial retaining ligaments. Arch Facial Plast Surg. 2012;14(4):289.

Budai M, et al. Relation between anthropometric and cepharometric measurements and proportions of the face of healthy young white adult men and women. J Craniofac Surg. 2003;14(2):154–61.

Carron MA, Zoumalan RA, Miller PJ, et al. Biochemical analysis of anchoring points in Rhitidectomy. Arch Facial Plast Surg. 2010;12(1):37–9.

Caruso MK, et al. An evaluation of mesotherapy solution for inducing lipolysis and treating cellulite. J Plast Reconstr Aesthet Surg. 2008;61(11):1321–4.

Castro CC, Boehm KA, Codner MA. Midface surgery. Edinburgh: Elsevier Saunders; 2009.

Chang H. Arterial anatomy of subdermal plexus of the face. Keio J Med. 2001;50(1):31–4.

Chen YS, et al. Evaluation of age-related intraorbital fat herniation through computed tomography. Plast Reconstr Surg. 2008;122(4):1191–8.

Choe KS, et al. The Korean American woman's face: anthropometric measurements and quantitative analysis of facial aesthetics. Arch Facial Plast Surg. 2004;6(4):244–52.

Coleman SR, et al. The anatomy of the aging face: volume loss and changes in 3-dimensional topography. Aesthet Surg J. 2006;26(Suppl):S4–9.

Cotofana S, et al. The anatomy of the aging face: a review. Facial Plast Surg. 2016;32:253–60.

Cotofana S, et al. An update on the anatomy of the forehead compartments. Plast Reconstr Surg. 2017;139:864e.

Cotofana S, et al. The relationship between bone remodeling and the clockwise rotation of the facial skeleton: a computed tomographic imaging–based evaluation. Plast Reconstr Surg. 2018;142:1447.

Cotofana S, et al. Arteries of the face and their relevance for minimally invasive facial procedures: an anatomical review. Plast Reconstr Surg. 2019;143:416.

Darcy SJ, et al. Magnetic resonance imaging characterization of orbital changes with age and associated contributions to lower eyelid prominence. Plast Reconstr Surg. 2008;122:921–9.

Davidge KM, et al. Naming the soft tissue layers of the temporoparietal region: unifying anatomic terminology across surgical disciplines. Neurosurgery. 2010;67:120–9.

DeFatta RJ, et al. Midface lifting: current standards. Facial Plast Surg. 2011;27:77–85.

Donofrio LM. Fat distribution: a morphologic study of the aging face. Dermatologic Surg. 2000;26(12):1107–12.

Doubt G, et al. Surgical anatomy relevant to the transpalpebral subperiosteal elevation of the midface. Aesthet Surg J. 2015;35(4):353.

Dumont T, et al. Anatomy and imaging of the deep fat of the face. Clin Anat. 2000;13:373–82.

El-Garem YF. Estimation of bony orbit depth for optimal selection of the injection technique to correct the tear trough and palpebromalar groove. Dermatologic Surg. 2015;41:94–101.

S. Oh et al., *The Art and Science of Thread Lifting Based on Pinch Anatomy and Moving Plane*, https://doi.org/10.1007/978-981-97-5516-5

Erdogmus S, et al. Anatomy of the supraorbital region and the evaluation of it for the reconstruction of facial defects. J Craniofac Surg. 2007;18:104–12.

Ezure T, et al. Involvement of upper cheek sagging in nasolabial fold formation. Skin Res Technol. 2012;18:259–64.

Farkas LG, et al. Anthropometric measurements of the facial framework in adulthood: age-related changes in eight age categories in 600 healthy white North Americans of European ancestry from 16 to 90 years of age. J Craniofac Surg. 2004;15:288–98.

Farkas LG, et al. International anthropometric study of facial morphology in various ethnic groups/races. J Craniofac Surg. 2005;16(4):615–46.

Farkas JP, et al. The science and theory behind facial aging. Plast Reconstr Surg Glob Open. 2013;1:e8–e15.

Fitzgerald R, et al. Update on facial aging. Aesthet Surg J. 2010;30(Suppl):11S–24S.

Furnas DW. Festoon, mounds, and bags of the eyelids and cheek. Clin Plast Surg. 1993;20:367–85.

Furnas DW, et al. The retaining ligaments of the cheek. Plast Reconstr Surg. 1989;83:11–6.

Gardetto A, et al. Does a superficial musculoaponeurotic system exist in the face and neck? An anatomical study by the tissue plastination technique. Plast Reconstr Surg. 2003;111(2):664–72.

Ghassemi A, et al. Anatomy of the SMAS revisited. Aesth Plast Surg. 2003;27:258–64.

Ghavami A, et al. The orbicularis retaining ligament of the medial orbit: closing the circle. Plast Reconstr Surg. 2008;121:994–1001.

Gierloff M, et al. Aging changes of the midfacial fat compartments: a computed tomographic study. Plast Reconstr Surg. 2012a;129:263–73.

Gierloff M, et al. The subcutaneous fat compartments in relation to aesthetically important facial folds and rhytides. J Plast Reconstr Aesthet Surg. 2012b;65:1292–7.

Goldberg RA. The three periorbital hollows: a paradigm for periorbital rejuvenation. Plast Reconstr Surg. 2005;116:1796–804.

Gosain AK, et al. Surgical anatomy of the SMAS: a reinvestigation. Plast Reconstr Surg. 1993;92:1254–63.

Gottfried R, et al. A classification of facial wrinkles. Plast Reconstr Surg. 2001;11:1735–50.

Gronovich Y. Innovative surgical approach using a mesh sling for the aging neck. Plast Reconstr Surg. 2018;141:1386.

Gruber RP, Levine SM, Levine JP. Facial topography: clinical anatomy of the face. Plast Reconstr Surg. 2013;132(1):249.

Guyuron B, et al. Factors contributing to the facial aging of identical twins. Plast Reconstr Surg. 2009;123:1321–31.

Ha RY, et al. Analysis of facial skin thickness: defining the relative thickness index. Plast Reconstr Surg. 2005;115:1769.

Haddock NT, et al. The tear trough and lid/cheek junction: anatomy and implications for surgical correction. Plast Reconstr Surg. 2009;123:1332–40.

Han HH, et al. Combined, minimally invasive, thread-based facelift. Arch Aesth Plast Surg. 2014;20(3):160–4.

Hartstein ME, Wulc AE, David EE, Holck. Midfacial rejuvenation. Cham: Springer; 2012.

Hastein ME, et al. Midfacial rejuvenation. Cham: Springer; 2012.

Hazani R, Chowdhry S, Mowlavi A, et al. Bony anatomic landmarks to avoid injury to the marginal mandibular nerve. Aesthet Surg J. 2011;31(3):286–9.

Hetzler L, et al. The brow and forehead in periocular rejuvenation. Fac Plast Surg Clin N Am. 2010;18:375–84.

Huang YL, et al. Clinical analysis and classification of the dark eye circle. Int J Dermatol. 2014;53(2):164.

Hussein S, et al. Surgical anatomy and blood supply of the fascial layer of the temporal region. Plast Reconstr Surg. 1976;77:17–24.

Hwang K, et al. Attachment of the deep temporal fascia to the zygomatic arch: an anatomic study. J Craniofac Surg. 1999;10(4):342.

Hwang K, et al. Origin of the lower orbicularis oculi muscle in relation to the nasojugal groove. J Craniofac Surg. 2015;26:1389–93.

Ioi H, Nakata S, Nakasima A, Counts A. Influence of facial convexity on facial attractiveness in Japanese. Orthod Craniofac Res. 2007;10(4):181–6.

Isse NG, et al. Elevating the midface with barbed polypropylene sutures. Aesthet Surg J. 2005;25:301–3.

Jackson JL, Kuriyama A, Hayashino Y. Botulinum toxin A for prophylactic treatment of migraine and tension headaches in adults: a meta-analysis. JAMA. 2012;307(16):1736–45.

Jang HJ, et al. Effect of cog threads under rat skin. Dermatologic Surg. 2005;31(12):1639–43.

Jones D. What lies beneath. Dermatologic Surg. 2011;37:387–90.

Kahn DM, et al. Overview of current thoughts on facial volume and aging. Facial Plast Surg. 2010;26:350–5.

Kikkawa DO, et al. Relations of the superficial musculoaponeurotic system to the orbit and characterization of the orbitomalar ligament. Ophthalmic Plast Reconstr Surg. 1996;12:77–88.

Kim YS, et al. The anatomical origin and course of the angular artery regarding its clinical implications. Dermatologic Surg. 2014;40:1070–6.

Kim HJ, et al. Clinical anatomy of the face for filler and botulinum toxin injection. Cham: Springer; 2016.

Kim H-S, et al. Topographic anatomy of the infraorbital artery and its clinical implications for nasolabial fold augmentation. Plast Reconstr Surg. 2018;142:273e.

Kleintjes WG. Forehead anatomy: arterial variations and venous link of the midline forehead flap. J Plast Reconstr Aesthet Surg. 2007;60:593–606.

Koh KS, et al. Branching patterns and symmetry of the course of the facial artery in Koreans. Int J Oral Maxillofac Surg. 2003;32:414–8.

Kpodzo DS, et al. Malar mounds and festoons: review of current management. Aesthet Surg J. 2014;34(2):235.

Kurita M, et al. Tissue reactions to cog structure and pure gold in lifting threads: a histological study in rats. Aesthet Surg J. 2011;31(3):347–51.

Lackey DE, et al. Contributions of adipose tissue architectural and tensile properties toward defining healthy and unhealthy obesity. Am J Physiol Endocrinol Metabol. 2014;306(3):E233–46.

Lambros V. Observations on periorbital and midface aging. Plast Reconstr Surg. 2007;120:1367–76.

Langevin HM, et al. Mechanical signaling through connective tissue: a mechanism for the therapeutic effect of acupuncture. FASEB J. 2001;15:2275–82.

Langevin HM, et al. Subcutaneous tissue fibroblast cytoskeletal remodeling induced by acupuncture: evidence for a mechanotransduction-based mechanism. J Cell Physiol. 2006;207:767–74.

Lee J-H, Hong G. Definitions of groove and hollowness of the infraorbital region and clinical treatment using soft-tissue filler. Arch Plast Surg. 2018;45:214–21.

Lee HB, et al. Evaluation of influence of individual facial aesthetic subunits on the cognition of facial attractiveness in public. J Korean Soc Plast Reconstr Surg. 2010;37(4):361–8.

Lee HJ, et al. Description of a novel anatomic venous structure in the nasoglabellar area. J Craniofac Surg. 2014a;25:633–5.

Lee JY, Kim JN, Yoo JY, Shin KJ, Song WC, Koh KS, Kim SH, Choi HG. Topographic relationships between the transverse facial artery, branches of the facial nerve, and the parotid duct in the lateral midface. Ann Plast Surg. 2014b;73:321–4.

Lee SH, Lee M, Kim HJ. Anatomy-based image processing analysis of the running pattern of the perioral artery for minimally invasive surgery. Br J Oral Maxillofac Surg. 2014c;52(8):688–92.

Lee JG, Yang HM, Choi YJ, et al. Facial arterial depth and relationship with the facial musculature layer. Plast Reconstr Surg. 2015a;135(2):437–44.

Lee JG, Yang HM, Hu KS, Lee YI, Lee HJ, Choi YJ, Kim HJ. Frontal branch of the superficial temporal artery: anatomical study and clinical implications regarding injectable treatments. Surg Radiol Anat. 2015b;37:61–8.

Lee CG, Jung J, Hwang S, et al. Histologic evaluation of bioresorbable threads in rats. Korean. J Clin Lab Sci. 2018a;50:217–24.

Lee HJ, Won SY, Hu KS, Mun SY, Yang HM, Kim HJ. The facial artery: a comprehensive anatomical review. Clin Anat. 2018b;31:99–108.

Lei T, Xu DC, Gao JH, Zhong SZ, Chen B, Yang DY, Cui L, Li ZH, Wang XH, Yang SM. Using the frontal branch of the superficial temporal artery as a landmark for locating the course of the temporal branch of the facial nerve during rhytidectomy: an anatomical study. Plast Reconstr Surg. 2005;116:623–9.

Liew S, Wu WT, Chan HH, et al. Consensus on changing trends, attitudes, and concepts of Asian beauty. Aesth Plast Surg. 2016;40(2):193–201.

Linden OE, et al. The relationship between age and facial asymmetry. Plast Reconstr Surg. 2018;142:1145.

Loukas M, et al. Gross anatomical, CT and MRI analysis of the buccal fat pad with special emphasis on volumetric variations. Sure Radiol Anat. 2006;28:254.

Lucarelli MJ, et al. The anatomy of midfacial ptosis. Ophthalmic Plast Reconstr Surg. 2000;16:7–22.

Macchi V, et al. Histotopographic study of the fibroadipose connective cheek system. Cells Tissues Organs. 2010;191(1):47–56.

Marur T, et al. Facial anatomy. Clin Dermatol. 2014;32:14–23.

Mendelson BC. In your face: the hidden history of plastic surgery and why looks matter. Richmond: Hardie Grant Books; 2013.

Mendelson BC. Submandibular gland reduction in aesthetic surgery of the neck: review of 112 consecutive cases. Plast Reconstr Surg. 2015;136:463–71.

Mendelson B, Wong CH. Changes in the facial skeleton with aging: implications and clinical applications in facial rejuvenation. Aesth Plast Surg. 2012;36:753–60.

Mendelson B, Wong CH. Anatomy of the aging face. In: Plastic surgery. 3rd ed. Philadelphia: Elsevier Saunders; 2013. p. 78–92.

Mendelson BC, et al. Surgical anatomy of the midcheek and malar mounds. Plast Reconstr Surg. 2002;110:885–96.

Mendelson BC, et al. Age-related changes of the orbit and midcheek and the implications for facial rejuvenation. Aesth Plast Surg. 2007;31:419–23.

Mendelson BC, et al. Surgical anatomy of the lower face: the premasseter space, the jowl, and the labiomandibular fold. Aesth Plast Surg. 2008a;32:185–95.

Mendelson BC, et al. Surgical anatomy of the midcheek: facial layers, spaces, and the mid cheek segments. Clin Plast Surg. 2008b;35:395.

Mendelson BC, et al. Surgical anatomy of the middle premasseter space and its application in sub-SMAS face lift surgery. Plast Reconstr Surg. 2013;132:57–64.

Meneghini F, et al. Clinical facial analysis (elements, principles, and techniques). Berlin: Springer; 2012.

Mitz V, Peyronie M. The superficial musculo-aponeurotic system (SMAS) in the parotid and cheek area. Plast Reconstr Surg. 1976;77:17–24.

Moore KL, Dalley AF, Agur AM. Clinically oriented anatomy. 8th ed. Philadelphia: Wolters Kluwer; 2018.

Moss CJ, et al. Surgical anatomy of the ligamentous attachments in the temple and periorbital regions. Plast Reconstr Surg. 2000;105:1475–90.

Munn L, et al. Changes in face topography from supine-to-upright position-And soft tissue correction values for craniofacial identification. Forensic Sci Int. 2018;289:40–50.

Muzaffar AR, et al. Surgical anatomy of the ligamentous attachments of the lower lid and lateral canthus. Plast Reconstr Surg. 2002;110:873–84.

Nakajima H, et al. Facial artery in the upper lip and nose: anatomy and a clinical application. Plast Reconstr Surg. 2002;109:855–61.

Nakajima H, et al. Anatomical study of subcutaneous adipofascial tissue: a concept of the protective adipofascial system (PAFS) and lubricant adipofascial system (LAFS). Scand J Plast Reconstr Surg Hand Surg. 2004;38(3):261–6.

Narins RS, Carruthers J, Flynn TC, et al. Validated assessment scales for the lower face. Dermatologic Surg. 2012;38(2):333–42.

O'Brien JX, et al. New perspectives on the surgical anatomy and nomenclature of the temporal region: literature review and dissection study. Plast Reconstr Surg. 2013;131:510–22.

Oh HS, et al. Correlations between cepharometic and photographic measurements of facial attractiveness in Chinese and US patients after orthodontic treatment. Am J Orthod Dentofacial Orthop. 2009;136(6):762.

Oh HS, et al. Changes in the layers of the temple during pinch manipulation: implications for thread lifting. Dermatologic Surg. 2019;10:1–6.

Park HS, et al. Harmonized profiloplasty using balanced angular profile analysis. Aesth Plast Surg. 2004;28:89–97.

Paul MD. Barbed sutures in aesthetic plastic surgery: evolution of thought and process. Aesthet Surg J. 2013;33(3):17–31.

Perrett D. In your face: the new science of human attraction. 2012.

Pessa JE. An algorithm of facial aging: Verification of Lambros's theory by three-dimensional stereolithography, with reference to the pathogenesis of midfacial aging, scleral show, and the lateral suborbital trough deformity. Plast Reconstr Surg. 2000;106:479–88.

Pessa JE, Garza JR. The malar septum: the anatomic basis of malar mounds and malar edema. Aesthet Surg J. 1997;17(1):11–7.

Pessa JE, Rohrich RJ. The cheek. In: Facial topography: clinical anatomy of the face. St. Louis: Quality Medical Publishing; 2012a. p. 47–93.

Pessa JE, Rohrich RJ. The lips and chin. In: Facial topography: clinical anatomy of the face. St. Louis: Quality Medical Publishing; 2012b. p. 251–91.

Pessa JE, et al. The malar septum: the anatomic basis of malar mounds and malar edema. Aesthet Surg J. 1997;17:11–7.

Pessa JE, et al. Double or bifid zygomaticus major muscle: anatomy, incidence, and clinical correlation. Clin Anat. 1998a;11:310–3.

Pessa JE, et al. Relative maxillary retrusion as a natural consequence of aging: combining skeletal and soft-tissue changes into an integrated model of midfacial aging. Plast Reconstr Surg. 1998b;102(1):205–12.

Pessa JE, et al. Variability of the midfacial muscles: analysis of 50 hemifacial cadaver dissections. Plast Reconstr Surg. 1998c;102:1888–93.

Pessa JE, Zadoo VP, Garza PA, et al. Double or bifid zygomaticus major muscle: anatomy, incidence, and clinical correlation. Clin Anat. 1998d;11(5):310–3.

Pessa JE, et al. Concertina effect and facial aging: nonlinear aspects of youthfulness and skeletal remodeling, and why, perhaps, infants have jowls. Plast Reconstr Surg. 1999;103:635–44.

Pilsl U, et al. The external nose: the nasal arteries and their course in relation to the nasolabial fold and groove. Plast Reconstr Surg. 2016;138(5):830e–5e.

Pinar YA, Bilge O, Govsa F. Anatomic study of the blood supply of perioral region. Clin Anat. 2005;18(5):330–9.

Prendergast P. Minimally invasive face and neck lift using silhouette coned sutures. In: Miniinvasive face and body lifts - closed suture lifts or barbed thread lifts. London: IntechOpen; 2013.

Radlanski RJ, et al. The face: pictorial atlas of clinical anatomy. Batavia: Quintessence Publishing; 2012.

Raskin E, et al. Why do we age in our cheeks? Aesthet Surg J. 2007;27:19–28.

Rawlani RJ, et al. Volumetric changes of the mid and lower face with animation and the standardization of three-dimensional facial imaging. Plast Reconstr Surg. 2019;143:76.

Reece EM, Rohrich RJ. The aesthetic jaw line: management of the aging jowl. Aesthet Surg J. 2008;28(6):668–74.

Reece EM, et al. The aesthetic jaw line: management of the aging jowl. Aesthet Surg J. 2008a;28:668–74.

Reece EM, et al. The mandibular septum: anatomical observations of the jowls in aging-implications for facial rejuvenation. Plast Reconstr Surg. 2008b;121:1414–20.

Rhee SC, et al. Balanced angular profile analysis. Plast Reconstr Surg. 2004;114(2):535–44.

Richard MJ, et al. Analysis of the anatomic changes of the aging facial skeleton using computer-assisted tomography. Ophthalmic Plast Reconstr Surg. 2009;25(5):382–6.

Rohrich RJ, Pessa JE. The fat compartments of the face: anatomy and clinical implications for cosmetic surgery. Plast Reconstr Surg. 2007;119:2219–27.

Rohrich RJ, Pessa JE. The retaining system of the face: histologic evaluation of the septal boundaries of the subcutaneous fat compartments. Plast Reconstr Surg. 2008;121:1804–9.

Rohrich RJ, Pessa JE. The anatomy and clinical implications of perioral submuscular fat. Plast Reconstr Surg. 2009;124(1):266–71.

Rohrich RJ, et al. The retaining system of the face: histologic evaluation of the septal boundaries of the subcutaneous fat compartments. Plast Reconstr Surg. 2008a;121:1804–9.

Rohrich RJ, et al. The youthful cheek and the deep medial fat compartment. Plast Reconstr Surg. 2008b;121:2107–12.

Rohrich RJ, et al. The anatomy of suborbicularis fat: Implications for periorbital rejuvenation. Plast Reconstr Surg. 2009;124:946–51.

Rubin LR, Mishriki Y, Lee G. Anatomy of the nasolabial fold: the keystone of the smiling mechanism. Plast Reconstr Surg. 1989;83(1):1–10.

Ruff G. Technique and uses for absorbable barbed sutures. Aesthet Surg J. 2006;26:620–8.

Ruff GL. The history of barbed sutures. Aesthet Surg J. 2013;33(3S):12S–6S.

Sadick NS, et al. A novel approach to structural facial volume replacement. Aesth Plast Surg. 2013;37:266–76.

Schaverien MV, et al. Vascularized membranes determine the anatomical boundaries of the subcutaneous fat compartments. Plast Reconstr Surg. 2009;123:695–700.

Sezgin B, et al. The effect of microneedle thickness on pain during minimally invasive facial procedures: a clinical study. Aesthet Surg J. 2014;34(5):757–65.

Shan XF, Xu H, Cai ZG, Wu LL, Yu GY. Botulinum toxin A inhibits salivary secretion of rabbit submandibular gland. Int J Oral Sci. 2013;5:217–23.

Shaw RB, et al. Aging of the facial skeleton: aesthetic implications and rejuvenation strategies. Plast Reconstr Surg. 2011;127:374–83.

Shin KJ, Shin HJ, Lee SH, Koh KS, Song WC. Surgical anatomy of the superficial temporal artery to prevent facial nerve injury during arterial biopsy. Clin Anat. 2018;31:608–13.

Shirakabe Y, et al. A new paradigm for the aging Asian face. Aesth Plast Surg. 2003;27(5):397–402.

Singer DP, Sullivan PK. Submandibular gland: an anatomic evaluation and surgical approach to submandibular gland resection for facial rejuvenation. Plast Reconstr Surg. 2003;112:1150–4.

Soh J, Chew MT, Wong HB. Professional assessment of facial profile attractiveness. Am J Orthod Dentofacial Orthop. 2005;128(2):201–5.

Spiegel JH, et al. Frontalis midline dehiscence: an anatomical study and discussion of clinical relevance. J Plast Reconstr Aesthet Surg. 2009;62:950–4.

Stutman RL, Codner MA. Tear trough deformity: review of anatomy and treatment options. Aesthet Surg J. 2012;32(4):426.

Stuzin JM, et al. Anatomy of the frontal branch of the facial nerve: the significance of the temporal fat pad. Plast Reconstr Surg. 1989;83:265–71.

Stuzin JM, et al. The relationship of the superficial and deep facial fascias: relevance to rhytidectomy and aging. Plast Reconstr Surg. 1992;89(3):441–9.

Suh DH, et al. Outcomes of polydioxanone knotless thread lifting for facial rejuvenation. Dermatologic Surg. 2015;41(6):720–5.

Sulamandidze MA, et al. Removal of facial soft tissue ptosis with special threads. Dermatologic Surg. 2002;28:367–71.

Sulamandidze MA, et al. APTOS suture lifting methods: 10 years of experience. Clin Plast Surg. 2009;36:281–306.

Sulamanidze M, Sulamanidze G. APTOS suture lifting methods: 10 years of experience. Clin Plast Surg. 2009;36:281–306.

Sundine MJ, et al. Analysis of the effects of subcutaneous musculoaponeurotic system facial support on the nasolabial crease. Can J Plast Surg. 2010;18(1):11–4.

Swift A, Remington K. BeautiPHIcation: a global approach to facial beauty. Clin Plast Surg. 2011;38(3):347–77.

Swift A, et al. Beautiphication: a global approach to facial beauty. Clin Plast Surg. 2011;38:347–77.

Tansatit T, Apinuntrum P, Phetudom T. A typical pattern of the labial arteries with implication for lip augmentation with injectable fillers. Aesth Plast Surg. 2014;38(6):1083–9.

Thaller SR, et al. The submuscular aponeurotic system (SMAS): a histologic and comparative anatomy evaluation. Plast Reconstr Surg. 1990;86:690–6.

Ugur MB, et al. A reliable surface landmark for localizing supratrochlear artery: medial canthus. Otolaryngol Head Neck Surg. 2008;138:162–5.

Villa MT, et al. Barbed sutures: a review of the literature. Plast Reconstr Surg. 2008;121:102–8.

Wan D, et al. The differing adipocyte morphologies of deep versus superficial midfacial compartments: a cadaveric study. Plast Reconstr Surg. 2013;133:615e–25e.

Wan D, Amirlak B, Rohrich R, et al. The clinical importance of the fat compartments in midfacial aging. Plast Reconstr Surg Glob Open. 2014;1(9):e92.

Watson S-W, Morales-Ryan C-A, Sinn D-P. Poster 14: internal midface lift: the foundation for facial rejuvenation. J Oral Maxillofac Surg. 2003;61(8S1):88.

Webster RC, et al. Supraorbital and supratrochlear notches and foramina: anatomical variations and surgical relevance. Laryngoscope. 1986;96:311–5.

Wong CH, et al. The tear trough ligament: anatomical basis for the tear trough deformity. Plast Reconstr Surg. 2012;129:1392–402.

Wong CH, et al. Facial soft-tissue spaces and retaining ligaments of the midcheek: defining the premaxillary space. Plast Reconstr Surg. 2013;132:49–56.

Wu WT. Barbed sutures in facial rejuvenation. Aesthet Surg J. 2004;24:582–7.

Wu WT. Nonsurgical face lifting with long barbed suture slings: the Woffles lift. J Aesthet Chir. 2013;6:13–20.

Wulc AE, et al. The anatomic basis of midfacial aging. In: Hartstein ME, et al., editors. Midfacial rejuvenation, vol. 2. New York: Springer; 2012. p. 15–28.

Yang C, et al. Tear trough and palpebromalar groove in young versus elderly adults: a sectional anatomy study. Plast Reconstr Surg. 2013;132:796–808.

Yang HM, et al. New anatomical insights on the course and branching patterns of the facial artery: clinical implications of injectable treatments to the nasolabial fold and nasojugal groove. Plast Reconstr Surg. 2014;133:1077–82.

Yi K-H, Oh SM. Lateral facial thread lifting procedure with temporal anchoring in deep temporal fascia: anatomical perspectives of superficial temporal artery. Skin Res Technol. 2024;30:e13587.

Yoon A et al. Absorbable thread: regenerative medicine using physical stimuli. MD world; 2012.

Yousif NJ, Gosain A, Matloub HS, et al. The nasolabial fold: an anatomic and histologic reappraisal. Plast Reconstr Surg. 1994;93(1):60–9.

Yousuf S, et al. A review of the gross anatomy, functions, pathology, and clinical uses of the buccal fat pad. Surg Radiol Anat. 2013;32:427–36.

Zadoo VP, Pessa JE. Biological arches and changes to the curvilinear form of the aging maxilla. Plast Reconstr Surg. 2000;106(2):460–6.

Zaruby J, et al. An in vivo comparison of barbed sutures devices and conventional monofilament sutures for cosmetic skin closure: biomechanical wound strength and histology. Aesthet Surg J. 2011;31:232–40.

Zhang HM, et al. Anatomical structure of the buccal fat pad and its clinical adaptations. Plast Reconstr Surg. 2002;109:2509–18.

Zhuang Z, Landsittel D, Benson S, et al. Facial anthropometric differences among gender, ethnicity, and age groups. Ann Occup Hyg. 2010;54(4):391–402.

Zufferey J. Anatomic variations of the nasolabial fold. Plast Reconstr Surg. 1992;89(2):225–31.

MIX
Papier aus verantwortungsvollen Quellen
Paper from responsible sources
FSC® C105338

If you have any concerns about our products,
you can contact us on
ProductSafety@springernature.com

In case Publisher is established outside the EU,
the EU authorized representative is:
Springer Nature Customer Service Center GmbH
Europaplatz 3, 69115 Heidelberg, Germany

Printed by Libri Plureos GmbH
in Hamburg, Germany